Jennie Fenstermacher

6 TH EDITION

SPEECH CORRECTION

PRINCIPLES
AND METHODS

Charles Van Riper

Department of Speech Pathology and Audiology
Western Michigan University
Kalamazoo, Michigan

Prentice-Hall, Inc., Englewood Cliffs, New Jersey 07632

Library of Congress Cataloging in Publication Data
VAN RIPER, CHARLES GAGE,
  Speech correction.

  Includes bibliographies and index.
  1. Speech, Disorders of. 2. Speech therapy.
3. Voice. I. Title.
RC423.V35 1978   616.8′554   77′21460
ISBN 0-13-829523-9

Printed in the United States of America

10 9 8 7 6 5 4 3 2 1

PRENTICE-HALL INTERNATIONAL, INC., *London*
PRENTICE-HALL OF AUSTRALIA PTY. LIMITED, *Sydney*
PRENTICE-HALL OF CANADA, LTD., *Toronto*
PRENTICE-HALL OF INDIA PRIVATE LIMITED, *New Delhi*
PRENTICE-HALL OF JAPAN, INC., *Tokyo*
PRENTICE-HALL OF SOUTHEAST ASIA PTE. LTD., *Singapore*
WHITEHALL BOOKS LIMITED, *Wellington, New Zealand*

To my wife,
the Earth Mother

CONTENTS

v

PREFACE

In this, the Sixth Edition of Speech Correction: Principles and Methods, we have sought not only to bring the text up to date but also to rewrite it with a wider readership in view. Students from many other disciplines are enrolling in the first course in speech pathology. Those who do intend to make a career in this field will take specialized courses dealing with each of the speech disorders. Accordingly, we have revised the book so that it is truly an introduction rather than a compendium. We have added chapters to provide more adequate background concerning the nature of speech and language. The contributions of linguistics and behavior modification to the field of speech pathology will be evident throughout. Nevertheless, we hope that another new generation of students, like those who have studied this text for almost forty years, will sense the challenge of trying to help those who cannot share our common heritage, the ability to communicate effectively. The author has been a working clinician all of his professional life and has enjoyed every bit of it. Hopefully, some of that enjoyment still permeates these pages.

C. Van Riper

1

INTRODUCTION

Welcome to the field of speech pathology. We wish we knew why you decided to explore it. Perhaps you are thinking about adopting it as a new profession full of promise. Perhaps you are taking the introductory course in speech pathology because you know that in your future work in special education, audiology, counseling, occupational or physical therapy, or classroom teaching you will encounter persons with serious communication problems. Or perhaps you are one of those individuals who just like to explore unknown lands. No matter. We are delighted to be your guide because we have roamed the peaks and valleys of this field for many years and know its fascinations and challenges. And because we know that those who have been deprived of that most fundamental of human rights, the ability to communicate, need all the help and understanding they can get. The author of this text, having been born at the age of thirty when he first managed to talk fluently enough to join the human race, knows that deprivation very personally and so his welcome is not simply an author's ploy. This text is a real invitation to those who want some meaningfulness in their lives by serving fellow human beings. You may or may not become a speech pathologist, but surely you can help some of those who cannot speak for themselves.

If there is any real hope for mankind in these troubled times it is to be found in the swelling tide of belief that somehow we must change this planet from a polluted sphere into one where man can fulfill his destiny with some grace. We are sickened from the ugliness in which we live and die. We are appalled by the way we have raped the good earth and anointed its wounds with human waste. We protest the human cruelty and exploitation we see all about us. We are angry with those who preceded us for handing down to us this heritage, and we are utterly determined to reverse this evil course, for we see very clearly where it will end.

This is a book about people troubled by the way they speak, about children and adults who stutter, or who cannot utter a sound because they have lost their vocal folds, or who possess some other speech disorder. At first glance, it might seem as though its contents could have no bearing on this generation's compelling need to make

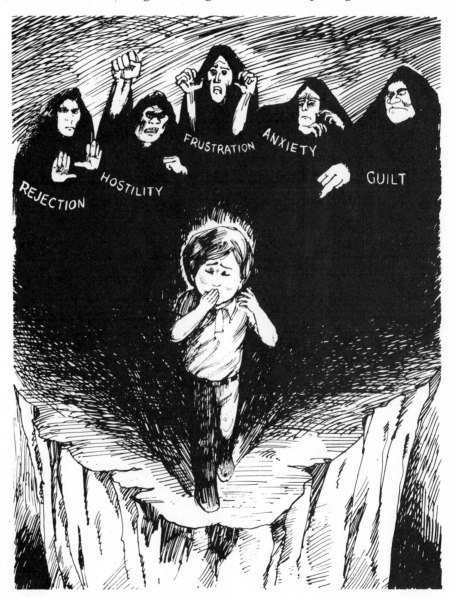

Figure 1   Sources of polluted lives.

the world a fit place for man to fulfill his infinite potential for something other than evil. But there are many kinds of pollution, and
some of the worst are those that reflect man's inhumanity to man.
Perhaps all other evils flow from this befouled spring. If so, the study
of speech pathology should help us discern what must be done.

It is important to realize that speech is the unique feature that
distinguishes man from animal. Had he not talked, man would still
be in Eden or the cave. In the dark mirror of speech pathology we
will find reflected his fears, his frustrations, his shame, and the way
he is treated by others; but the profession of speech therapy also provides the hope that somehow, someday, we can solve our problems.
The author has been privileged to spend his life seeking to reduce,
prevent, and heal that special kind of human misery found in defective speech, and it has given him a sense of meaningfulness he hun-
gers to share. He is under no illusions about the extent of his own
personal contribution. By any measure it is infinitesimal, but at least
it has been directed toward eliminating some of the human pollution
that surrounded the people who have felt his impact. Each of us must
do what we can so that our children's children will find a better
world and better individuals to inhabit it.

Sometimes it seems that there are so many human ills and evils
that anyone who dedicates his life to their diminishing is dooming
himself to a life of futility and frustration. We have not found it so.
Though our individual efforts may seem at times to have no more effect than those of an ant carrying a grain of sand away from the sea-
shore, we have before us the example of atomic fission in which one
active particle triggers those about it, and these then fire others until
incredible forces are released. Each human being has within his lifetime a host of opportunities to trigger forces for good or evil which
lie latent in his fellows. We believe that it is therefore possible for
any one of us to start chain reactions which may finally result in the
kind of world and the kind of men we hope for.

Speech Deviancy   All societies develop value systems and a corresponding set
of controls to insure that their members respect them. These
value systems vary widely from culture to culture, and so do the controls that implement them. While all human societies place a pre-
mium upon effective communication as a primary bond holding
them together, certain societies seem to prize it more than others. In
our own, a highly competitive, upwardly mobile one, verbal skill is
greatly rewarded. We swim in a vast ocean of words all of our lives.
Effective speech in such a society is of the utmost importance if one

is to gain and maintain membership or to get the status and material possessions which are constantly held up to us as goals to be desired.

It is very hard for normal speakers to comprehend how difficult it is to live in a culture such as ours without possessing the ability to speak in an acceptable fashion. Perhaps a few glimpses into the lives of the speech-handicapped may help. Here are some excerpts from autobiographies:

> After they found out I had cancer the doctors took out my voice box, and suddenly I was in a new, terribly strange world. I'd open my mouth to talk and nothing came out, just a rush of air out of the hole in my neck. I was mute. I could move my mouth and tongue but only silence came. And I got terribly afraid and depressed and wanted to die. How was I ever to work again? How was I to have friends? I was a stranger even to my wife and to myself. I tried to pray for strength and my mouth moved but no words came.

> My friends tell me I'm attractive, but at twenty-four years of age I can count all the dates I've had on the fingers of one hand. Boys don't want to go out with girls who talk through their nose like I do. The doctors fixed my cleft lip so you can't hardly see the scar, but my voice is nasal and they say they can't help with that. In grade school the kids called me "Honker" or "Nosey" and mocked the way I talked. People don't do that now that I'm grown up, but they look at me funny and shy away. Or they are extra kind to me and that's worse. I don't want pity. I just want to live like everybody else. I wonder how many nights I've cried myself to sleep over these miserable years.

> Maybe the best way I can tell you how my stuttering covers my life is by writing some of what happened today. I was OK until I had breakfast, because I didn't talk. Then I went down to the corner drugstore because I had overslept, or rather just lay there in bed, dreading the day. I wanted coffee and rolls, but I ordered milk and oatmeal because I knew I'd stutter hard on those other words and I didn't want the old lady who waited on me to feel sorry for me. I hate oatmeal, and I had a little block on it anyway, dammit. Then I walked back to school and once went over to the other side of the street so I wouldn't have to say hello or to talk to a girl in my class who knows me. I remembered the times I've stopped someone in their tracks waiting for me to get the hello out. In my first class the instructor called on

me out of the blue, and although I knew the answer, I played dumb and shook my head no, and then felt like a dog. A cur, a mongrel! After class I hurried away up to the library, got a book, and pretended to study hard when anyone I knew passed by. I also had to tie my shoestring which then broke and broke again when I fixed it. I thought of going downtown to get a new pair of shoestrings, but I didn't know where I could just point to them without saying anything. Maybe at Kresge's, but maybe not. So I finally tied enough knots to hold, though it looked lousy. Felt ashamed that I didn't even have the guts to ask for shoestrings. Put it off like I always do. I'm broke and wrote a letter to my Dad asking for money. Wanted to put a special delivery stamp on it, but remembered the last time I tried to buy one at the post office, and the sp-spsp-sp-sp-sp just kept going forever, and the clerk got impatient and the people in line behind me too, and well, I couldn't face it, so I got a regular stamp out of the machine and mailed it. Got thirty cents left to eat on and hope Dad isn't as slow as he often is in answering. Maybe I can borrow from my roomie—but God, that'll mean a mess of stuttering too. Hate to ask favors. I'll be making faces and jump around. I've got over about fifteen ways of saying it to him but can't find one combination that has any chance of being said without stuttering. . . .

This glimpse into the inner world of a stutterer as he reacts to his speech deviancy may seem to present an exaggerated and distorted picture. Unfortunately, it is not distorted. We have heard literally thousands of similar tales in one form or another. These people have been hurt deeply and repeatedly because they did not and could not conform to the speech standards of our society. The tragedy lies in the fact that they *could not.* They were not responsible for their defective speech, but those who hurt them acted as though they were, as though they had a choice. This assumption is the core of the problem not only of the person with a speech disorder but also of the poor, the insane, and most of the other kinds of deviancy.

Once, on Fiji in the South Pacific, we found a whole family of stutterers. As our guide and translator phrased it: "Mama kaka; papa kaka; and kaka, kaka, kaka, kaka." All six persons in that family showed marked repetitions and prolongations in their speech but they were happy people, not at all troubled by their stuttering. It was just the way they talked. No hurry, no frustration, no stigma, indeed very little awareness. We could not help but contrast their attitudes and the simplicity of their stuttering with those which would have been shown by a similar family in our own land, where the pace of living is so much faster, where defective communication is rejected, where stutterers get penalized all their lives. To possess a marked speech disorder in our society is almost as handicapping as to be a physical cripple in a nomadic tribe that exists by hunting. Lemert, the sociologist, found a similar contrast in the way stutterers were treated among Polynesians as compared to the Japanese. He writes, "In common with the Hawaiians and Samoans, Manganians neither laugh at nor ridicule the stutterers. The individuals who stutter are not socially rejected and are under no handicap as to marriage or occupation. No attempt is made by the Manganians to treat or correct stuttering since it is accepted as an inborn characteristic." Lemert (1962) showed that the Japanese, on the other hand, reacted to stuttering much as we do.

All societies demand a certain amount of conformity of their members. Only in anarchy could all members theoretically "do their own thing." The patterning of this conformity varies, of course, from culture to culture, and the demands change within any specific one from time to time. One needs only observe the variance in fashion or dress to understand that this is true. The hemlines go up and the hemlines come down. Beards disappear only to reappear after a generation or two. Moral values ebb and flow, a Reformation yielding to a Restoration. When the tyranny of conformity becomes too onerous, there are always a few mavericks to lead a revolt. They usually take a beating, but their impact sets off a counter reaction that spreads throughout the society until a new set of rules and demands predominates. Some societies are more rigid than others and change slowly, but ours seems to oscillate rather easily. The current youth movement may be viewed as the culmination of a fairly long trend against the excessive controls for conformity which dominated the value systems of preceding generations. Certainly our society is now in flux, and many of the old values are being strongly challenged. If this is disturbing, it is also exciting in its prospect that we may yet create a world in which men can live not only in harmony with a less polluted environment but with themselves.

If so, the major change must come in the way we interact with others. We must come to have concern for those less fortunate than ourselves. In our emerging affluent society in which machines do most of the work and leisure time becomes increasingly available, our energies must find creative outlets. If we merely use that leisure and affluence to indulge our appetites, we shall become decadent and corrupt, thereby inviting our inevitable extinction. If, on the other hand, we seek to alleviate human misery wherever and in whatever form it exists, we shall flower beyond all vision. It is with these thoughts in mind that we present the problems of those handicapped by disordered speech, for, in a small way, in speech therapy we find a minor model of things to come, a template of the future.

The speech pathologist dedicates himself to the reduction of a special kind of misfortune. There are other human ills, of course: poverty, hunger, disease, war, intolerance, injustice. When the whole pool of human misery is surveyed, it might seem that those who are handicapped in communication must represent little more than an adjacent and insignificant puddle. How can we have the nerve to present the field of speech pathology as the shape of things to come, as a possible promise of a better future? All we can answer is that those who have concerned themselves with the untangling of tongues do seem to feel this way. They are concerned about the unfortunate; they devote their lives to the relief of human distress. But there is something more—and it is difficult to put into words. When we deal with speech, we deal with the essence of man. Only human beings have mastered speech. It is what sets us apart from all other species. Because we can speak, we can think symbolically; and it is this which has enabled man to conquer the world and space and every other creature. Dimly we believe, or at least hope, that someday it may enable us to master ourselves.

We who have spoken so much so easily and for so long find it hard to comprehend the miraculous nature of speech—this peculiarly human tool. It seems as natural and as easy as breathing. But those of us who try to help those who have been deprived of normal communication soon come to know how utterly vital and necessary speech is to human existence. Not only do we use it in thinking and in the sending and receiving of messages, we also build our very sense of self out of word-stuff. We need speech to command and restrain ourselves. Our words are our means for controlling others. Verbally we express our loves and hates. It is the safety valve of our emotions, the medicine of psychotherapy. Only those who come to know the problems of those who have been denied the magical power of the spoken word can realize the tremendous scope of this marvelous instrument that man has invented. Indeed, there are times when it seems that man has just began to exploit the latent powers inherent in his speech. Someday he may learn to employ all those powers, but now he is like an ape using a flute to scratch himself. We who deal with the speech-handicapped do not take speech for granted. We are constantly aware of the extent of their deprivation. Our task is no small one; it is to help these persons gain the tools they need to fulfill their potential; it is to help them to join or rejoin the human race.

What the Speech Pathologist Does[1]   Since we felt it would be appropriate here to give you an immediate glimpse of the kind of work speech pathologists do, we wrote to a number of our former students now practicing their profession in various settings and asked them to send us brief descriptions of some of the casework they had done that day.

Our first account came from a young speech pathologist,[1] who works in the public schools—mainly with children whose speech sounds are incorrectly produced:

> I'd like to tell you about Sammy, a little fourth grader, who said his name today correctly for the first time in his life. He has a severe slushy lateral lisp on all the sibilant sounds, and even on the *ch* and *j* sounds and sometimes they bubble with saliva. The other kids mock him and make his life pretty miserable. They call him Drunken Sammy among other things, and when they do, he cries. Really suffers, Dr. Van! Worse yet, he's had speech therapy from my predecessors for three years. The last one left me a note saying that she had tried hard to help him but had failed and she felt there must be some organic basis for his problem. She also suggested that perhaps Sammy should be given a year or two of vacation from speech therapy for he was beginning to feel like a total failure.
>
> After our first few sessions I was tempted to take her advice because this is my first year on the job and I hated to begin with a chronic failure but after I saw how unhappy the boy was I decided to take him out of the group and work with him alone during the noon hour. The first thing I did was to give him the Deep Test of Articulation to see if there was any combination of sounds in which the *s* or *z* were made correctly. All but two of them were errors, but the *ks* (as in X) and the *gz* (as in *exam*) were ok. I asked myself, "Why these?" and the only answer I could come up with was that if the tongue was down against the lower teeth as it is in the *k* and *g,* then the *s* and *z* when they followed these sounds might also be made with a lowered tongue tip. Perhaps Sammy had to make his sibilants this different way if he were to make them correctly, using a groove along the blade of the tongue rather than along the tongue tip to create the hissing sound he needs. So I got a little peanut butter,

---

[1] We use the terms *speech pathologist* and *speech clinician* in this text rather than *speech therapist* because the latter term tends to imply an auxiliary service to the medical profession and because the American Speech and Hearing Association has so decreed.

pasted it on the back of his lower teeth, and told him to keep tasting it as he tried to say his name. Believe it or not, it worked. The *s* was perfect and he knew it too for he kept saying "Sammy, Sammy, Sammy," over and over till I thought he'd never stop. And then he cried—and I guess I almost did too. Oh, I know there's a lot more to do, to make the new sound stronger and to get it into other words and combinations, but the kid has hope at last. He finally was able to say his own name. Made my day!

Among the many evidences that speech pathology is a rapidly growing profession is the continuing increase in community speech and hearing centers. These are funded by charitable agencies such as the United Way or Easter Seal or other organizations and are usually supported in part by fees. Here is the report of a worker in such a center:

My duties are varied and depend upon the particular caseload we have at any one time. At present I usually have one or two diagnostic sessions each morning or application interviews with parents. Then I may see a stutterer or an aphasic for therapy. In the afternoons, most of my work is with small groups. One of these consists of pre-school deaf children but the one I enjoy most is the group of three laryngectomees.[2] Let me tell you a bit about them. Mr. J. has been with us the longest and has the best esophageal speech of any of them. Very intelligible! Yesterday he managed to say a thirteen syllable sentence with good intensity on a single burp. I mean intake, of course, but my patients call it burping and I forget to be professional, we have so much fun. He's working mainly on trying to get more loudness and more inflections. The second man is Mr. F. who is just beginning to string a series of words into phrases without having to stop and gulp before every syllable. Our third member is a fifty-year-old woman who is having a very hard time. The only way she can get any sound at all is by the tongue-pumping air injection procedure. Mrs. W. fails often, especially when trying to start the syllable with the /p/, /b/, /t/, or /d/ sounds. She wrote me a note saying that she hates the sound of the burp— that it sounds vulgar, ugly. Mrs. W. is very depressed most of the time and until we put her with the two men I was pretty sure she'd quit. But they've really helped her, Mr. J. especially, for he's a gay spirit and a fine example. And he's a pretty good

[2] These are persons who have had their larynxes removed surgically because of cancerous growths on or in the area of the vocal cords.

teacher of esophageal speech too. Even better than I am, though I'm much better than when you coached me four years ago. When I demonstrate, they kid me about feeling sorry for me because my larynx gets in the way. I'm not as good as Mr. J. but I'm better than the other two and all in all it's a learning experience for all of us. Oh, by the way . . . did you ever hear something like this? They all confessed to lighting a cigarette and putting the end of it into the hole in their necks and trying to smoke. Lord, wouldn't you think they'd have more sense? Don't think they tried it more than once, though. All of them said that they'd been two-pack-a-day smokers.

Here's the report from a speech pathologist in another kind of job setting:

As you know, I work in a child guidance clinic. Our clientele consists mainly of children with severe emotional problems and I work closely with our psychiatrists, social workers, and psychologists both in diagnosis and treatment. But you asked for the most interesting thing I did today. I guess it was the recheck of a child we have seen three times. The girl, aged four-and-a-half, first came to us about six months ago with echolalia.[3] She simply repeated anything that anyone else said to her. Automatically and with the same inflections! Weird! To express her own wants she used gesture language. The psychologist surprisingly found her not to be at all retarded. The social workers felt that although she was an only child and the parents were overly perfectionistic and anxious, the family situation was really pretty healthy.

The psychiatrist made a tentative diagnosis of childhood schizophrenia. My own initial examination revealed no difficulty in comprehension, and surprisingly no articulation errors when she repeated what was said to her. Her mother told me that the girl had been ill a lot during the first two years and had said her first words about the time of her third birthday, that she had begun using phrases and sentences rather than individual words from the very beginning. The echolalia had showed itself first when talking to the father but soon was being used consistently with anyone. Well, to make a long story short, I felt that the child had been taught to be echolalic by her anxious parents. They had drilled her in speech too much, you know, in

---

[3] You will find a definition of this and other unfamiliar words in the Glossary on page 455.

the "Say this . . . and say that" fashion. Their demands for speech had been too great. Constant questioning, naming, repeating. No wonder the girl became echolalic.

Anyway, I had two sessions with the child, demonstrating to the observing parents how to interact without any speech demands at all, giving examples of simplified speech and parallel talking (verbalizing what the child was doing, or seeing, or feeling). I showed them samples of my own self-talk as I played with her. Short and simple utterances only, and no questions or requests that she say anything. Anyway, it worked out pretty well, for Mary once said a few spontaneous words right in front of them. After the second demonstration session I outlined to the parents how they should follow this program in the home and in our recheck conference today, a month later, they reported that the girl was using more spontaneous speech and that the echolalia was fading out. This job is sure challenging.

Some speech pathologists work in hospital clinics. This is how one of them described her work:

You asked for a description of my professional activities on a typical day but there seem to be no typical days. They all are very different; each new one brings new problems which is why I like working in the medical setting of a hospital speech and hearing clinic. That, and the chance to work closely with physicians, physical therapists, occupational therapists, and even with our medical social worker. There are so many different kinds of patients and so many disorders that I have never seen before.

But the bulk of my cases are stroke patients or patients whose aphasias resulted from traumatic head injuries that required neurosurgery. Besides doing therapy with these, I also have to do repeated assessments of their speech and language to provide the attending physician with the information he needs about their progress or lack of it. He needs this so that he can make the necessary decisions. I've found that the usual formal tests for aphasia must be supplemented by a lot of informal observation and interaction with these patients because they tire so fast or get so emotional when they fail some test item. In the testing situation they rarely show how much speech and language ability they really possess. Let me give you an example.

This afternoon one of the nurses complimented me on my "bed-side manner" after hearing a young male patient laugh for the first time in many weeks. This man had been in a deep depression and with plenty of reasons for it. He'd been in a bad automobile wreck that killed his wife and child and left him a hemiplegic wreck too. When he did try to talk, all that came out was compulsive jargon. Not all of my aphasics know when they talk gibberish but he did, and it devastated him. Almost every time he tries to talk, he starts crying and does not seem to be able to stop. But today I got him to be able to count aloud up to twenty with only one mistake. Trying to establish some imitation, I got him to mimic some communicative gestures like nodding yes and head shaking for no and then trying to read my lips and mimic them silently.

After some of this I then began to count aloud and so did he. It surprised and shocked him to hear himself saying those numbers and that's when the nurse heard him laugh. Of course, when he started laughing, he couldn't stop and then he was laughing and crying at the same time. Took me a long time to calm him down and he didn't want me to leave so I had to make sure he understood that I'd be back tomorrow at the same time. Pretty hard to do because my words didn't seem to sink in so I acted out my leaving the room and then returning, pointing to the clock and a calendar and saying something like this over and over again slowly and with plenty of pauses: "Miss Peterson (pointing to myself) go now . . . Miss Peterson come back (turn one page of desk calendar). Miss Peterson (pointing) see John (pointing) tomorrow . . . This time (I showed him the time on the clock). John eat . . . John eat (pointed to five o'clock feeding time). Then John sleep (I acted out sleeping as I pointed to 10 o'clock) and so on. Somehow, something got through to him and I feel he understood I'd be back for he waved the fingers of his non-paralyzed hand to indicate goodbye and smiled when I left. For the first time John and I have a tiny ray of hope but I've got my fingers and legs crossed. Poor devil.

Still another facet of the field of speech pathology is the rapidly growing opportunity to do private practice. Those who undertake to set up a private clinical practice have to be very competent, experienced, and able to establish close relationships with the medical profession. And they must be prepared to undergo an initial period of financial insecurity. Nevertheless, the number of private practitioners is growing yearly and we submit a portion of a letter from one of them:

> When I last wrote you some years ago I had just retired from my job in the hospital speech and hearing clinic so that I could raise a family. Now, two babies later, both of whom are now in school, I am back in the profession — this time in private practice full time and I love it, though often at the end of a day I'm pretty worn out. Private practice is much more demanding than any other job in the field and I've worked, as you know, in the public schools, in the hospital clinic, and for a time supervised students in a college training center. It all started when my own pediatrician asked me to help with two of his patients, a child with severe language delay and a young stutterer. I worked with them in my own home while my children were in school and it was good to be using my brain and skills again after seven years of being just a housewife and mother. Well, one thing led to another and pretty soon I was so swamped with requests for help that I knew I either had to expand or quit. Fortunately, I had an audiologist friend in much the same situation, so we decided to join forces.
>
> So here we are in a two-room suite in the Medical Arts building with physicians, dentists, and other professionals, working harder but making more money than we ever did on our old jobs. The worst part is the paper work, for the secretary we share part time with a physical therapist is as overworked as we are. But it's fascinating. You have to be professionally competent to survive in private practice and I think I've learned more these last few years that I ever did in my life. About a third of our clients are on Medicare or Medicaid and we have several hospitals that contract for our services. Occasionally we even make home calls, usually after office hours and we always take one or two patients who cannot pay our regular fees. But, Dr. Van, I've found that when people have to pay for my services they work harder — and, heaven knows, so do I. We'd starve if we didn't produce results.
>
> Sometimes this is not easy to achieve — as with the man who missed the appointment which enables me to write you now. He has Parkinson's disease, and the L-dopa medication which seemed to help at first is now becoming less effective so the prognosis is not good. Why would I accept a client with such a degenerative disease? Why not? I gave him six months of usable

speech that was not present when he came and I gave him back his human dignity. I'm sure he feels our sessions were worth the money he paid me. Luckily, most of our clients make gains and hold them. All I can say is that it sure is good to be back at work and to be able to use my professional skills again. I'm happier and so is my husband and family even though at times things get a bit hectic.

These brief pictures of the field of speech pathology just sketch the surface of the topography. You have seen just a few of the many opportunities that exist within its boundaries and only a few of the many kinds of speech disorders that need help. Moreover, for some workers, speech pathology provides an initial stepping stone to other fields of service. The public school speech pathologist, because he comes into close contact with many teachers and principals, and because he works with so many children with other handicaps, may end up administering programs in special education. Because such a person is also qualified as a teacher, he may shift into that occupation. Since much of the work in clinical settings involves testing and diagnosis as well as counseling, some speech pathologists go into clinical psychology.

And here we should mention our sister profession of audiology. All speech pathologists must take some course work concerned with the problems of the deaf and hard of hearing, just as all audiologists must have some preparation in dealing with speech disorders. Indeed, they have a common professional organization, the American Speech and Hearing Association, to which they both belong. Accordingly, some of our students begin as speech pathologists, then change to audiology if they find the communication problems due to hearing loss more attractive.

Like speech pathologists, audiologists work in a variety of settings. We even find them in industry trying to prevent noise-induced hearing loss, conducting noise surveys to reduce noise pollution, testing ear damage, and doing many other things. One of our former students, a clinical audiologist in a hospital speech and hearing clinic, gives this picture of his professional day:

I spent the eight o'clock hour on correspondence and reports of yesterday's hearing testing. Then at nine o'clock I examined a patient with otosclerosis referred to me by the otologist who is considering performing a stapedectomy.[4] For various reasons,

[4]See Glossary.

this took longer than I expected and I was late for my next appointment with a patient I had previously tested and who was ready for hearing-aid selection and orientation. She found it very hard to decide on the aid that seemed to help her the most. She said they all sounded "too noisy". She's been so hard of hearing for so long, she's forgotten what the world of sound is like. And I guess she expected, like most of my clients, that the hearing aid would not be just an aid but would restore her hearing completely. Took a lot of delicate counseling. Then in the afternoon I was scheduled to conduct two lipreading groups. Next I tested a man who had been in an industrial accident who claimed it had deafened him totally. It hadn't; he was malingering. Then I examined the eardrum of a teen-ager with a complaint of fullness in her ear and ended my day by using the artificial ear to calibrate one of our audiometers. Every day is different, but that's the way this one went.

Many of you who read this book are not planning to become professional speech pathologists but all of you are certain to encounter men, women, and children who cannot speak normally for there are at least 18,000,000 such persons in our country alone. Will you turn away from their need for help and understanding? Will you add one more rejection to the many they have already endured? Or will you do what you can? Here is an excerpt from a letter written us by a former student who is a classroom teacher, not a speech pathologist or audiologist.

Although I've only had the introductory course in speech pathology, I've often been able to help a few children with speech problems right in my classroom. I've been teaching third grade now for three years and love it. Wouldn't do anything else. I've steered clear from the severe speech disorders because we have a speech therapist who visits our school twice each week and who knows a lot more than I do but I've been able to help the gains she gets become more permanent by following her suggestions with my children who lisp or cannot pronounce their *r* or *l* sounds.

Well, today at lunch hour I asked her why she didn't take Joe for therapy. Joe's a very bad stutterer when he recites, which is seldom. Her answer was that Joe's mother had refused permission to let him have any speech help this year so her hands were tied. She said that Joe's mother was a mild stutterer herself and perhaps that was why, though it didn't make sense. I told the speech therapist that Joe never volunteered in class and usually answered my questions in as few words as possible or said he didn't know when I was pretty sure he did. And when I told her too that Joe rarely went out with the other children to play at recess time, the therapist asked me to find out why. So today, when again he stayed in, I just up and asked Joe about it when we were by ourselves. Tears came in his eyes as he said it was because he "talked funny" and the other kids mocked him. And he even asked me if I would teach him to talk better. Of course I said yes and we made a date to begin after school tomorrow. Anyway, I put in a frantic call to the speech therapist and she will coach me and help out indirectly. She said that there was lots that I could do and I'm sure there is. At least I can make it easier for him. Poor little kid! I was really touched when, just before he left to get on the bus, he came up to my desk and shyly touched my hand. That's all—just a touch, and then he ran out.

Now that you've had a few brief glimpses of some speech pathologists at work, let us turn to the problems of their clients so that you can understand why people enter this profession. The basic reason is that they want to relieve a special kind of human misery.

The Emotional Fraction of a Speech Handicap   The pollution of human misery comes from many wells, but its composition is the same. Abnormal speech is no asset to anyone. It invites penalty from any society which prizes the ability to communicate effectively. Normal speech is the membership card that signifies that its owner belongs to the human race. Those who do not possess it are penalized and rejected. Even the abnormal speaker himself often feels this rejection is justified.

Moreover, the inability to communicate, to get the rewards our society offers to those who can talk effectively, results in great frustration. To be unable to say the word when he desires to do so, as in the case of the stutterer; to say "think" when he means "sink," as in lisping; not to be able to produce a voice at all, as in the aphonic; to try to say something meaningful only to find that gibberish emerges, as in the aphasic—all these are profoundly frustrating. Anxiety, guilt, and hostility are the natural reactions to penalty and frustration. You too have known these three miseries transiently when you have been punished or met frustration, but many individuals with defective speech spend their lives immersed in these emotions.

Penalties   Let us look at some illustrative penalties culled from the auto-biographies of stutterers, remembering that similar tales could be told by individuals with other varieties of defective speech:

Most clerks look away when I get stuck and begin to force. It always infuriates me that they don't even have the decency to look at me. Once I even went to the manager of a store about it, and he looked away too.

My father wouldn't ever listen to me when I stuttered. He always walked off. I finally got so I'd say everything to him by having mother give him the message.

People do not usually laugh at my other kinds of stuttering, but when I begin to go up in pitch, they always smile or laugh right out loud. I was phoning a girl today and hung up when I heard her snickering.

My mother always hurried to say the word for me whenever company was in the house. I often asked her not to, but she couldn't help herself. It used to shame me so, I'd go up in my room and cry; and I never went visiting with them. Sometimes I'd eat in the kitchen when we had strangers come for dinner.

The other boys in the school used to call me "stuttercat" and imitate me whenever I came to school. At first I always managed to be tardy and stay after school to avoid them, but my folks got after me, and then I began to fight with them. I got to be a pretty good fighter, but the bigger boys always licked me, and the teacher punished me when I hit the girls. I still hate girls.

After I came to high school from the country, everybody laughed at me whenever I tried to recite. After that, I pretended to be dumb and always said "I don't know" when the teacher called on me. That's why I quit school.

Every time I'd ask for a job, a funny look would come over their faces, and some of them would say no right away even before I finished what I was going to say. Some of the others, and one of them was a stutterer too, just waited till I finally got it out and then they'd shake their heads. One storekeeper was so sympathetic I could hardly get out of there fast enough.

> The worst time I ever had was when a hotel clerk saw me jumping around and called a doctor. He thought I was having a fit.

These are but a few of the many penalties and rejections which any individual with an unpleasant difference is likely to experience. Imitative behavior, curiosity, nicknaming, humorous response, embarrassed withdrawal, brutal attack, impatience, quick rejection or exclusion, overprotection, pity, misinterpretation, and condescension are some of the other common penalties.

The amount and kind of penalty inflicted on a speech defective are dependent on four factors: (1) the vividness or peculiarity of the speech difference; (2) the person's attitude toward his own difference; (3) the sensitivities, maladjustments, or preconceived attitudes of the people who penalize him; and (4) the presence of other personality assets.

First of all, in general, the more frequent or bizarre the speech peculiarity, the more frequently and strongly it is penalized. Thus a child with only one sound substitution or one that occurs only intermittently will be penalized less than one with almost unintelligible speech, and a mild stutterer will be penalized less than a severe one. Second, the speech deviant's own attitude toward his deviancy often determines what the attitude of the auditor will be. If he considers it a shameful abnormality, his listeners can hardly be expected to contradict him. Empathic response is a powerful agent in the creation of attitudes. Third, the worst penalties will come from those individuals who are sensitive about some difference of their own. Since some of them have parents or siblings with similar speech differences, they are often penalized very early in life by those persons.

> You ask why I slap Jerry every time he stutters? I do it for his own good. If my mother had slapped me every time I did it I could have broken myself of this habit. It's horrible going through life stuttering every time you open your mouth, and my boy isn't going to have to do it even if I have to knock his head off.

Moreover, many individuals have such preconceived notions or attitudes concerning the causes or the unpleasantness of speech handicaps that they react in a more or less stereotyped fashion to such differences, no matter how well adjusted the speech deviant himself may be. Finally, as we have pointed out, the speech deviant may possess other abilities or personal assets which so overshadow his speech difference that he is penalized very little.

Even though some children with a speech disorder are fortunate enough to be brought up in a family and an environment where they meet little punishment for their difference, eventually they will meet the rejection that society reserves for the person who has an unacceptable difference. Indeed, some of these protected children are more vulnerable than those whose lives have been full of penalty. Let us give a few examples from our own practice:

> A second-grade boy had been receiving speech therapy for over a year and had made excellent progress in mastering many of his defective sounds. In the third grade he met a teacher who was old and uncontrolled, who had had to return to teaching after her husband had died, and who hated the whole business. She used the boy as a scapegoat for her own frustrations. Under the guise of helping him, she ridiculed his errors and held him up to scorn before his fellows. Shortly after the fall term began, this boy's speech began to get worse, and within a few months it had lapsed to its former unintelligible jargon.

> We had been working for three years with Ted, an eight-year-old youngster. His cleft palate had been repaired surgically; but the muscles were very weak, and there was scar tissue which made it a bit difficult to close off the rear opening to the nasal passages with speed. He had improved greatly, however, and only a few bits of nasal snorting or excessive nasality remained when he talked carefully. Then one day his associates on the playground, led by the inevitable bully, began to call him "Nosey–Nosey." Within one week his speech disintegrated into a honking, unintelligible jargon, and he refused to come to the clinic for any more therapy.

Covert Penalties   Not all of the penalties bestowed upon the person who talks queerly are so obvious. Perhaps the worst ones are those that are hidden, the covert kind. One of our stutterers said this:

> In my whole life, never did my parents ever say a single thing about my stuttering, no matter how hard or badly I stuttered. Sometimes they might blink an eye or become transfixed or look away or change the conversation, but we never talked about it. It was a black shadow that always followed me, but no one looked at it. It was unmentionable, unspeakable. Mustn't talk about such dirty things. Sometimes I wanted to shout, "I'm hav-

ing trouble. Can't you see? I'm stuttering. Help me! Help me!''
But I couldn't break that wall of silence.

Most of the more obvious penalties are felt by children. After a
speech-handicapped person becomes an adult, few people mock him,
laugh at him, or show disgust. Instead, he now finds that they shun
him. Their distant politeness may hurt worse than the epithets he
knew when he was young. One of our cases, a girl with a paralyzed
tongue and very slurred speech who was desperately in need of work
so she could eat and have a place to sleep, contacted forty-nine different prospective employers before she found one who would give
her a chance to exist. ''Not one of them ever said anything about my
speech,'' she told us. ''Some were extra kind, some were impatient,
some were rude, but all of them had some other reason besides my
speech for saying no. I could tell right away by seeing how they
changed the moment I began to talk. Like I was unclean or something.''

Why do such things happen? Why do we punish the person
who is different? Why must he punish himself? Surely Americans are
some of the kindest people who have ever lived on this earth. We
show our concern for the unfortunate every day. No nation has ever
known so many agencies, campaigns, foundations, and private charities. One drive for funds follows another. Muscular Dystrophy, the
Red Cross, the United Fund, the Heart Association, Seeing Eye dogs,
the coin bottle in the drugstore, the pleading on radio and television.
Surely all of these activities seem to show that we help rather than
punish our handicapped, but perhaps we find it easier to give our
money than ourselves.

Cultural anthropologists have regarded this altruism with more
than academic interest. They point out that our culture is one that
features the setting up of a constant series of material goals and possessions which are highly advertised. Prestige and status seem often
to be based upon winning these possessions and positions in a
highly competitive struggle. We fight for security and approval, but
in the process we trample underfoot the security of others. Some psychologists have felt that our need to help the handicapped is a prod-
uct of the guilt feelings we possess from this trampling. Others at-
tribute our concern for the underprivileged to fear lest someday we
too will be the losers in the battle for life. They claim that we tend to
say to ourselves, ''There, but for the grace of God, go I,'' when we
meet someone who has failed to find a place for himself in the world
for reasons beyond his control. These organized charities do much
good, but they cannot fulfill the needs of the handicapped for per-

sonal acceptance. Until we understand those needs and find ourselves able to care for each other on a person-to-person basis, the
pollution of human misery will continue to exist.

Aggressive or
Protest Behavior
as a Reaction
to Penalty

Penalty and rejection by his associates may lead an individual to react aggressively by attack, protest, or some form of
rebellion. He may employ the mechanism of projection and
blame his parents, teachers, or playmates for his objectionable difference. He may display toward the weaknesses of
others in the group the same intolerant attitude which they have
manifested toward his own. In this way he not only temporarily min-
imizes the importance of his own handicap, but also enjoys the re-
venge of recognizing weaknesses in others. He may attempt to shift
the blame for rejection. He will say, "They didn't keep me out because I stutter—they just didn't think I had as nice clothes as the rest
of them wore." In this way he will exaggerate the unfairness of the
group evaluation and ignore the actual cause. Another attack reaction
may be to focus all attention upon himself. He can refuse to cooperate wtih the group in any way, can belittle its importance openly,
and can refuse to consider it in his scheme of existence. Finally, he
may react by a direct outward attack. A child, or an adult with an
easily provoked temper, may indulge in actual physical conflict with
members of the group that has not accepted him.

> Ivan, whom we straightway named "The Terrible," was a very
> agile little boy of six with completely unintelligible speech. He
> was a holy terror. Other mothers would sweep their children
> back into the house when Ivan came tricycling up the sidewalk.
> No baby-sitter ever sat twice at his house. His mother worked
> days, probably in self-defense; and the boy was cared for by his
> grandfather and grandmother, who lived upstairs. Only the
> grandfather could control Ivan, and when he left the house to go
> to the store the grandmother would flee to her bedroom and
> lock the door because Ivan would occasionally swarm up her
> and bite her, preferably on the nose. She was hard-of-hearing
> and found Ivan's garbled jargon quite impossible to com-
> prehend. Ivan demanded that people understand him. If they
> did, he was well behaved and cooperative. But when they
> didn't, he went berserk; he scratched, bit, and attacked the ob-
> ject of his hatred. It took two years before Ivan was tamed and
> talking, and our speech clinic still bears certain scars as an en-
> during memorial to Ivan. So do this therapist's hands.

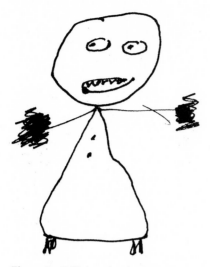

Figure 2   Self-drawing by Ivan the Terrible.

A rejected individual may spread pointed criticism of the group in a resentful manner. In any of these methods, the object of the rejection does not retreat from reality—he reacts antagonistically and attacks those who made his reality unpleasant. The more the speech-deviant person attacks the group, the more it penalizes him. Often such reactions interfere with treatment, for many of these persons resent any proffered aid. They attack the speech pathologist and sabotage his assignments. The inevitable result of these attack reactions is to push him even further from normal speech and adequate adjustment.

Frustration

Frustration is always experienced when human potential is blocked from fulfillment. It is the ache of the giant in chains. All lives are full of frustrations. We cannot live together without inhibiting some of our impulses and desires. Circumstances always place barriers in the paths we desire to take. But for some persons, the cup of frustration is filled to the brim and more is added every day. Frustration breeds anger and aggression, and these corrupt everything they touch. Those who cannot talk normally are constantly thwarted. Consider, then, how a person must feel if he cannot talk intelligibly. Others have difficulty in understanding the messages of the stutterer, the jargon-talking child, or the person who has lost his voice forever due to cancer. Others listen, but they do not, they cannot, understand. The aphasic tries to ask for a cigarette and says, "Come me a bummadee. A bummadee! A bummadee!" This is frustration.

Or even when the listener can understand the words, he finds himself distracted by the odd contortions of the spastic's or stutterer's face, the twitching of the cleft-palate case's nostrils; and he forgets what has been said and asks that it be repeated. This is frustration too. Communication is the lifeblood of a society. When it cannot flow, the pressure builds up explosively. The worst of all legal punishments short of death is solitary confinement where no one can talk to the prisoner, nor can he talk to anyone else. There are such prisoners walking about among us, sentenced by their speech and hearing disorders to lives of deprivation and frustration.

> One young stutterer diagnosed his own problem for us. His speech was full of irregular and forced repetitions. He hesitated. He seldom was able to utter even a short sentence without having wide gaps in it. One day, after he had just beaten up our plastic-clown punching bag he confided in us. "Y-y-y-you know . . . y-y-you know whuh-whuh-what's wrrrrrong with me? I-I-I-I'm the lllllittlest . . . child." He was. He was the runt of the litter, the weakest, smallest, most unattractive of the eight children in that family. The others were an aggressive bunch, yelling, fighting, arguing, talking. His mouth never had an ear to hear it. When his sentences were finished, it was some brother's or sister's mouth that finished them. He was constantly interrupted or ignored. He had learned a broken English, a hesitant speech.

The good things of life must be asked for, must be earned by the mouth as well as the hands. The fun of companionship, the satisfaction of earning a good living, the winning of a mate, the pride of self-respect and appreciation, these things come hard to the person who cannot talk. Often he must settle for less than his potential might provide, were it not for his tangled tongue. Speech is the "Open Sesame," the magical power. When it is distorted, there is small magic in it—and much frustration.

We need safety valves for emotion. When we can express the angry evils within us, they subside; when we can verbalize our grief, it decreases. A fear coded into words and shared by a companion seems less distressing. A guilt confessed brings absolution. But what of the poor devils who find speaking hard, who find it difficult even to ask for bread? This wonderful function of speech is denied them. The evil acids cannot be emptied; they remain within, eating their container. For many of us it comes hard to verbalize our unpleasant emotions, even though we know that in their expression we find relief. How much more frustrating it must be for those who feel that they have only the choice of being still—or being abnormal.

Perhaps most frustrating of all is the inability to use speech as the expression of self. One of the hardest words for the average stutterer to say is his own name. Most of us talk about ourselves most of the time. We talk so people will notice us, so we can feel important. This egocentric speech is highly important in the development of the personality. Until the abnormal child begins to use it, he has little concept of selfhood, according to Piaget, the famous French psychologist. If you will listen to the people about you or to yourself, you will discover how large a portion of your talking consists of this cock-a-doodle-dooing. When we speak this way we reassure ourselves that all is well, that we are not alone, that we exist and belong. The person with a severe speech defect finds no such reassurance when he speaks. He exposes himself as little as he can. In this self-denial, too, lies much frustration.

One very severe frustration is the deprivation from social interaction which persons with speech disorders experience. It is not hard to understand why this occurs. Speech is the vital prerequisite for human interaction. It is the bond that unites us together. When it is impaired, that bonding is disrupted. Long ago the author spent a week once in a school for the deaf where all the students used sign language and did very little lipreading. He felt isolated, rejected, excluded from that miniature society; and it was with relief that he re-

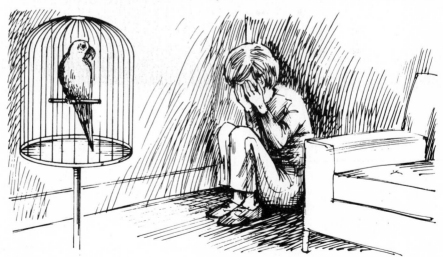

Figure 3 Even birds can talk.

entered a speaking world. Those who cannot talk feel much the same way. They are rejected from membership. They find it hard to belong. The worse they talk the more isolated they become. Here again we find in speech pathology a miniature model of a basic evil that pollutes mankind, the same rejecting exclusion that plagues the crippled, the poor, the insane, the old, and the minority groups.

Anxiety

It should not be difficult to understand why people who meet rejection, pity, or mockery would experience anxiety. When one is punished for a certain behavior, and the behavior occurs again, fear and anxiety raise their ugly heads. If penalty is the parent of fear, then we might speak of anxiety as the grandchild of penalty, for the two are not synonymous. The stutterer may fear the classmate who bedevils him, or he may fear to answer the telephone since fear is the expectation of approaching evils which are known and defined. But anxiety is the dread of the unknown, of defeats and helplessness to come. In its milder form, we speak of "worrying." There is a vague nagging anticipation that something dangerous is approaching. To observe a person in an acute anxiety attack is profoundly disturbing. Often he can find no reason for his anxiety, but it is there just the same. At times it fades, only to have its red flare return when least expected. Few of us can hope to escape it completely in our lifetimes, but there are those for whom anxiety is a way of life. It is not good to see a little child bearing such a burden.

One of the evil features of anxiety is that it is contagious. When parents of a handicapped child begin to worry about his speech, the child is almost bound to reflect and share their feelings. "Will he ever be able to go to school, to learn to read, to earn a living, to get married? Who will hurt him? Will he ever learn to talk like the fellows?" Such thoughts may never leave the parents' lips, but somehow they are transmitted to the child, perhaps by tiny gestures or facial expressions or even the holding of the breath. Once the seeds of anxiety are planted, they sprout and grow with incredible speed.

Another of the evils of anxiety is that it usually is destructive. It does not aid learning or speech therapy. It distracts; it negates. It undermines the self-esteem. The person seeks to contain it, to explain it. Sometimes he invents a symptom or magnifies one already there. When speech becomes contaminated with anxiety, the way of the speech pathologist is hard. One of the first things a student must learn is to create a permissive atmosphere in which speaking is not painful, over which no threat hangs darkly. The speech therapy room of the public school must be a gay, pleasant place, so much so that some little children hang on to their defective speech sounds so they will not have to leave. All of us need a harbor once in a while; *these* children need a haven often, one where for once they can feel free from penalty and frustration, where defective speech is viewed as a problem instead of a curse. In the presence of an accepting, understanding clinician, they can touch the untouchable, speak the unspeakable. There they can learn. Anxiety does not help in learning or relearning.

Reactions to Anxiety   Anxiety is invisible, but it has many faces. By this we mean that it shows itself in different ways.

Edward had undergone many operations for his cleft palate, but the scars on his face and the speech that came from his mouth bore testimony of his difference. Throughout his elementary and secondary school years, he had appeared a carefree, laughing, mischievous child. He was the happy clown, the gay spirit, and by this behavior, he had managed to gain much acceptance. When other people laughed at him, he laughed with them. His grades were poor, although he was bright. Then suddenly, in the final semester of his senior year in high school, he underwent a marked personality change. He laughed no longer; he became apathetic, quiet, and morose. Formerly very much the extrovert, he now withdrew from contacts with others. He daydreamed. He walked alone. Our intensive study of this boy revealed that he had always lived with anxiety, that his gay behavior was adaptive but spurious. Underneath he had always ached. The compensatory pose of gaiety had brought him rewards, but it had not allayed the anxiety. When faced with the necessity for leaving school and earning a living, the anxiety flared up too strongly to be hidden, and the change of personality took place. Not until we were able to provide some hope through the fitting of a prosthesis (a false palate) and some information about the possibility of plastic surgery, did the anxiety decrease sufficiently to enable us to improve his speech.

One of the common methods used to ease anxiety is the search for other pleasures. By gratifying other urges we seem to be able temporarily to diminish anxiety's nagging. Some of the people with whom we have worked are compulsive eaters of sweets; they grow fat and gross. And then they worry about their weight. Others relieve their anxiety by sexual indulgences. There are others who find a precarious and temporary peace by regressing to infantile modes of behavior, trying to return to the period of their lives when they did not need to worry about speaking. We also find a few sufferers who attach themselves to a stronger person like leeches, hoping for the security of dependency. Yes, there are many ways of reducing anxiety; but unless the spring from which it flows is stopped, it always returns. That is why people with defective speech need speech pathologists.

When the anxiety clusters about speaking, one way of reducing it is to stop talking. Some persons with speech disorders merely become taciturn; some lose their voices; others contract what is called *voluntary mutism* and do not make an attempt to communicate except through gestures. We knew a night watchman once who claimed that he averaged only two or three spoken sentences every twenty-four hours. "It's easier on me than stuttering." We've also known several hermits; they had either speech defects or woman trouble.

There is also a curious mechanism called "displacement," which most of us use occasionally to reduce our anxiety. We start worrying about something else besides the real problem that is causing us such distress. The shift of focus seems to bring some relief, much as a hot water bottle on the cheek can ease a toothache. The scream of a little child in the night may reflect such a displacement, but perhaps a better example can be found in Andy.

Andy stuttered very severely when he came to us at the age of seven. He blinked his eyes, jerked and screwed up his mouth, and sometimes cried with frustration when he was unable even to begin a sentence. At times he spoke very well. But what struck us most about Andy was his furrowed brow. Whether he stuttered or not, he seemed to be constantly worried. His face always had an anxious expression. Finally we were able to get him to tell us what he was worrying about. Surprisingly, it was not about his stuttering or his parents' very evident concern about his speech. Andy said he was worrying about the moon hitting the sun. He said that if this happened, everything would blow up. He said that on those nights when there wasn't any moon, and both sun and moon were down under there someplace, that they might crash together. Andy said he could never sleep on those nights. His mother and father had told him this couldn't happen, but Andy said they had lied about Santa Claus; and how did they know, anyway, that it wouldn't happen? It took a lot of play therapy, speech therapy, and parent counseling before Andy was able to surrender his solar phobia and express his real anxiety, which concerned his speech.

We wish to conclude this section with a caution. Let us remember that some children with abnormal speech have no more anxiety than children who speak normally. All of us have some anxiety, probably need some. A bit of anxiety in the pot of life is like a bit of salt in a stew. It makes it tastier. But too much salt and too much anxiety ruin both. We have had to describe the anxiety-fraction of a speech handicap so that you will not add to it, perhaps so that you may relieve it. Those of us who come in contact with handicapped children or adults may unwittingly make their burdens heavier if we do not understand. But there are some fortunate persons with speech disorders who are lucky in their associates and ability to resist stress, who seem to manage to get along with a minimum of anxiety. They may find themselves loved and accepted. They may possess philosophies or compensating assets that make the speech problem minor in importance. Let us just give one example.

> At thirty-two, a very talented singer developed cancer of the larynx, and it was removed surgically. She reacted to the challenge with courage, mastered esophageal speech, and began to specialize in the history of musical instruments, playing the lute, the Irish harp, and many other ancient stringed instruments. She said, "I would have been only a second-best vocalist, and I would have spent my life in self-love, self-exhibition, and frustration. Now I have many more friends and acquaintances. I have things to give. I hardly ever think of myself. It's a good thing I lost my voice."

So let us state our caution again. If there is excessive anxiety, recognize its face where you find it, no matter how it is disguised; but do not invent or imagine its presence if it is not there!

Guilt

Like anxiety, guilt also contributes a part of the invisible handicap that often accompanies abnormal speech. We have long been taught that the guilty are those who are punished. Intellectually we can understand that the converse of this proposition need not be true, that those who are punished are not always those who are guilty. But let affliction beset us, and we find ourselves in the ashes with Job of the Old Testament. "What have I done to deserve this evil?" We have known many persons deeply troubled by speech disorders and other ills, and most of them have asked this ancient question. Parents have asked it; little children have searched their souls for an answer. Here's an excerpt from an autobiography.

> Even when I was a little girl I remember being ashamed of my speech. And every time I opened my mouth, I shamed my mother. I can't tell you how awful I felt. If I talked, I did wrong. It was that simple. I kept thinking I must be awful bad to have to talk like that. I remember praying to God and asking him to forgive me for whatever it was I must have done. I remember trying hard to remember what it was, and not being able to find it.

It seems to be the fashion now to blame parents for many of the troubles of their children, for juvenile delinquency, for emotional conflicts, for defective speech. We can blame the school if Johnny cannot read, but few parents of a child who comes to school with un-intelligible speech have escaped the blame of their neighbors. The father of a cleft-palate child often feels an urge to accuse the mother, and the mother the father, for something that is the fault of neither. When guilt enters a house, a home is in danger. Children who grow up in such an atmosphere of open or hidden recrimination are prone to blame themselves. Thus the emotional fraction of a speech disorder may grow.

Reactions to Guilt Feelings Guilt is another evil that eats its container. In its milder forms of regret or embarrassment, most people can handle it with various degrees of discomfort. However, when shame and guilt are strong, they can become almost unbearable. To protect himself, the person may react with behavior that produces more penalty or more guilt. We have seen children deliberately soil themselves, throw temper tantrums, break things, steal things, even set fires so that they could get the punishment they felt their guilt deserved. After the punishment comes a little peace!

Other children punish themselves. We have stutterers use their stuttering to hurt themselves, using it in much the same way as the flagellants of the Middle Ages flogged and tortured their bodies for their sins. We have known children with repaired harelips and cleft palates who could not bear to watch themselves in a mirror even to observe the action of the tongue or soft palate. We have heard children cry and strike themselves when they heard their speech played back from a tape recorder. We who deal with such children must always be alert to this need for punishment lest they place the whip in our hands.

Here is what one adult with cerebral palsy painfully typed for us:

> Sometimes when I lie in bed pretty relaxed I almost feel normal. In the quiet and the darkness I don't even feel myself twitching. I pretend I'm just like everybody else. But then in the morning I have to get up and face the monster in the mirror when I shave. I see what other people see, and I'm ashamed. I see the grey hairs on my mother's head and know I put them there. I eat but I know it isn't bread I can earn. Oh there are times when I get interested in something and forget what I am, but not when I talk. When I talk to someone, he doesn't have a face. He has a mirror for a face, and I see the monster again.

We who must help these people must also expect at times to find apathy and depression as reactions to the feelings of guilt. It is possible to ease the distress of guilt a little by becoming numb, by giving up, by refusing to try. Again, we may find individuals who escape some of their guilt by denying the reality of their crooked mouths or tangled tongues. They resist our efforts to help them because they refuse to accept the *fact* of abnormal speech. Somehow they feel that the moment they admit the existence of abnormality, they become responsible. And with responsibility comes the guilt they cannot bear. So they resist our efforts to help them. Finally, we meet persons who absolve themselves from guilt by projection, by blaming others for their affliction, by converting their guilt into hostility or anxiety. But this brings us to the next section.

Hostility

Both penalty and frustration generate anger and aggression. We who are hurt, hate. We who are frustrated, rage. Here is an example to help you understand. It was written by an aphasic veteran who had been shot in the head.

> The worst feature of my brain injury was the frustration. I would know exactly what I wanted to say, but it would come

out of my mouth differently. If I wanted to say "Please pass the cake," my mouth might say, "Please part the ice," which didn't make sense to anyone else or even to my own ears. A hundred times a day this would happen. I'd find myself crying or cursing or frozen into some stiff posture or making some meaningless movements with my leg, and I knew that these were just my ways of trying to handle the complete feeling of inability that characterized my life.

Reactions to Hostility   Hostility, like anxiety and guilt, ranges along a continuum all the way from momentary irritation through anger to intense hatred. Some children with severe speech problems show little hostility; yet we have known some with mild and minor disorders to show much. One child may have much anxiety or guilt but little hostility; another may reveal quite an opposite state of affairs. Some children just seem to roll with the punches and the frustrations and manage to get along with a minimum of emotional response. But often hostility and aggression are found, and so we must understand them.

History of the Handicapped

There are times, when we survey the extent of human distress, that it seems that this dream of creating a better world is so unrealistic that it would be foolish to try to do anything to make it come true. Why seek to make one's own life meaningful in this way when there is such an immense amount of misfortune all about us? Why pick up a few beer cans when millions are discarded each day? Why try to help those who are less fortunate than we are when the powerful forces of our own culture keep generating more unhappiness? Is there any hope for mankind?

The history of the way society has treated the handicapped, sad and sorry as it is, may give us the glimmerings of that hope. Although we have some way to go before we can call ourselves civilized, the contrast between the present and past treatments of the retarded, the deaf, the blind, the crippled, the insane, the poor, and those who cannot talk normally shows very clearly that we have made gains. We find in this cultural history a hopeful progression from considering the handicapped persons as intolerable nuisances, then as objects of mirth, then as pitiful beggars, and now as challenging problems. Though these attitudes are still in evidence today, they are surely less prevalent.

Rejection   Primitive society tolerated no weakness. Tribes struggled hard for survival, and those members who could not aid materially were quickly rejected. The younger men killed the leaders when they had lost their teeth or their energies had abated. The inhabitants of ancient India cast their cripples into the Ganges; the Spartans hurled theirs from a precipice. The Aztecs regularly sacrificed deformed persons in times of famine or when one of their leaders died. The Melanesians had a simple solution for the problem of the handicapped: they buried them alive. Among the earlier Romans, twins were considered so abnormal that one of them was always put to death, and frequently both were killed. They left their malformed children on the highways or in the forests. If the children survived, they were often picked up by those who always prey upon the handicapped and were carried to the market place to be trained as beggars. They were not even valuable enough to be slaves.

The Bible clearly reflects these early rejection attitudes. Remember Job? The prevailing belief in Old Testament times was that man's physical state was determined by his good or bad relationship with his deity. Disabilities were regarded as divine punishment for sin. A normal person could invoke similar punishment merely by associating with those who had thus incurred the wrath of God. Consequently, the blind and the crippled wailed with the lepers outside the city wall.

During the Middle Ages the physically disabled were frequently considered to be possessed by evil spirits. They were confined to their own homes. They dared not walk to the market place lest they be stoned. Even in this century, elimination of the handicapped has been practiced. The Kaffir tribes in South Africa clubbed sickly or deformed children. The Nazis kept only the best of their civilian prisoners for slaves; the others died in the gas chamber.

In this country we might hang the man who killed his crippled son. We have come far in our journey toward civilization, but perhaps not far enough. Rejection takes many other forms. Spirits, too, can be killed. This is what one handicapped person has to say:

> We think the inhabitants of old Sparta cruel for putting to death the weak, those who would be unable to compete or to contribute much to their society; but were they, after all, much more inhuman than we who nurse the weakling, keep it alive, yet as

much as possible keep it from normal persons, especially the children, for fear its contact will contaminate them; then throw it out to compete with normal adults? (McKnight, 1936)

How many of those reading this book would unhesitatingly accept an invitation to a dance if it were tendered by a hunchback?

Humor   It did not take the promoters long to discover that the handicapped provided a rewarding source of humor. One history of the subject states that before 1000 B.C. the fool or buffoon became a necessary part of feast-making and "won the laughter of the guests by his idiocy or his deformity." In Homer's *Odyssey*, comic relief from tragedy was illustrated by the vain effort of the one-eyed Polyphemus to pursue his tormentors after they had blinded him. For a thousand years thereafter every court had its crippled buffoons, its dwarf jesters, its stuttering fools. Attila the Hun held banquets at which "a Moorish and Scythian buffoon successively excited the mirth of the rude spectators by their deformed figures, ridiculous dress, antic gestures, and absurd speech." Cages along the Appian Way held various grotesque human disabilities, including "Balbus Blaesus" the stutterer, who would attempt to talk when a coin was flung through the bars. In Shakespeare's *Timon of Athens*, Caphis says, "Here comes the fool; let's ha' some sport with 'im." Often this sport consisted of physical abuse or exposure of the twisted limb. These handicapped fools accepted and expected ridicule. At least it provided a means of survival, a livelihood, and it represented an advance in civilized living.

Gradually, the use of the handicapped to provoke mirth became less popular in continental Europe, and the more enterprising had to migrate to less culturally advanced areas to make a living. At one time Peter the Great had so many fools that he found it necessary to classify them for different occasions. When Cortez conquered Mexico he discovered deformed creatures of all kinds at the court of Montezuma. On the same continents today you may find them used to provoke laughter only in the circus sideshows, in the movies, on the radio, and in every schoolyard.

Pity   Religion is doubtless responsible for the development of true pity as a cultural reaction to the handicapped. James Joyce said that pity is the feeling which arrests the mind in the presence of whatsoever is grave and constant in human suffering and unites it with the human sufferer. It was this spontaneous feeling that prompted religious leaders to give the handicapped shelter and protection. Before 200 B.C. Asoka, a Buddhist, created a ministry for the care of unfortunates and appointed officers to supervise charitable works. Confucius said, "With whom should I associate but with suffering men?" Jesus preached compassion for all the disabled and made all men their brothers' keepers. In the seventh century after Jesus' death the Mohammedan religion proposed a society free from cruelty and social oppression and insisted on kindliness and consideration for all men. A few hundred years later Saint Francis of Assisi devoted his life to the care of the sick and the disabled. Following this, the "Mad Priest of Kent," John Ball, was so aroused by the plight of the crippled and needy left in the wake of the Black Death that he publicly pleaded their cause, often at the risk of his own life. With the rise of the middle class, true pity for the handicapped became much more commonplace. The oppression which the merchants and serfs had suffered left them more sympathetic to others who were ill used. The doctrine of the equality of man did much for the handicapped as well as for the economically down-trodden.

However, many crimes have been committed in the name of charity. The halt and the blind began to acquire commercial value as beggars. Legs and backs of little children were broken and twisted by their exploiters. Soon the commercialization of pity became so universal that it became a community nuisance. Alms became a conventional gesture to buy relief from the piteous whining that dominated every public place. True pity was lost in revulsion. Recognizing this unhappy trend, Hyperius of Ypres advocated that beggars be classified so that work could be provided according to their capacities. His own motives were humanitarian, but he cleverly won support for his cause by pointing out that other citizens "would be freed of clamor, of fear of outrage, or the sight of ugly bodies." His appeal was successful; and asylums and homes for the handicapped began to appear, if only to isolate the occupants so that the public need not be reminded of their distress. Another motive which improved the position of the handicapped was the belief that one could purchase his way into heaven or out of hell by charity. The coin thrown to the cripple has been impelled by many motives. The longing for religious security, the heightening of one's own superiority by comparison with the unfortunate, the social prestige of philanthropy, and the desire to be freed from embarrassment have all contributed to the welfare of the handicapped. Pseudopity has accomplished much, but true compassion would have ended the tragedy.

Present Treatment of the Speech Handicapped

We have sketched the treatment accorded the handicapped at some length because the speech-deviant person is diagnosed immediately as belonging to that unfortunate group. The moment the cleft-palate child or stutterer speaks he joins his brethren, the crippled, the deaf, the spastic, the blind, and perhaps the fool. He is different. He possesses an abnormality. A little child hesitates in his speech; his parents diagnose him as a stutterer; he reacts to his hesitations as though they were unpleasant; his playmates accept his evaluation or his parents' evaluation, and so he joins the unhappy tribe of the million stutterers who exist in this country today.

It may seem strange to learn that the primitive attitudes of rejection, humor, and pity are still very common reactions to the perception of speech defects today. Listen to these:

> They got me inside a circle of them, and every time I tried to break out and go home, they pushed me back. "Make a speech. Make a speech." I tried to tell them I had to get my groceries home. My mother had to have them for supper, but the men would just laugh all the harder and push me back. They told me to say different things if I wanted to get out, things like "She sells sea shells" and dirty words. I was crying and I got mad and swore at them, and then they let me go but I can hear them yet.

> I asked the girl for a dance and had a hard time getting it out. She flushed, then blurted out, "Well, I'm not that hard up yet."

> I can take almost anything but that pitying glance. It's sort of as if I have a cup in my hand every time I talk and people feel they ought to put some pennies in it. I can't explain it, but when they look away or down at their feet I feel like something unclean. I can't help it that my operation tore loose, and I talk through my nose, but I can't even explain it to them.

We no longer keep our "Balbus Blaesuses" in cages, but the song about "K-K-K-Katy" is still being sung although "Stuttering in the Starlight" and "You-you-you tell 'em that I-I-I stutter" have been forgotten. Cartoons and comic strips do not fail to exploit the impediments of speech.

Nevertheless, we end this chapter on a hopeful note. Throughout our society we discern a need for change. We are beginning to reduce exploitation and pollution. We no longer accept selfishness as the basic law of human interaction. We are beginning to care for those less fortunate than we are, realizing that the unhappiness of others diminishes our own good fortune. We cannot continue to live in a world polluted by misery, injustice, and cruelty. We must do what we can.

References

BREWER, S. C. "A Personal Look at Cleft Palate." *Language, Speech, Hearing Services in the Schools*, IV (1973), 203–06.

BROWN, C. and C. VAN RIPER. *Speech and Man*. Englewood Cliffs, N.J.: Prentice-Hall, Inc., 1966.

CAMERON, C. C. *A Different Drum*. Englewood Cliffs, N.J.: Prentice-Hall, Inc., 1973.

CLARK, L. *Can't Read, Can't Write, Can't Talk Too Good Either*. New York: Walker and Company, 1973.

CURRY, F. K. W. "Speech Maturation." in A.S.H.A. Reports, No. 7. *Orofacial Function: Clinical Research in Dentistry and Speech Pathology*, 1972.

EMERICK, L. "A Clinical Success: Mark; and a Clinical Failure: Sherrie." in M. Fraser, ed., *Stuttering, Successes and Failures in Therapy* (Memphis, Tenn.: Speech Foundation of America, 1968), pp. 21–39.

———, *The Parent Interview*. Danville, Ill.: Interstate, 1969.

GREENBERG, J. *I Never Promised You a Rose Garden*. New York: Holt, Rinehart & Winston, 1964.

LAUDER, E. "The Laryngectomee and the Artificial Larynx." *Journal of Speech and Hearing Disorders*, XXXIII (1968), 147–57.

LEMERT, E. M. "Stuttering and Social Structure in Two Pacific Societies," *Journal of Speech and Hearing Disorders*, XXVII (1962), 3–10.

LUKENS, K. and C. PANTER. *Thursday's Child Has Far to Go*. Englewood Cliffs, N.J.: Prentice-Hall, Inc., 1969.

McDONALD, E. T. *Understanding Those Feelings*. Pittsburgh: Stanwix House, 1962.

McKNIGHT, R. V. "A Self-Analysis of a Case of Reading, Writing, and Speaking Disability." *Archives of Speech*, I (1936), 43–47.

MOSS, C. S. *Recovery with Aphasia—The Aftermath of My Stroke*. Urbana: U. Illinois Press, 1972.

PEDREY, C. "Letter to the Editor." *Journal of Speech and Hearing Disorders*, XV (1950), 266–69.

RITCHIE, D. *Stroke*. New York: Doubleday & Company, Inc., 1961.

ROLNICK, M. and A. R. HOOPS. "Aphasia as Seen by the Aphasic." *Journal of Speech and Hearing Disorders*, XXXIV (1969), 58–63.

SIES, L. F. and R. BUTLER. "A Personal Account of Dysphasia." *Journal of Speech and Hearing Disorders*, XXVIII (1963), 261–66.

SILVERMAN, F. H. "Concern of Elementary School Stutterers about Their Stuttering." *Journal of Speech and Hearing Disorders,* XXXV (1970), 361–63.

SLUTSKY, H. "Maternal Reaction and Adjustment to the Birth and Care of Cleft-Palate Children." *Cleft Palate Journal,* VII (1967), 425–29.

STRANDBERG, T. E., J. GRIFFITH, and M. W. HOLLOWELL. "A Case Study of Psychogenic Hoarseness." *Journal of Speech and Hearing Disorders,* XXXVI (1971), 281–86.

TRAVIS, L. E. and L. D. SUTHERLAND. "Psychotherapy in Public School Speech Correction." in L. E. Travis, ed., *Handbook of Speech Pathology and Audiology.* (Englewood Cliffs, N.J.: Prentice-Hall, Inc., 1971).

VAN RIPER, C. "Success and Failure in Speech Therapy." *Journal of Speech and Hearing Disorders,* XXXI (1966), 276–79.

WEDBERG, C. F. *The Stutterer Speaks.* Boston: Expression Co., 1937.

WEINER, P. S. "The Emotionally Disturbed Child in the Speech Clinic: Some Considerations." *Journal of Speech and Hearing Disorders,* XXXIII (1968), 158–66.

ZEDLER, E. "Social Management." in J. V. Irwin, and M. Marge, eds., *Principles of Childhood Language Disabilities* (Englewood Cliffs, N.J.: Prentice-Hall, Inc., 1972), pp. 381–89.

2

SPEECH DISORDERS

Speech therapy begins with diagnosis. If we are to help a person who seems unable to talk normally, we must first answer some preliminary questions: *Is his speech really abnormal? In what ways?* The first of these questions demands that the person who assesses the speech must know the normal range of differences which all normal speakers demonstrate. You probably do not lisp but you too probably would distort some of your *s* sounds were you to try to say this sentence swiftly: "He thrusts his fists against the posts but still insists he sees the ghosts." Most normal speakers have trouble saying such a tongue twister, and so any errors would not indicate a real speech problem. Similarly, all of us hesitate, falter, or repeat words and syllables at times—usually under communicative stress—but this does not mean that all of us stutter. The boy whose larynx suddenly almost doubles in size at the beginning of adolescence will often show pitch breaks and a falsetto but these should only be considered deviant when they persist too long. All of us have had the experience of temporarily being unable to find a word such as a person's name even though it may be very familiar. We say that it is "right on the tip of the tongue" and sometimes the more we search for it the harder it is to locate. Stroke patients with aphasia have such word-finding difficulties too, but you don't have to worry that you are becoming aphasic if you can't find that particular name or word once in a blue moon. To know if speech is abnormal one must know what the normal variations are.

There are dangers in misdiagnosis, as the following example demonstrates:

We once had to solve the problem of voluntary mutism in a four-and-a-half-year-old girl. She had not spoken a word for six

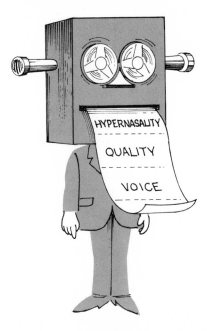

Figure 4   The speech clinician diagnoses a speech disorder.

months. Although previously she had been as verbal as any other child her age, gestures were now her only means of communication and her parents were very worried. We interviewed them at length and the picture that finally evolved was this. Sally's parents had married late and Sally was the only child. (It has been said that being an only child is a disease in itself.) Her first words had appeared a little later than usual, and the mother who had had a severely retarded sister was concerned that Sally's speech delay might have been a sign of similar retardation. So the mother pulled the onion to make it grow. She drilled Sally constantly on the correction of the articulatory errors such as *th* for *s,* or *w* for *r,* which most children normally show during this stage of speech development. A perfectionist herself, and highly anxious, the mother made such exorbitant speech demands upon the child that the girl just quit talking in self-defense. Moreover, through her voluntary mutism, Sally found that she could control and manipulate the big people who previously had been over-controlling and manipulating her. She enjoyed her discovery of the fact that you can lead a horse to water but you can't make it speak. Almost every time someone

asked her to say something, she would shake her head negatively—but as she did so, there was always a tiny smile.

This is not the place to give a detailed account of how we successfully enabled Sally to talk again, but we can sketch the major outline of the therapy. The program involved some play therapy with
puppets who acted out her parent's excessive demands and verbalized her own feelings. We developed a system of progressive reinforcements for gesture, then for pantomime, then for whispering, and
finally, for vocalized speech. But most important of all, we counseled
her parents, helping them to understand how their own needs and
anxieties had created the excessive demands that led to Sally's voluntary mutism, and to realize that the girl's speech errors were not abnormal at all—that they just reflected the normal course of speech development.

Teachers of the mentally retarded, or the cerebral palsied, and
certain other children enrolled in special education will need to recognize that the usual developmental norms of speech performance
may not always apply to these children. Each child must be assessed
in terms of his own history and his other disabilities before a judgment of speech abnormality is made. Flexible, elastic yardsticks must
be used, not rigid ones.

But speech pathologists too must have these yardsticks if they
wish to avoid dangers of misdiagnosis. Here is an account from
Wendell Johnson, one of the pioneers in the field:

> All through his previous years at school he had been known,
> not merely as a normal speaker, but as a definitely superior
> speaker. He had won a number of speaking contests, had served
> as chairman of several student groups. Then one day a "speech
> correction teacher" examined him in the course of a school sur-
> vey, and for some reason, told him that he was a stutterer, and
> advised him to "watch" his speech and be careful when he
> talked. Within a few months he would have been regarded as a
> stutterer and a fairly severe one by anyone professionally famil-
> iar with this type of speech problem. In reacting to the diag-
> nosed characteristics of his speech, to the interruptions of one
> sort or another which are normally found in the speech of ev-
> eryone, but which in his case had been called stuttering—he de-
> veloped muscular tensions, facial contortions, and apprehensive-
> ness about speaking. In short, that teacher made him into a
> stutterer.[1]

[1] W. Johnson, "Letter to the Editor," *Journal of Speech and Hearing Disorders,* XIV
(1949), 175–76.

Definition   Our first question *(Is this person's speech really abnormal?)* de-
             mands a definition of deviancy, and here is the way we define it:
*Speech is abnormal when it deviates so far from the speech of other
people that it calls attention to itself, interferes with communication, or
causes the speaker or his listeners to be distressed.*

We can condense this definition into three adjectives. Speech is
defective when it is *conspicuous, unintelligible,* or *unpleasant.* The first
adjective refers to the fact that abnormal speech is different enough
to be noted. It varies too far from the norm. A child of three who
says "wabbit" for "rabbit" has no speech defect, but the adult of fifty
who uses that pronunciation would have one because it would be a
real deviation from the pronunciation of other adults. If you said
deze, doze, and *dem* for *these, those,* and *them* in a hobo jungle, none
of the other vagrants would notice. If you used the same sounds in a
talk to a P.T.A. meeting a good many ears would prickle. Many of us
force the airstream down too broad a tongue groove to produce the
high-pitched *s* sound characteristic of our English speech. Because we
do so does not necessarily mean that we have lateral lisps. Only
when our *s* is so slushy and low in pitch that it calls attention to itself can we be said to have that type of speech defect.

How wide a variation is required before we should be concerned about a speech difference? Only the cultural norms can answer this question. Among the Pilagra Indians no attention is ever
paid to baby-talk or peculiar speech until the child is at least seven
years of age. Many Indian tribes do not even have a word for stuttering, although many of their membership no doubt have hesitant
speech. According to the famous anthropologist Sapir, who worked
among the Nootka, repetitive and hesitant speech seems to be more
common than fluent rhythmic speech in this tribe of Indians. One
would have to stutter badly indeed to have a speech defect in such a
culture. In England the dropping of an *h* or the flatting of a vowel
would cause instant social penalty in upper class society, whereas the
same behavior would be quite unnoticeable in Australia. Excessive
assimilation nasality would not be noticed by a Tennessee mountain-
eer, but the same voice quality in an Eastern girls' school would send
its owner to the speech clinic. A speech defect, then, is one which is
so different from the normal speech of the social group that it is
highly conspicuous. The individual who refers a case to the speech
pathologist should evaluate its context accordingly.

The second part of the definition refers to intelligibility. When a
speech difference interferes with communication it tends to be labeled as defective.

When you listen, not to what a stranger says, but to his peculiar voice or hesitations or distorted consonants, communication is broken. If his face suddenly jumps around as he struggles to utter an ordinary word, all communicative content is lost in amusement or amazement. Many stutterers habitually lower their eyes to escape the shock of observing the expression of incredulity and surprise on the faces of their auditors. Cleft-palate adults have been known to pretend to be deaf and dumb and to beg for a pencil so that their communication could be accomplished without interruption.

If, as one of our eighteen-year-old cases illustrated, you heard someone reciting "Poh koh an tebbuh yee adoh ow pohpadduh baw poh uhpah dih kawinaw a new naytuh" you might find it very hard to understand him — unless you knew he was saying the first lines of Lincoln's "Gettysburg Address." Speech is defective when it is difficult to understand, when its intelligibility is poor.

That communication is impaired when a person loses his voice (aphonia) is obvious. The person whose larynx has been removed is pretty helpless until he learns to "swallow" air and speak on the expelled burp. But even then, the monotone is difficult to listen to or understand. The cleft-palate child's teacher finds great difficulty in fathoming what he is trying to recite. A falsetto voice distracts attention from what is being said. The more conspicuous the vocal abnormality, the more unintelligible the speech becomes.

Many a stutterer has had to ask for a paper and pencil in order to make his simplest wants known. The words emerge from such contortions and broken garblings of utterance that frequently both the stutterer and the listener give up.

A speech defect, then, is one which calls attention to itself and interferes with communication.

The final part of our definition deals with the maladjustment and emotional handicap which the speech deviant adds to his disability. Sometimes this maladjustment is the dominant feature of the disorder. We worked with a woman who claimed to have stuttered actually only once in her life — during a high-school graduation speech. Her speech was certainly not fluent, since it was marked by numerous hesitations, pauses, and avoidances of certain words. She was badly handicapped socially and vocationally. Her listeners were constantly puzzled and confused by her peculiar speech behavior. And yet she had actually "stuttered" only once. This case, of course, is an extreme instance of the importance of maladjustment in producing a speech defect. Usually, the abnormality of rhythm, voice, or articulation is sufficiently bizarre to provoke so many social penalties that maladjustment is almost inevitable.

Classification of Speech Disorders

There are many ways in which we could classify the various speech disorders, but if we look at the behavior itself we find that they seem to fall into four major categories: *articulation, time, voice,* and *symbolization* (language). This fourfold classification, it should be understood, refers to the *outstanding* features of the behavior shown. Thus, even though his stuttering causes certain sounds to be distorted, we place the stutterer in the second category because the major feature of his disorder is the broken timing of his utterance. The person with aphasia often shows articulation errors, broken rhythm, inability to produce voice; but the outstanding feature of aphasia is the inability to handle symbolic meanings and language. Therefore, we would place aphasia under disorders of symbolization or language. Certain individuals show more than one of these disorders. A child with severe cerebral palsy, for example, may show all four.

In What Ways Is the Speech Abnormal? This, the second of our three preliminary diagnostic questions, requires that we get an adequate sample of the person's verbal output, scan it, and compare it against the standard patterning of normal speech. It is not enough merely to discover that the speech is deviant. We must know which features of that speech are abnormal. Far too often we have received phone calls

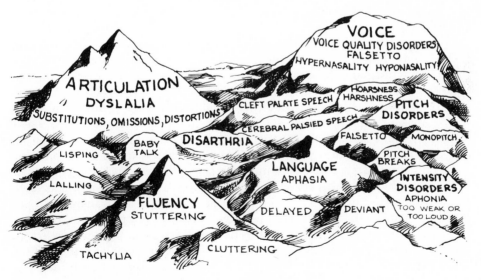

Figure 5 The field of speech pathology.

or letters from parents or teachers who tell us only that the child "doesn't talk right" and who then ask us the impossible question "What can I do to help?"

What we must do, of course, is to watch and listen to that child as we set our internal diagnostic computers to whirring. And we must feed into them all the information we can obtain by scanning his speech in four sweeps. We repeatedly scrutinize it: (1) for errors in speech sound production (*articulation*); (2) for abnormalities in pitch, intensity, and quality (*voice*); (3) for deviancies in the flow of utterance (*fluency*); and (4) for difficulties in encoding or decoding (*language*).

Each of these four aspects of human speech (articulation, voice, fluency, and symbolization or language) has its own criteria of normality, and each has a range of acceptable differences. The *s* sound in *Sue* is not the same sound as it is in the word *see*; it is lower in pitch, but this variation is within normal limits. But when that *s* is too slushy as in a person with a lateral lisp we would diagnose abnormality. *A difference to be a difference must make a difference.* If it calls attention to itself, interferes with the receiving of the message, or is unpleasant to the speaker or his listener, we then have a speech problem.

One of the common mistakes made by beginners in this field is the failure to scan all these four features of the speech of a person who obviously had some communicative abnormality. One of our former students wrote:

> I learned another lesson today and I don't know why it took me so long. I have been working with a junior-high-school boy whose speech is full of distorted speech sounds due to the fact that he keeps his tongue flat in his mouth. Often he is unintelligible. I suppose you'd call it lalling. Yet he could make every sound perfectly in isolation and often in single words if I said them first. Well, I began therapy by working to mobilize the lifting of the tongue tip and to disassociate it from any jaw movement and by stimulating him strongly with the sounds on which the distortions occurred. He was immediately successful in anything I asked him to do yet there was no transfer into real communication. Then just by chance I happened to overhear him talking to a girl in the hall and saw him have a very severe stuttering block, so of course we discussed this at our next session. Come to find out, he doesn't have any articulation problem at all. He just uses this lalling kind of speech as a way to keep from stuttering. Says he's only been using it for a few

months and that though it helped at first because it was so novel and distracting, it was beginning to lose its effectiveness. After he told me this I realized that I had noticed many hesitations and gaps in his speech but had ignored them. The abnormal articulation had just been too conspicuous. Anyway, now we can begin to tackle the real problem.

Experienced speech pathologists do not make this mistake. Their diagnostic computers do not stop until they have scanned enough speech samples for deviancy not only in articulation but in voice, fluency, and language. They know the normal ranges of differences for each, and bells ring in their heads when they find behaviors that are beyond the normal boundaries.

Workers in the field of special education must be alert to the necessity for recognizing the multiple features of speech that may show deviancy. The child who is deaf, deafened, or severely hard of hearing will show not only articulatory errors, inappropriate vocal inflections, or a monotonous voice; he also often may have a language disability or the rhythm of his fluency will be broken by pauses in the wrong parts of a sentence. Similarly, the child with cerebral palsy may show deviancy in all four features. So may the child with mental retardation or deficiency. The emotionally disturbed child may present the picture of a strange voice quality along with infantile kinds of articulatory errors. Though the speech of a child with a cleft palate is often conspicuously nasal, he will also tend to show speech sound errors, one of which may be the use of the glottal stop (similar to a tiny cough) for his *k* sounds. It is not enough merely to recognize that a person does not speak normally. We must know what features of his speech are abnormal.

The Disorders of Speech   Again, it is not enough merely to recognize that the deviancy exists in articulation, voice, fluency, or language. We must be able to analyze that deviancy so as to identify exactly what the person is doing that makes his speech conspicuous, hard to understand, or unpleasant. If a person has an articulation problem, we must know what sounds are produced incorrectly, for all of them are not defective. If the voice is abnormal, the speech pathologist will survey the pitch, loudness, and vocal quality aspects of that voice before he zeroes in on the targets of his therapy. It is not enough just to say that the person stutters, for there are literally thousands of different stuttering behaviors, though certain ones are demonstrated most frequently. If a person is aphasic (dysphasic is the more precise word), his language disability must be carefully analyzed if it is to be remedied.

Articulation Disorders

How does one learn to do this diagnostic analyzing? The answer lies in training and experience. We begin that training by providing some word pictures of individuals with disorders of articulation.

> Robert was in the third grade when we first met him. No one called him "Bobby." He was a loner, preferring to stay in his seat at recess, and when forced to leave, stood shyly at the school entrance watching the other children. They did not penalize him; they just ignored him. Although of normal intelligence and doing well in arithmetic, he had marked disabilities in reading and spelling; and the teacher felt that this was probably due to his many defective sounds. With some difficulty it was possible to understand what he said when he did offer a few words, but often a word or phrase would be completely unintelligible. When asked to repeat, he would say it over and over again in a sad little voice, and always in the same fashion. In analyzing a fair sample of his speech we found that he consistently produced all the vowel sounds correctly and also the *m, n, p, b, w, t, d,* and *f* sounds. Most of the other sounds were either omitted or replaced with these sounds, although on a few words such as "can" and "gum" we heard him say the *k* and the *g* very normally. His mother reported that he had not really begun to talk until the year before he entered kindergarten, and the school records indicated that he had not improved in the four years since he entered school. We enrolled him in the clinic, enlisted the aid of his teacher and his parents, and gave him intensive speech therapy for an hour each day. By the end of six months he was speaking almost normally, and a year later showed no sign of any articulatory problem. He had also made great gains in reading and spelling. But what was even more important, he began to participate in the play activities of his schoolmates and changed from being an isolate to a member of their groups.

> Mrs. M. was referred to us by her dentist whom she had threatened to sue for malpractice. She was a big belligerent woman, a high-school teacher of speech who spoke in highly conscious,

pear-shaped tones. She gestured with the hand supine, the hand prone, and the ictus. Mrs. M. also had conducted an interview program over the local TV station once a week but had recently been replaced. She felt that this had occurred because of the change in her speech subsequent to the fitting of an upper dental plate. Our examination revealed that her sibilants, the *s, z,* and *sh* sounds, were distorted by a very obvious, high-pitched whistle. The dentist informed us that he had varied the appliance in every way possible to alter this unpleasant whistling and had brought in consultants from his own field to help, but without success. He had hoped that as she became accustomed to the denture, the whistle would disappear; but it had now persisted for three months and, if anything, was getting worse. It was evident that Mrs. M. had become morbidly conscious of these whistled sibilants; and so, in our trial therapy, we piped in masking noise through earphones as we asked her to attempt *s* sounds while anchoring the tip of her tongue against her lower teeth. The whistle disappeared immediately, and we tape-recorded Mrs. M.'s speech to show her that it did so. She was delighted and worked hard to eliminate the abnormality, and within a month was speaking normally again. We suspect that prior to the fitting of the denture she had habitually used this lower tongue position to produce the sibilants and had developed the whistle by constantly exploring tongue contacts with the unfamiliar appliance in her mouth.

We do not wish to leave the impression that disorders of articulation present little difficulty to the clinician. Some of them have been our toughest cases. Somehow we remember our failures much more vividly than we do our successes. They haunt us. What did we do wrongly or what did we fail to do? One of them was Joe.

Joe was in the fifth grade when we first worked with him. Only one of his sounds was defective—the vowel *r* sound as in *fur.* He was able to make the consonantal *r* perfectly, articulating it correctly whenever it occurred as the initial consonant of a syllable. He could say "run," "radio," or any other word beginning with *r* without error. Even the consonant blends, *pr, tr, gr,* etc., were uttered normally. But when the *r* occurred as a vowel as in *church,* he said "chutch." He said "theatuh," "mothuh," "guhl." When the *r* was part of a diphthong as in *ar, or, ir,* not only was the *r* distorted but the preceding vowel was often misarticulated. Instead of "far," he said "foah," and in these distorted diphthongs we heard sounds that we had never heard before. We worked hard with Joe and initially felt that the prognosis was good, that we could probably effect a transition from the consonantal to the vowel *r* with ease. We failed completely. He tried and we tried with all our might. We used every technique known to us. We vainly explored every possible reason for the persistence of the errors. We tried different therapists. They failed. When Joe was a senior in high school we tried again with the same result. We still wonder what else we might have done.

As we have seen from our scrutiny of the preceding examples, the basic problem shown by a person with a disorder of articulation is that he has failed to master the speech sounds of his language. Each of these three persons could be characterized as having a *phonemic* disorder rather than one of voice or of fluency or of symbolization. Although they differed one from the other in the pattern of their phonemic errors, they all showed one or more of the following types: (1) substitution of one standard English phoneme for another; (2) a distortion of a standard sound; (3) an omission of a sound that should be present; or (4) an addition or insertion of an irrelevant sound. These are the kinds of articulatory errors which these people show. Most young children during the course of their speech development show all of these at one time or another; but some children persist in their usage, having failed to perceive the contrasting features of the correct sound as compared with the defective one, or having been unable to achieve its correct production.

Articulatory errors often appear in clusters, and some of these clusters have acquired common names. *Lisping* is one such cluster. It consists of defective sibilant sounds such as the *s* and *z*, the *sh* and *zh* and others that are characterized by the friction of air escaping through a narrow opening. Names have also been given to subvarieties of the lisp. Thus we have the *interdental* or *frontal* lisp in which the voiced or unvoiced *th* sounds are substituted for the *s* and *z* respectively: "Thum people like thum thingth and other people like other thingth but ath for me, I like thpitting. I can even thpit in thirclth and thpiralth," said one of our lispers and proceeded to do so. Another common variety of lisp is the *lateral* lisp in which the sibilants are distorted. The *s* and *z*, and even the *ch, j,* and *th* sounds are spoken mushily. When older people are first fitted with dentures, they tend to show some of this lateral omission of air, and so do college students when intoxicated. Some little children learn this sort of a sibilant and never master the correct ones. There are also other lisps: the occluded type in which the *s* may be prefaced by a short *t* sound or the *z* by a *d*. Such a person would say, "TSally had a dzipper that wouldn't open." In cleft-palate speakers we often find nasal lisps in which the airstream is emitted through the nose instead of through the teeth. Nasal lispers snort their sibilants.

Another term which is fortunately fading from the speech pathologist's professional vocabulary is *lalling*. It refers to a cluster of errors, primarily upon the *r* and *l* sounds, in which the tongue tip fails to lift sufficiently to produce the contact or contour necessary for correct production. If you will anchor your tongue tip below your bottom teeth and refuse to lift it as you say, "Lulu was a lallapalooza of a laller" you will recognize the kind of speech which some still prefer to call lalling.

You doubtless have heard the term *baby-talk,* which was dignified by the synonymous phrase "infantile perseveration" some years ago. The term does not have a precise referent, but usually it means that the person seems to be using the kinds of substitutions, distortions, and omissions common in early childhood. "Muvver, the doddie (doggie) want to dow owdoh" might represent the kind of speech which the lay person would call baby-talk.

Actually these names do not denote different types of disorders. They are not mutually exclusive. Lallers often lisp, and lispers talk baby-talk, and all of them show oral inaccuracy. The important feature of all articulatory disorders is the presence of defective and incorrect sounds. The forty-year-old farmer who wept when he heard his voice on a recording of a children's rhyme did so because of the defective and incorrect sounds he had produced. A six-year-old said this:

> Tinko Tinko itto tah,
> How I wondah wheh you ah,
> Up abuh duh woh soh high
> Yike a diamon' in duh kye.

As the above selection indicates, most articulatory cases have more than one error and are not always consistent in their substitutions, omissions, insertions, or distortions. This is not always the case, however. Thum lingual lithperth merely thubthitute a *th* for the *eth* thound. Othershshkwirt the airshtream over the shide of the tongue and are shed to have a lateral lishp. Others thnort the thnound (nasal lisp). Many children have been know to buy an "ites tream toda" or an all-day "tucker."

It would be impossible to portray the acoustic characteristics of some of the distortions used by clients with misarticulation, even if we used the phonetic alphabet. Seldom does an adult substitute a true *w* for the *r* as he attempts such a phrase as "around the rock." He usually produces a sound "something like a *w* and something like the velar *r* made with the back of the tongue elevated and the tip depressed." In some lateral lisping, the sound produced is more of a salivary unvoiced *l* instead of the *s*, a sloppy slurping sound which disgusts not only its hearers but its speaker too.

Many of the omissions heard in articulation cases are merely weakly stressed consonants. In a noisy room, an eighteen-year-old boy in describing a winter scene would seem to say, "The 'ky and 'no in wintuh." The missing sounds, however, were evident in quiet surroundings and were perfectly formed; but their duration was so brief that any noise seemed to mask their presence. Many cases, however, do entirely omit sounds they cannot produce. Additions of linking sounds are frequently found in blends ("the buhlue-guhreen color of spuhruce trees"); and when a child adds *ee* to every final *r* sound, as one of our cases did, the peculiarity is very noticeable.

To many persons, articulatory defects seem relatively unimportant. But severe articulation cases find the demands of modern life very difficult. We knew a woman who could not produce the *s, l,* and *r* sounds and yet who had to buy a railroad ticket to Robeline, Louisiana. She did it with pencil and paper. A man with the same difficulty became a farmer's hired hand after he graduated from college rather than suffer the penalties of a more verbal existence. Many children are said to outgrow their defective consonant sounds. Actually, they overcome them through blundering methods of self-help, and far too many of them never manage the feat. One man, aged sixty-five, asked us bitterly when we thought he would outgrow his baby-talk.

Some of these articulation cases have a great deal of difficulty communicating. Mothers cannot understand their own children. Teachers and classmates fail to comprehend speech when it is too full of phonemic errors. Try to translate these familiar nursery rhymes:

> Ha ta buh, Hah ta buh,
> Wuhnuh peh, two uh peh,
> Ha ta buh.
>
> Tippo Tymuh meh a pyemuh,
> Doh too peh,
> Ted Tippo Tymuh to duh pyemuh
> Yeh me tee oo weh.*

*Hot Cross Buns and Simple Simon

Many children who are severely handicapped by unintelligible speech also find it very difficult to express their emotions except by screaming or acting out their conflicts. Most of us relieve ourselves of our emotional evils by using others as our verbal handkerchiefs or wastebaskets. We talk it out. But when a child runs to his mother crying "Wobbuh toh ma tietihtoh" and she cannot understand that Robert stole his tricycle, all he can do is to fling himself into a tantrum. The same frustration results from his inability to use speech for self-exhibition. Often penalized or frustrated when he tries to talk, he soon finds it better to keep quiet, to use gestures, or to get attention in other ways. Many people tend to regard articulatory errors as being cute or relatively unimportant. Some of the most handicapped people we have ever known were those who could not speak clearly enough to be understood.

Thusfar, because we have had to use the ordinary alphabet to indicate deviancy in speech sound production, we aren't sure that you know how these people really talked. The professional speech pathologist, because he recognizes that it is impossible to use the regular orthographic *abc's* of English spelling in recording abnormal articulatory errors, uses a different alphabet, the IPA (International Phonetic Alphabet), which has a special symbol for each distinctive sound (*phoneme*). Some of these symbols are identical with those of our standard alphabet; others are different. This alphabet also has certain diacritical marks which can be used to show the characteristics of the errors. Anyone preparing to become a professional speech pathologist must take some coursework in phonetics to help him analyze and record abnormal articulation.

Since our purpose in this text is to acquaint you with the field of speech pathology we feel that you should at least have an opportunity to see this alphabet and to find out how it would be used in diagnosing the problems of a child whose speech sounds are faulty. The same key to the phonetic alphabet will be found on the back cover of this book.

Table I is a chart showing how all the consonant speech sounds of our language are articulated, and alongside each sound are some key words to help you recognize the referents of the strange symbols. The speech pathologist would do more than simply encircle or underline or record the symbols of the phonemes that were abnormally produced, though this would probably be one of his first diagnostic processes. In addition, he would also try to identify the characteristics of the errors and the contexts in which they occur, and do a lot of other things which we will consider in a later chapter. Here we wish merely to demonstrate that it is necessary to analyze deviant articulation in some detail. The child doesn't simply "not talk right".

We've got to know exactly what he does incorrectly if we are to help him.

TABLE I The Phonetic Alphabet

Phonetic Symbol	Key Words English	Phonetic	Phonetic Symbol	Key Words English	Phonetics
CONSONANTS					
b	back, cab	bæk kæb	p	pig, sap	pɪg sæp
d	dig, red	dɪg, rɛd	r	rat, poor	ræt pʊr
f	feel, leaf	fil lif	s	so, miss	so mɪs
g	go, egg	go ɛg	t	to, wit	tu wɪt
dʒ	just, edge, angel	dʒʌst ɛdʒ	ʃ	she, wish	ʃi wɪʃ
h	he behaves	hi bɪhevz	tʃ	chin, itch	tʃɪn ɪtʃ
k	keep, track	kip træk	θ	think truth	θɪŋk truθ
l	low, ball	lo bɔl	ð	then, bathe	ðɛn beð
l̩	simple, fable	sɪmpl̩ febl̩	v	vest, live	vɛst lɪv
m	my, aim	maɪ em	w	we, swim	wi swɪm
m̩	kingdom madam	kɪŋdm̩ mædm̩	hw	where, when	hwɛr hwɛn
n	not, any	nɑt ɛnɪ	j	yell, young	jɛl jʌŋ
n̩	action, mission	ækʃn̩ mɪʃn̩	ʒ ʒ	measure, version	mɛʒɚ vɝʒn
ŋ	sing, uncle	sɪŋ ʌŋkl̩	z	zebra, ozone	zibrə ozon
ʔ	oh oh!	ʔo ʔo			

(margin notes: "not tested for" pointing to m̩, n̩; "glottal stop" pointing to ʔ; "angel" written near dʒ; "no beginning" written near oh oh!)

VOWELS					
a*	far, sad	far sad	ɒ*	law, wrong	lɒ r ɒŋ
ɑ	father, mop	fɑðɚ mɑp	ɝ	early, bird	ɝli bɝd
e	great, ache	gret ek	ɜ*	early bird	ɜli b ɜd
æ	sad, sack	sæd sæk	ɚ	perhaps, never	pɚhæps nɛvɚ
i	intrigue, me	ɪntrig mi	u	to, you	tu ju
ɛ	head, rest	hɛd rɛst	ʊ	pudding, cook	pʊdɪŋ kʊk
ɪ	his, itch	hɪz ɪtʃ	ʌ	mother, drug	mʌðɚ drʌg
o	own, bone	on bon	ə	above, suppose	əbʌv səpoz
ɔ	all, dog	ɔl dɔg			

DIPHTHONGS					
aɪ	my, eye	maɪ aɪ	ɔɪ	toy, boil	tɔɪ bɔɪl
aʊ	cow, about	kaʊ əbaʊt			

CENTERING DIPHTHONGS					
ɛr	wear, fair	wɛr fɛr	ɪr	beer, weird	bɪr wɪrd
ɑr	barn, far	bɑrn far	aɪr	wire, tire	waɪr taɪr
ʊr	lure, moor	lʊr mʊr	aʊr	hour, flower	aʊr flaʊr
ɔr	shore, born	ʃor bɔrn			

*These vowels are heard in Eastern and Southern speech.

Fluency Disorders

About two million persons in this country suffer from disorders of fluency, primarily from the disorder called *stuttering*. A severe stutterer's speech abnormality may be very conspicuous, and it certainly can be very distressing. When the flow of speech is excessively fractured its meaning is hard to grasp. The contortions and struggling, the backing up and starting again, the prolongations of sounds, the compulsive repetitions of syllables, the difficulty in initiating utterance bother both the speaker and the listener alike.

Stuttering It is difficult to find typical illustrations for this disorder since it is characterized by a high degree of variability. Nevertheless, we present some examples from our practice:

William was brought to us by his concerned parents. They were especially worried because the father had stuttered as a child and a grandfather and uncle had been stutterers. When he was introduced to us, he said, "I'm nnnnot Wuh-Wuh-Wuh-Wuh-W-W-William. I-I-I-I'm Billy. Thuh-Thuh-that's my name." He seemed to be unaware of his repetitions and showed no reluctance to talk. Indeed, he jabbered easily and constantly. Billy was an extrovertive, outgoing child, and a very active one. We had to do most of our analysis of the problem on the wing as he explored every corner of our office, opening drawers, playing with our instruments, even going through the pockets of our overcoat in the closet. All this was accompanied by a verbal commentary on what he was doing or perceiving and much of what he said either to us or to himself was full of short syllabic repetitions or the prolongations of sounds. Only rarely would he say an entire phrase or short sentence without them. He just burbled, bubbled, and bounced without any signs of frustration. His parents said that this was the way he talked most of the time except when saying his prayers. Then he was fluent. Although many children show some of this sort of disfluency between the second and fourth years as they master speech, Billy had much more than the normal amount. He almost seemed to be speaking a stuttering language. What concerned us more was that the number of syllabic repetitions per word averaged four or five, whereas in normally speaking children they seldom exceed two per word. Moreover, Billy was using the "schwa" or neutral vowel ("uh") on many of his repetitions. He was not saying "bo-bo-bo-boat" but "buh-buh-buh-boat." He was also prolonging certain sounds. Once he said, "fffffffor," with the *f* being prolonged for over two seconds. Finally, these "stutterings" did not seem to reflect variations in communicative stress. They were too consistent. We accepted him for treatment.

Peter was an eleven-year-old stutterer. Speaking, to him, was hard labor. Although he stuttered on other words also, it was on the first words of his utterances that he had the most trouble. He would open his mouth and nothing would come out. You could see him forcing and struggling. His face was contorted. Sometimes he would just give up and tears came to his eyes. Not all of his blockings were of this type, however. On certain words he would drawl out the vowel ("Caaaaaaan"), and the pitch would rise. On others he would repeat a syllable compulsively many times, and these syllables too would show the same fire-siren effect. When relaxed or distracted Peter could be very fluent, the stuttering occurring in volleys; yet he did not seem to avoid speaking nor did he attempt to disguise his trouble. The more he stuttered, the more he seemed to feel a need to talk. He was hurt and frustrated by his stuttering and was highly aware of it when it happened, but he showed no signs of fear.

Cynthia was sixteen, a very attractive girl, popular with her classmates and the boys, an excellent student. Outwardly she stuttered very little so far as repetitions or complete blockings were concerned. She talked very fast, but her speech was full of postponement tricks, avoidances, and disguise reactions. She feared certain sounds and words and would substitute synonyms for those she thought she might stutter on, or pretend to think or cough or revise her sentences or say "ah-ah-ah-ah" or "well" or "Oh, you know" to gain time or hide her stuttering. She was very skillful in using these disguise reactions in her ordinary, casual speech. When she had to read aloud however, as she did in French class, some severe repetitive stuttering was very evident. It also showed up when she had to introduce herself or someone else. Although outwardly she was a gay, almost scatterbrained girl, this was a facade. She worried greatly about her stuttering and was very despondent in private. Her word, sound, and situation fears were very intense. She was very ashamed to be a stutterer.

In considering this disorder, let us observe its various aspects. The stutterer shows breaks in the usual time sequence of utterance.

The usual flow is interrupted. There are conspicuous oscillations and fixations, repetitions and prolongations of sounds and syllables. There are gaps of silence that call attention to themselves. If you ask a stutterer a question, the answer may not be forthcoming at the proper time. The stutterer's speech sometimes seems to have holes in it. Some sounds are held too long. Syllables seem to echo themselves repeatedly and compulsively. Odd contortions and struggles occur which interfere with communication. The stutterer may show marked signs of fear or embarrassment. He fits our definition because his speech behavior deviates from the speech of other people in such a way that it attracts attention. All of us hesitate and repeat ourselves, but the stutterer hesitates and repeats himself differently than we do, and more often.

One of the interesting features of stuttering is that it seems to be a disorder more of communication than of speech. Most stutterers can sing without difficulty. Most of them speak perfectly when alone. Usually, it is only when they are talking to a listener that the difficulty becomes apparent. Stuttering varies with emotional stress and increases in situations invested with fear or shame. When very secure and relaxed, stutterers often are very fluent. In extreme cases even the thinking processes seem to be affected — but only when they are thinking aloud, and again in the presence of a listener.

Stuttering takes many forms; it presents many faces. The only consistent behavior is the repetition and prolongation of syllables, sounds, or speech postures. It changes as it develops, for stuttering usually grows and gets worse if untreated.

Initially, and for some time thereafter, the child's speech is broken by an excessive amount of repetitions of syllables and sounds or, less frequently, by the prolongation of a sound. He does not seem to be aware of his difficulty. He does not struggle or avoid speaking. He does not seem to be embarrassed at all. Indeed, he seems almost totally unconscious of his repetitive utterance. He just bubbles along, trying his best to communicate. An excerpt from a parent's letter may illustrate this early stuttering:

> I would appreciate some advice about my daughter. She is almost three years old, and has always been precocious in speech. Four weeks ago she recovered from a severe attack of whooping cough, and it was immediately after that when she began to show some trouble with her speech. One morning she came downstairs and asked for orange juice, and it sounded like this: "Wh-wh-wh-where's my orange juice?" Since then, she has repeated often, and sometimes eight or nine times. It doesn't seem to bother her, but I'm worried about it as it gets a lot

worse when she asks questions or when she is tired, and I'm afraid other children will start laughing at her. One of her playmates has already imitated her several times. No one else in our family has any trouble talking. What do you think we should do? Up to now we have just been ignoring it and hoping it will go away.

Unfortunately, stuttering does not always remain so effortless. The child begins to react to his broken communication by surprise and then frustration. The former effortless repetitions and prolongations become irregular, faster, and more tense. As the child becomes aware of his stuttering and is frustrated by it, he begins to struggle. Finally, he becomes afraid of certain speaking situations and of certain words and sounds. Once this occurs, stuttering tends to become self-perpetuating, self-reinforcing. The more he fears, the more he stutters, and the more he stutters, the more he fears. He becomes caught in a vicious circle.

In the older stutterer, stuttering occurs in many forms, since different individuals react to their speech interruptions in different ways. One German authority carefully described ninety-nine different varieties of stuttering (each christened with beautiful Greek and Latin verbiage), and we are sure that there must be many more. Stutterers have been known to grunt or spit or pound themselves or protrude their tongues or speak on inhalation or waltz or jump or merely stare glassily when in the throes of what they call a "spasm" or a "block." The late Irvin S. Cobb described a certain Captain Joe Fowler who manifested his stuttering through the use of profanity. Captain Joe was able to speak very well under ordinary circumstances; but when he got angry or excited, his speech stopped entirely, and he was able to get started again only through the use of a stereotyped bit of cursing. Some of the imitations of stuttering heard in the movies and on radio may seem grotesque, yet the reality may be even more unusual.

Some stutterers develop an almost complete inability to make a direct speech attempt upon a feared word. They approach it, back away, say "a-a-a-a" or "um-um-um," go back to the beginning of the sentence and try again and again, until finally they give up communication altogether. Many stutterers become so adept at substituting synonyms for their difficult words, and disguising the interruptions which do occur, that they are able to pose as normal speakers. We have known seven severe stutterers whose spouses first discovered their speech impediments after the wedding ceremony. Stutterers have preached and taught school and become successful traveling salesman without ever betraying their infirmity, but they are not happy individuals. The nervous strain and vigilance necessary to avoid and disguise their symptoms often create stresses so severe as to produce profound emotional breakdowns.

This general picture of stuttering gives you a general overview of the disorder, but it does not show you how a speech pathologist would analyze the problem of a specific client. First he would ask the question: "What behaviors does this person show that are unlike those of a normal speaker?" In his analysis, he would be interested in the overt, visible and audible manifestations of the problem such as repetitions, prolongations, tremors, inappropriate mouth postures, or abnormal foci of tension. He would note how the stutterer avoids or postpones the speech attempt. He would try to determine how the latter seeks to release himself from the verbal oscillations and fixations that break up the flow of speech. Through interview and observation the speech clinician would probe the stutterer's inner world. What speaking situations are most feared? What words and sounds are viewed as difficult? How much frustration does he feel? How much shame and embarrassment? Is the disorder getting worse? How fluent can he be in certain situations? These and a host of other questions and scannings provide the diagnostic information needed to plan appropriate therapy. Stutterers badly need help but unfortunately far too few ever get any, except from the ignorant, and these harm more than they help. We are determined that you will not be one of them.

Cluttering   Another disorder in which the time sequence is disturbed is called cluttering. It is frequently confused with stuttering because it too shows many repetitions. However, the major features of cluttering are first, the excessive speed of speaking; second, the disorganized sentence structure; and third, the slurred or omitted syllables and sounds. The clutterer can speak perfectly when he speaks very slowly, but it's almost impossible for him to do so except for short periods. They truly have "tangled tongues." The speech is cluttered speech; it is disorganized, pell-mell speech, sputtered speech. The true clutterer has no seeming awareness of his excessive speed or garbled utterance. He is always surprised when others cannot understand him. He has no fears or shames. He does not struggle or avoid. Some clutterers become stutterers as well; most do not. Clutterers speak by spurts, and their speech organs pile up like keys on a typewriter when a novice stenographer tries for more speed than her skill permits. An old text in speech correction has this description: " . . . a

torrent of half-articulated words, following each other like peas running out of a spout"; but the torrent is also irregularly interrupted in
its flow. People constantly ask the clutterer to repeat. They are em-
pathically irritated by his uneven volleys of hasty syllables. They find
themselves interrupting during his panting pauses and then in turn
being interrupted by a new overwhelming rush of jumbled words.

Voice Disorders

The first thing a professional speech pathologist does when he becomes convinced that the speech deviancy involves phonation or
voice is to scrutinize the client's voice for abnormalities in *pitch* or
intensity (loudness) or *quality*. He knows that more than one of these
three dimensions may show significant differences from the normal
range of variation. Moreover, he knows that this range is wider than
those for normal articulation or fluency, so he is careful not to diagnose abnormality if it is not there.

Disorders of Pitch   The normal range of pitch variations depends upon sex, age,
and several other factors. The voices of men are generally
lower in average pitch than those of women. A deep-voiced male
would have no voice disorder; the woman who speaks with a bass
voice is conspicuous. A six-year-old boy with a high-pitched treble
voice would incur no penalty from society; a thirty-year-old man
would find raised eyebrows if he began to speak in such tones. Under conditions of great excitement, many of us have voices which
crack or show pitch breaks. But when an adult shows these same
pitch breaks upward into the falsetto when he orders a hamburger or
says goodbye, we suspect the abnormal. Again, there are times when
it is appropriate to speak with a minimum of inflection, but a person
who consistently talks on a monopitch will find his listener either irritated or asleep. In deciding whether a person has a pitch disorder
we must always use the normal yardstick.

The above discussion has anticipated our listing of the pitch
disorders. They are as follows: *too-high pitch, too-low pitch, monotone*
or *monopitch, pitch breaks, stereotyped inflections,* and *diplophonia*.

The following description was uttered by a two-hundred-pound
football player in his high, piping, shrill, child's voice:

Yes, I was one of those boy sopranos and my music teacher
loved me. I soloed in all the cantatas and programs and sang in

the choir and glee clubs, and they never let my voice change. I socked a guy the other day who wisecracked about it, but I'm still a boy soprano at twenty-two. I'm getting so I'm afraid to open my mouth. Strangers start looking for a Charlie McCarthy somewhere. I got to get over it, and quick. Why, I can't even swear but some guy who's been saying the same words looks shocked.

A high-pitched voice in a male is definitely a handicap, communicative, economic, and social.

When a woman's voice is pitched very low and carries a certain type of male inflection, it certainly calls attention to itself and causes maladjustment. The following sentence, spoken by a casual acquaintance and overheard by the girl to whom it referred, practically wrecked her entire security: "Every time I hear her talk I look around to see if it's the bearded lady of the circus."

On every campus some professor possesses that enemy of education, a monotonous voice. A true monotone is comparatively rare, yet it dominates any conversation by its difference. To hear a person laugh on a single note is enough to stir the scalp. Questions asked in a true monotone seem curiously devoid of life. Fortunately, most cases of monotonous voice are not so extreme. Many of them could be described as the "poker voice"—even as a face without expression is termed a "poker face." Inflections are present, but for fear of revealing insecurity or inadequacy they are reduced to a minimum.

By stereotyped inflections we refer to the voice which calls attention to itself through its pitch patterning. The sing-song voice, the voice that ends every phrase or sentence with a falling inflection, the "schoolma'am's voice" with its emphatic dogmatic inflections, are all types of variation which *when extreme,* may be considered speech defects.

Pitch Breaks   These may be upward or downward, usually the former. The adolescent boy, learning to use his adult voice, often experiences them. Often they can be very traumatizing. To have your voice suddenly flip-flop upward into a falsetto or child's voice is to lose control of the self. When you want to speak you don't wish to yodel. Often individuals who fear this experience use a monopitch or too low or too high a pitch level to keep the flip-flopping from occurring. Pitch breaks wreck communication; they define the speaker as one who cannot control himself or who is very emotional. They often interfere with the person's ability to think on his feet since he must forever be monitoring his voice. They may sound funny to others, but we have not found them so.

A curious pitch disorder, a rare one, is found in *diplophonia*. The person uses two pitches at the same time, producing a fluttering sort of voice which is very noticeable. We wish we could play for you the tape that would demonstrate it. One of our clients, a very attractive girl, developed diplophonia as the result of having discovered that she could speak in a deep bass by adjusting her larynx in a certain way. She played with this deep voice, shocked her roommates in the shower or bedroom, and generally used it for kicks. Then she found that she could use both her own voice and the deep voice at the same time, even being able to sing simple tunes in harmony with herself. About the time that she had decided to use it to go into show business, she found that she could no longer shift back and forth at will between the two voices but instead had the double voice, the diplophonia, all the time. Terrified, she came to us for help.

Another disorder, the *tremulous voice,* is not solely the voice of old age, though certainly we often find it in the aged. It appears in the voices of individuals with cerebral palsy, especially in those with athetosis. Persons with one paralyzed vocal cord are likely to show it too. We find it reflecting the tremors of Parkinson's disease and the muscular difficulties of multiple sclerosis. And we have worked with a few individuals who were neither aged nor sick, yet whose tones wobbled abnormally when they spoke. The fluctuations of pitch in the tremulous voice are slower and larger than we find in the normal vibrato, and they are not as regular. A good vibrato enhances a voice; the tremorous shakiness of the tremulous voice impairs its effectiveness in communication.

Disorders of Intensity   Most of us, if we have abused our voices by excessive shouting or yelling, or have suffered from a severe cold, have experienced *dysphonia.* For a time we cannot talk loudly enough or can speak only in a breathy whisper. In the latter case, we can be said to have *aphonia,* the complete loss of phonation. Dysphonia, therefore, is the more general term.

When the speech pathologist confronts dysphonia he knows he will have a tough diagnosic problem. He must try to identify the causes of the loss of voice through interviewing the client and try to sort out the predisposing from the preciptating causes, as well as identify the factors that may be maintaining the disorder. Is there a long history of vocal abuse, of regularly having to speak in an environment with high noise levels, of having to communicate too often with a family member who has become deafened? Does the client have a long history of chronic laryngitis? Is he a college cheerleader? How many packs of cigarettes does he smoke each day? Has there been a history of previous loss of voice and under what conditions? Speech pathology involves a lot of detective work, and these questions are only a few of those which are helpful in understanding the nature of the problem.

Again, the behavior itself interests us. How does this person with dysphonia attempt the production of voice? We may observe his thyroid cartilage, (his "Adam's apple"), to see if it assumes the position for swallowing at the moment he begins to phonate. We note any evidences of excessive tension in the area of the throat. We look for the mis-timing of the breath pulse or for other breathing abnormalities. And, knowing that the dysphonia may be one of the first signs of organic abnormalities, such as growths on the vocal cords, benign or cancerous, or the reflection of paralysis, the speech pathologist perhaps may save a life by insisting that his client be seen by a laryngologist before he will work with him.

Most dysphonias, however, do not have such an organic pathology. Our voices are the barometers or our emotional states. They reflect our feelings of anxiety, guilt, or hostility. When these acids begin to eat their human containers too often, voice disorders may ensue. Here is an illustration:

> Miss J. was a kindergarten teacher who shouldn't have been any kind of teacher. If at one time she had loved little children that affection had long gone. She screamed at the kids, tried vainly to establish order in the chaos which prevailed in her room, and at the end of each afternoon was so fatigued she had to go to bed as soon as she came home from school. We got to know her well, because every March for several years she would get aphonia (lose her voice) and come to us for treatment. There were no growths (nodules) on her vocal folds, nor any organic pathology of significance, though her throat was usually inflamed. She could only speak in a strained whisper. The symptoms, of course, were convenient in that she could not teach. March is a long wait from either Christmas or summer vacation. Most of our therapy was palliative (time-gaining) and consisted of various exercises in breathing and soft phonation. Finally, we were able to persuade her to get the psychological counseling which

had been our main goal all along. With this and our help in getting her a position as a receptionist in a medical clinic, her
voice returned, this time permanently as our five-year follow-up
revealed. We felt we had done a good deal, not only to alleviate
her own misery, but also that of many small children.

Speech pathologists, as well as physicians, may use certain adjectives before the term *aphonia* to indicate the presumed cause of the
disorder. In our preceding illustration, Miss J. might be said to have
the hysterical type of *aphonia* because of its evident neurotic nature.
Someone whose loss of voice seemed to be due to vocal abuse and
strain would have a *functional aphonia,* but not an hysterical one. On
the other hand, when the loss of voice is due to paralysis or growths
upon the vocal folds, it would be called an *organic aphonia* or *dysphonia,* depending upon whether the loss was complete or incomplete.

One strange vocal intensity disorder that presently defies labeling as organic or functional is termed *spastic (or spasmodic) dysphonia.*
A person with this disorder may begin to speak with good voice,
then tense the laryngeal and throat muscles so tightly that she or he
almost chokes in the act of speaking and the rest of the sentence
comes out in little bursts of squeezed sound or whispered air flow. It
is very difficult to describe in words but very easy to recognize when
heard. At times the spastic dysphonic also has trouble getting started,
showing behaviors that have caused it to be called by some authorities by the term "vocal stuttering." Like stuttering it varies in severity with communicative stress. The research seems to indicate that
there may be some neurological involvement in spasmodic dysphonia, and it is very difficult to treat and usually gets worse. There
are many puzzles that remain to be solved in the field of speech pathology, and this is one of them.

Another voice problem, *ventricular dysphonia,* has been classified
among the intensity disorders because the speech produced often
fades in its loudness enough to impair comprehension. People with
ventricular dysphonia produce phonation with their false vocal folds
which are located and have their constriction point just above the
level of the true vocal folds. The sound seems strangled. You have
probably used ventricular (or false vocal fold) phonation when grunt-
ing on the toilet or when lifting a heavy object. The voice so produced is also harsh in quality. It often resembles spastic dysphonia
but differs from it by not showing the spasmodic breaks in phonation or the complete loss of tone. This disorder is fortunately rare because it can be very handicapping.

Disorders of   When the speech pathologist has to diagnose the problem of
Voice Quality   a person whose voice quality is conspicuously unpleasant
(rarely does such a voice problem impair intelligibility) he
knows that he has a hard task. First of all, he faces the fact of human
variability. We have almost as many characteristic voice qualities as
we have faces—which is why it is so easy to identify a speaker by
the voice alone. And the quality or timbre of a voice is often very
difficult to describe in words. In novels, voices have been called
thick, thin, reedy, shrill, sweet, round, brilliant, rich, and even metal-
lic, but these adjectives are rarely used by speech pathologists (except
derisively). Yet even the terms used by professionals, with some exceptions, are imprecise. Only a few of them are descriptive enough to
have gained any real currency.

One of the exceptions is the voice quality disorder termed
hypernasality. The lay person would say that a speaker with such a
disorder seems to be talking through his nose too much. When most
of the vowels or the voiced continuant sounds as well as the nasal
sounds, /m/, /n/, and /ŋ/, have so much excessive nasality in them
that the voice is conspicuously unpleasant, most speech pathologists
would agree on the diagnosis of hypernasality. No one should have
to whine when he passionately says "I love you." Not all hypernasality gives the impression of whining, however. To whine you
also usually show the upward inflection patterns of complaint combined with the excessive nasality. And some of our clients, the more
neurotic ones who bathe constantly in self-pity, show this combination of pitch and quality deviations. But there are others, as we have
said who do not whine, yet show too much nasality.

In certain sections of this country there are dialectal ways of
speaking which show more nasality than we find generally. Providing the Hoosier who speaks this way stays on his Indiana farm, he
certainly would not possess any voice disorder at all, but he would
have to reduce that nasality were he to become an actor or radio announcer in some other part of our land. (Again, here we find the
need always to define abnormal speech in terms of norms.) Persons
from certain rural parts of New England are also said to have a nasal
twang which we would hate to classify as abnormal. Indeed, most of
this dialectal hypernasality seems to be due to what is termed *assimilation nasality* which refers to the nasalization of only those sounds
which precede or follow the /m/, /n/, or /ŋ/. Most of us show some
assimilation nasality in saying such words as name, man, or mangle,
the vowels being nasalized, especially in swift speech.

Another voice quality disorder which is fairly easily recognized
is the *harsh* or *strident* voice. People would describe it as raspingly

unpleasant, as "grating upon the ear." There is tension in it, an abrupt beginning of phonation, an unevenness rather than smoothness, and bits of that scratchy noise called the *vocal fry*. Try speaking aloud very harshly to see how well this description fits.

A third disorder of voice quality is the *breathy* voice. Hot Breath Harriet had one and used it as a Maine guide uses a birchbark horn to bring a lovelorn moose to the gun. In our culture, for some esoteric reason, a low-pitched, husky voice in a woman sounds sexy to the vulnerable male, even though it may merely be the result of asthma or a paralyzed vocal cord or a post-nasal drip. It certainly can call attention to itself and impair intelligibility in a noisy environment.

These three, the hypernasal, the harsh, and the breathy voices, can be labeled with some precision. But how about the hoarse voice? Is it an entity in itself, or is it a combination of the harsh and breathy voice qualities? Our research has not clearly provided the answer to these questions but you should know that when a person doesn't have the flu or a cold and yet has shown a hoarse voice for a month or more, he should be referred immediately to a speech pathologist or laryngologist because growths may be forming on the vocal folds or some other unpleasant consequences may lie in wait. Even when the hoarse voice is merely the temporary result of vocal abuse and strain, it is a signal that something should be done.

The *falsetto* voice, when it is the only voice used by a speaker who is not a professional yodeler, has also been included among the disorders of voice quality, though often the pitch is abnormally high. A Mickey Mouse sort of voice, it turns the heads of anyone within earshot. Some of our most troubled voice cases have been adult males who told us their voices never changed at puberty. They suffered many penalties from society until we showed them how to find their real voice (which often was a very low-pitched bass.) The falsetto is produced by a different kind of vocal fold vibration and most of us, male or female, can speak in a falsetto if we try. Besides the different laryngeal action, we also tend to use different resonating cavities when using the falsetto voice, and this creates the characteristic voice quality accompanying the pitch change. It is also possible for some speakers to use a very low-pitched falsetto, and when they do the voice is described as *throaty* or *pectoral.*

Finally, we have the disorder of *denasality,* another one that is difficult to describe or define. Sometimes called the adenoidal voice because it is characterized by a lack of nasality (hyponasality), when you hear it you want to swallow or clear your throat and are impelled to get out of range of suspected cold germs. Denasality has also been classified among the articulation disorders because the /m/, /n/, and

/ŋ/ lose some of their nasality and turn into /b/, /d/, and /g/ respectively, and other consonants are also distorted. If you will pretend that you have a very bad cold and say this sentence, you will probably show the picture of denasality: "Mary doesn't know if she can come."

The speech pathologist soon comes to recognize that few voice quality disorders are free from deviancies in pitch or intensity and that their abnormality is increased when these other vocal features differ from the norm. For example, an excessively harsh and also excessively strident voice is more noticeable and more unpleasant than one which is not as loud. When we find a voice which is both hypernasal and is too high in its pitch levels, we can sometimes bring it closer to normality by lowering the pitch. In spastic dysphonia we hear harshness and breathiness combined. Again, we find deviant voices wherein several abnormal vocal quality differences are apparent, as in the harsh nasal voice. In helping our students to sort out and to remember all these features of abnormal voice, we ask them to try to produce them before applying the diagnostic labels. Why don't you?

Nancy's nasal voice was also so harsh that it repelled anyone who had to listen to her for any length of time. She was unattractive in face, figure, and personality. She had never dated in all her nineteen years and was a very unhappy person. The mother, an attractive woman of forty, who brought her to the clinic, had the same sort of voice quality. Examination revealed no organic pathology, though at times Nancy sounded almost as nasal as a person with a cleft palate. We even probed and used transillumination to see if a submucous cleft existed, but there was none. None of her consonants was accompanied by nasal airflow. The soft palate seemed to function adequately in whispering; but when she produced vocalized vowel sounds, it and the walls of the throat showed little movement. Tests of her hearing revealed a moderate hearing loss in the low frequencies. When we played back to her a tape of her voice with amplification, Nancy was shocked and appalled. She had never known how she sounded. It would take too long to describe her therapy. It required the fitting of a hearing aid and over a year of clinical sessions twice weekly in which we taught her to speak more softly, more breathily, and at a lower pitch. We separated her from her mother by helping her get a college scholarship. We arranged it so that she was placed in a dormitory suite with several of our majors in speech pathology, who took her under their wing, reinforced her new voice, improved her grooming, and in general created a new personality. Speech therapy involves more than the mouth or throat.

Language Disorders

One of the chief fascinations about the field of speech pathology is the opportunity it presents for exploration and discovery. Man, like the bear, must go over the mountain to see what he can see. The baby discovers his toes and babbles with delight; the child roams the fringes of his neighborhood; the adult walks gingerly on the moon. At this very moment all over the world there are people testing the boundaries of the known in astronomy, physics, chemistry, biology, and a hundred other sciences. In speech pathology, because it is a relatively new field, the unknown is very near. Every speech disorder has its puzzles, unanswered questions, and problems to be solved.

Of all the disorders of communication, those of language disability most urgently need exploration. Although humans have been talking for thousands of years, language itself still holds many mysteries and the disorders of language have many more. There are two major language disorders: *aphasia* (dysphasia) and *delayed or deviant language development.*

Dysphasia   Again, as in aphonia and dysphonia, the term aphasia if used precisely would refer to the complete inability to comprehend or use language symbols, a condition which fortunately is rarely found, while *dysphasia* refers to a lesser degree of disability. (Since most working speech clinicians are too busy to be precise, they tend to use either term and so shall we). It is impossible to give you a "typical" description of an aphasic because the disorder appears in many forms. He might show impairment in comprehending or formulating his messages or in finding ways to express them. His disability may be shown in reading, writing, or silent gesturing as well as in speaking. His speech may be so garbled as to be incomprehensible to others, or merely broken by a search for words that momentarily he cannot find. He may say "bread" when he wants to ask for "butter" or "jugga" for soup. He may nod his head affirmatively when he wants to say no. He may hold a pencil in his hand and yet not be able to copy the triangle placed before him. Dysphasia as a disorder has a thousand faces and the speech pathologist's first job is to analyze the features of the disability presented by the person before him. So let us here confine ourselves to two brief symptomatic pictures: Here's what R. V. McKnight wrote (after her recovery) about her difficulty in comprehending what the word "your" meant:

> "I mentally heard it, but it had no meaning. I felt that it was related to the word 'you' but I could not figure out the relationship between the two. I continued to puzzle over this until the speaker had finished his lecture and sat down ... More generally, when I do not recognize the meaning, I do not recognize the sound. The word is a jumble of letters."(McKnight, 1936)

Some of our aphasics have told us that when trying to read, they see "a line of meaningless squiggles or scribbles" and haven't the slightest idea as to what they mean. Some of them cannot even recognize the snapshots of their own faces or those of their friends.

In these last two examples, we see the receptive problems of aphasia, the difficulties in comprehending language symbols whether they are spoken or written. More dramatically visible is the impairment shown when the aphasic tries to express himself in speech. Here is what one of our clients told us after he had made a partial recovery:

> It was like ... it was like the alphabet ... No I mean words ... words were in my face, no, I mean (points to his head) you know, but I couldn't find. No. I got them but ... but they won't come, you know. Gone. Then come back and go again. Forget but they in ... they in mouth, yes. I know, yes, but they won't come. And I get ... sleep ... no, not sleep ... sleep, No! Get awful slired ... tired ... tired, yes. Oh my!

Often the speech pathologist is just one member of the rehabilitation team when dealing with the patient who has dysphasia. He must work closely with the physician, and with occupational and physical therapists. Often he is the person who must work most closely with the families of the stroke victim, helping them to understand the nature of the sufferer's communication difficulties, and seeing to it that they help rather than hinder the rehabilitation process so that he may be given back his human dignity. No work in speech pathology is more challenging than helping an aphasic to become able to communicate effectively again.

Delayed or Deviant Language Development   This problem will be faced sooner or later by every worker in the field of special education as well as by the speech pathologist. A child who, for one reason or another (and there may be many reasons), does not understand what others say to him or who does not know the basic rules by which our language is structured is truly handicapped indeed, for he cannot send the messages that must be sent in a society that demands constant communication. The child with language delay is pretty helpless in a world of words.

Moreover, it is not a minor problem even for the speech pathologist, a recent survey showing that over 21 percent of the caseload of public-school speech pathologists now consists of children with language disabilities. Because of the prevalence of this disorder, in many school systems, the worker in speech pathology[3] is no longer called a speech therapist but instead he is referred to as the "speech and language clinician."

Although the child with delayed language development usually shows many articulation errors (sometimes to the point of unintelligibility), his major difficulties often lie in vocabulary deficits which restrict his speech output, in grammatical deficits which prevent him from expressing himself according to the hidden rules of communication (appropriate plurals, tense, subject-predicate, etc.), or in his inability to handle transformations, such as being able to know the difference between a statement and a question or to be able to express himself in both ways.

Anyone who wants to help a child with such a language disability must not only determine that his language competence and performance are inferior to other children of his chronological, mental, or physical age levels; he must also analyze the child's specific difficulties in encoding and decoding. Let us provide an illustration:

> Mrs. P. had asked for an appointment because her son, John, age five, was "slow in talking." Despite the fact that her physician had told her not to worry and that he would outgrow "it", she was very concerned. The boy should be entering kindergarten next year and she knew he would not be ready. She said that he had been ill a lot until he was three, at which time he began to say his first words—with simple sentences or phrases appearing a little later. He now talked a lot but she was about the only person who could understand most of what he did say.

---

[3] W. R. Neal, "Speech Pathology Services in the Secondary Schools," *Language, Speech and Hearing Services in the Schools,* 7, 1976, 6–10.

She made it very clear that Johhny understood everything said to him, however, could follow directions, etc.

Our diagnostic session went poorly. The boy refused to be separated from the mother and refused to say anything no matter how hard she tried to get him to respond. Johnny was an only child and she told us he'd been "spoiled rotten" because he'd been ill so much. It was our impression that Johnny enjoyed being able to thwart her attempts to get him to say this and say that.

Since the mother was so anxious and so insistent that the boy did a lot of talking at home, we made arrangements to send one of our students there with a cassette tape recorder to procure the samples we needed. Here is one brief sample with the translation and her analysis. (The mother had happened to mention to the student that she would have to go to the grocery.)

Language sample:
"Donny doh toe . . . Mummy tay Donny toe?"
(Johnny go to the store) (Mother take Johhny to the store)
"Donny doh tah . . . Deh eye-tee-toe"
(Johnny go in the car) (Get ice cream cone)

Articulatory analysis:
Vowels OK. Distinction between voicing and unvoicing of cognate consonants OK. Nasal consonants OK. Limited repertoire of consonants: /t/ and /d/ plosives used for all other plosives and for affricates. Omission of most other sounds.

Language analysis:
Subject-predicate OK; phrase structuring basically OK, but boy omits all pronouns and prepositions and adverbs; inflections appropriate for statements, commands, and questions; syllabification OK.

We were not too happy with this student's analysis and report, but they do indicate in a crude way what we do when we attempt to diagnose the communication problems of a child who shows delayed language development.

These, then, are the disorders of communication with which the speech pathologist must cope. If at the moment you feel a bit overwhelmed by their number and variety, be reassured. We shall discuss them one at a time in later chapters. Our purpose here is merely to acquaint you with the scope of speech pathology.

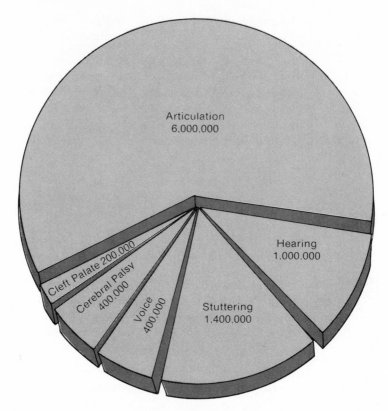

Articulation
6,000,000

Hearing
1,000,000

Cleft Palate 200,000

Cerebral Palsy
400,000

Voice
400,000

Stuttering
1,400,000

Figure 6 Estimated prevalence of speech disorders. (From *Human Communication and its Disorders: An Overview,* National Advisory Neurological Diseases and Stroke Council Report, 1969.)

References

BERMAN, M. and E. LEACH. *Identifying Speech Disorders* New York: Harper & Row, 1974. (A series of four 16 mm. films in black and white showing disorders of language, stuttering, articulation, and voice.)

BERRY, M. L. *Language Disorders of Children.* Englewood Cliffs, N.J.: Prentice-Hall, Inc., 1969.

BLAKE, J. N. "A Therapeutic Construct for Two Seven-Year-Old Nonverbal Boys." *Journal of Speech and Hearing Disorders,* XXXIV (1969), 363–69.

BOONE, D. R. *An Adult Has Aphasia.* Danville, Ill.: Interstate, 1965.

BURKOWSKY, M. B. "Vocal Ulcers in a Seventy-One Year Old Male." *Journal of Speech and Hearing Disorders,* XXXIII (1968), 268–69.

DENES, P. and E. PINSEN. *The Speech Chain.* Baltimore: Waverly Press, 1969.

DUBER, H, W. "A Speech Pathologist Talks to the Parents of a Nonverbal Child." *Rehabilitation Literature,* XXX (1969), 360–62.

EGLAND, G. O. *Speech and Language Problems.* Englewood Cliffs, N.J.: Prentice-Hall, Inc., 1970.

FISHER, H. B. and J. LOGEMANN. "Objective Evaluation of Therapy for Vocal
Nodules: A Case Report." *Journal of Speech and Hearing Disorders,*
XXXV (1970), 227–85.

GERSTMAN, H. L. "A Case of Aphasia." *Journal of Speech and Hearing Disorders,* XXIX (1964), 89–91.

HALL, P. K. and J. B. TOMBLEN. "Case Study: Therapy Procedures for Remediation of a Nasal Lisp." *Language, Speech, Hearing Services in the
Schools,* VI (1975), 29–32.

HALPERN, H. "A Case Report of Elective Mutism." *Journal of Communication
Disorders,* II (1969), 69–71.

KASTEIN, S. and B. TRACE. *The Birth of Language: The Case History of a Non-
verbal Child.* Springfield, Ill.: C. C. Thomas, 1970.

KILLILEA, M. *Karen.* Englewood Cliffs, N.J.: Prentice-Hall, Inc,. 1962.

KOBITCH, L. "What It Is To Be a Laryngectomee: A Specific Case Study." *Human Communication,* IV (1975), 45–47.

KNOX, D. *Portrait of Aphasia.* Detroit, Mich.: Wayne State U. Press, 1971.

LUKENS, K. and C. PANTER. *Thursday's Child Has Far To Go.* Englewood Cliffs,
N.J.: Prentice-Hall, Inc,. 1969.

LUPER, H., ed. *Stuttering: Successes and Failures in Therapy.* Memphis, Tenn.:
Speech Foundation of America, 1968.

McBRIDE, C. *Silent Victory.* Chicago: Nelson-Hall, 1969.

McKNIGHT, R. V. "A Self-Analysis of a Case of Reading, Writing, and Speaking Disability," *Archives of Speech,* I (1936) 43–47.

ROSENBEK, J. C. "Treatment of Developmental Apraxia of Speech: A Case
Study." *Language, Speech, Hearing Services in the Schools,* V (1974), 13–
22.

WOLSKI, W. and J. WILEY, "Functional Aphonia in a Fourteen-Year-Old Boy:
A Case Report." *Journal of Speech and Hearing Disorders,* XXX (1965),
71–75.

WYLIE, D. "Tommy Tunes In." *Exceptional Children,* XXXII (1965), 259–61.

3

SPEECH AND LANGUAGE

Before we begin to describe the ways that speech pathologists treat the various speech disorders it is necessary to provide you with some essential information about the speech mechanism, the nature of the speech sounds, the basic structure of our language, and how speech develops normally.

During your first few years, you and a million other babies accomplished something that you could not possibly do now, not even if you spent the rest of your life at the task. You learned to understand a strange new language and to speak it like a native. Moreover, you learned that language easily. Without any formal instruction you perfected your pronunciation of its sounds, acquired a large number of meaningful words, and mastered the hidden linguistic rules that appropriately link those words together in phrases and sentences of incredible variety.

Present linguistic theory claims that this incredibly difficult achievement is due to an inborn trait of all human beings—the potential capacity for language acquisition. Attempts to explain the phenomenal rapidity of that acquisition solely in terms of learning theory have not been very satisfactory, though learning, of course, must be involved. Otherwise, some of us wouldn't be speaking English while others are talking Swahili. Linguists distinguish language *competence* from language *performance,* the former referring to the knowledge of the features and structure of language, and the latter to its use in communication. They speak of a "universal language competence" as being innate in all human beings and a "particular language competence" which reflects how well a person knows a particular language such as Spanish or Thai or English. Although it is possible to teach a parrot or a mentally-retarded child to echo "Polly wants a cracker," that bird will not have any true language and the child may have very little. Without competence one cannot generate new sentences. Though the parrot may have said that one sentence a thousand times, it could never transform it into such an utterance as "Polly wants a drink" no matter how thirsty it was. Nor could the mentally-retarded child express a desire for water if his teachers had merely asked him to repeat that same utterance about crackers over and over again. He needs language, not just the facsimile of speech. Some of the most difficult clients with whom the speech clinician must work are those with echolalia. These children parrot the speech of others, often with remarkable fidelity, but they do not know what they are saying and they cannot communicate their wants. They lack the particular language competence they need. They can "speak" but they cannot speak our language, for they have not discovered the basic structure of that language.

We are not sure how a human infant acquires his competence in a particular language. Certainly he must be exposed to it. Kaspar Hauser, imprisoned when a child and isolated for sixteen years, acquired no speech at all and remained almost mute despite intensive training by the best teachers of his time. Kamala, the Wolf Girl of India, Victor, the Wild Boy of Aveyron, and Lucas, the Baboon Boy of Africa, were physically normal but not one of these abandoned children raised by animals ever acquired meaningful speech. Evidently the propensity of human beings to acquire language (universal competence) must be triggered by close contact with other humans.

Moreover, the contact must be a significant, meaningful one. A child exposed only to the constant chatter of a radio or television screen would not master our language though he might be able to repeat a few commercials. *He must be spoken to by someone important to him and encouraged to respond.* There must be both models and involvement. There must be identification both ways. When a speech pathologist finds a child with very deficient language ability, he knows that somehow he must provide for that child another involved human being with whom the child can identify. Usually that person is the clinician himself.

The human miracle—the acquisition of speech and language—becomes even more astounding when we consider the complexity of the task. Even the instrument that the infant must master if he is to speak a language is so complicated in its structure and manipulation that it seems impossible that a baby could ever learn to play it at all, let alone be required to become a virtuoso. If you were given a trumpet and told to play the overture to Wagner's *Tannehauser,* you'd be in a similar situation. Let us examine the human instrument.

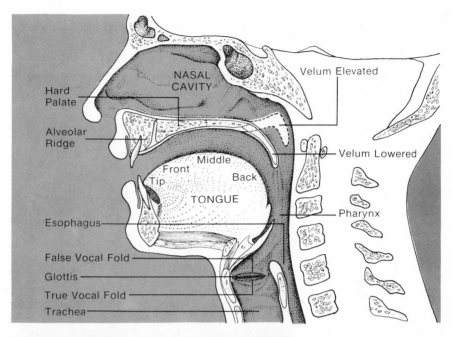

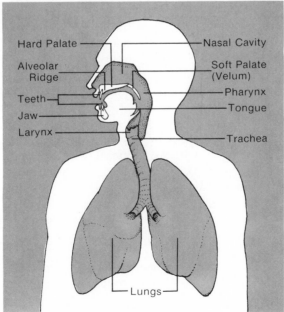

Figure 7   The speech mechanism.

The Speech Mechanism

In Figure 7 we find an illustration of this instrument—the speech-producing mechanism. As with the trumpet, the infant must use the air pressure from his lungs to produce the necessary air pressure and airflow for speech. If you were to produce a sound from a trumpet, you'd also have to learn to hold your lips together on the mouthpiece with just the correct amount of tension as you blow. Similarly, the human tone is produced in the larynx by a lip-like structure called the *true vocal folds.* (We also have some *ventricular* folds, called the false vocal cords or folds, just above the true ones, which are useful in other functions such as swallowing or defecation, but using these false folds can produce a rare voice disorder called ventricular phonation.)

Then in the airway just above the larynx is the throat cavity or *pharynx* which, when unduly and excessively tensed or squeezed, will make a harsh voice worse. Again going upward, we find the *velum* or soft palate, a valve-like mechanism. The child must learn that when his velum is lifted and squeezed his voiced or unvoiced airflow will go into the mouth cavity while on the other hand, if it is lowered and relaxed, some of the airflow will go upward into the nasal cavities and then out through the nostrils. Unlike a trumpet, the human instrument that babies must master has not one horn but two, one above the other, two chambers, the oral and the nasal cavities, each with an outlet. If a baby's velum was defective at birth (as in cleft palate) and the surgery was unsuccessful, too much of the sound and airflow will leak out of that upper opening. But even when the velum (soft palate) is not cleft, some persons never learn to operate this "back door to the nose" appropriately and so they come to the speech pathologist with hypernasal or denasal (not nasal enough) speech. All who speak our language properly must learn to lower the soft palate when making our /m/, /n/, and /ŋ/, the nasal sounds, and to raise it for all others.[1]

When we watch a skilled trumpet player's fingers we see an impressive display of coordination, but those who have witnessed x-ray motion pictures of the tongue in action, or who have watched it directly through a plastic window in the cheek of a cancer patient, have observed the ultimate in motor coordination. The precision of

---

[1] The /ŋ/, is the phonetic symbol for the last sound in the word *thing,* is a separate sound, not a combination of /n/ and /g/. (Compare "thin-g" with "thing".) A table of these phonetic symbols will be found on the back cover of this book. [ðə mæstɚɪ əv fonɛtɪks ɪznt æz hɑrd æz ju maɪt θɪŋk fɔr mɛnɪ ɪf nɑt most əv ðɛm ɑr sɪmɪlɚ tu ðə lɛtɚz əv aʊr ɔrdɪnɛrɪ ælʃəbɛt ‖ jul sun rɛkəgnaɪz ðɛm ‖

the tongue contacts, the constant shift of contours, and the rapidity of sequential movements are almost unbelievable. And it seems impossible that a little child could possibly learn to move that tongue—a tongue that he cannot even see—so skillfully!

How Our Speech To produce the /t/ or /d/ plosive sounds the tongue must
Sounds are Produced move upward and forward to make contact with the upper
gum (or alveolar) ridge; to make the /k/ or /g/ plosives its rear portion must be lifted to touch the soft palate, so that just for an instant the airflow is dammed up, and then the tongue comes down to release it. For the /s/ and /z/ sibilant fricative sounds, the upper surface of the tongue must be grooved narrowly to produce the necessary hissing or buzzing sounds; for the *sh* /ʃ/ and *zh* /ʒ/ sibilant fricatives a slightly wider groove must be employed.

The contours of our tongues vary with each vowel for there are front, middle, and back vowels, each vowel family having several members distinguished by the height of the tongue bulge and the amount and rounding of the mouth opening. Thus the /u/ vowel as in *flute* /flut/, for example, is the highest back vowel and has the narrowest lip rounding while the *ee* /i/ is the highest front vowel.[2]

Most children learn all these different postures, contours, and coordinations with very little difficulty, and they learn them very early, but deaf children may never get some of them right in a lifetime.

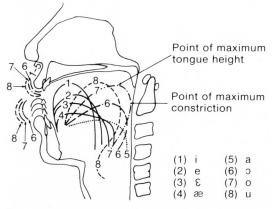

(1) i   (5) a
(2) e   (6) ɔ
(3) ɛ   (7) o
(4) æ   (8) u

Figure 8 Tongue and lip positions for the vowels. (From *Normal Aspects of Speech, Hearing, and Language,* Minifie, Hixon, and Williams. Englewood Cliffs, N.J.: Prentice-Hall, Inc., 1973, p. 187.)

[2] The central vowels such as "uh" (/ə/ or /ʌ/) are produced with the tongue lying in an almost neutral, or nearly relaxed, position on the floor of the mouth cavity. The contours of all the different vowels are shown in Figure 8.

Moving still further forward in the airway we come to the real lips. These also modify the airstream to produce the significant changes that come to be recognized as different labial (lip) sounds When held together they can dam up the airflow, which, when suddenly released, creates our /p/ and /b/ plosive sounds. When the lower lip is lifted to maintain a light contact with the upper teeth and the airflow is forced through this opening, we hear the friction noises of the /f/ or /v/ *fricative* sounds. Another pair of fricative sounds, the /θ/, as in *thin* /θɪn/, and the /ð/, as in *them* /ðɛm/, find the airstream forced through a narrow slit between the tongue tip and the teeth. Most children confuse these fricatives early in their speech development. They say *fum* for *thumb,* and some children need professional help once these errors become habituated and part of their language.

To make it even more difficult for the child, our English language has a lateral sound, the /l/, half consonant and half vowel, in which the tongue makes a sustained contact with the hard palate while the voiced air stream flows around its sides. It's often a very hard sound to master but another semi-consonant and semi-vowel, the /r/, requires a camel-like double hump on the tongue for its identification, and its production is even more difficult to learn. No wonder so many of the children seen by the speech pathologists have articulation errors on these /r/ and /l/ sounds.

To add further to the burden of learning English, we have consonant combinations. In the *ch* /tʃ/ of *choke* /tʃok/ and the *j* /dʒ/ of *joke* /dʒok/ the child must learn to link a plosive and a fricative sequentially. (Try saying *it* and *she* swiftly and you'll be uttering "itchy" before you know it.) These consonant combinations are called *affricates* and many children need help if they are to learn to combine their components. Also, besides these affricates, there are consonantal clusters or blends such as /gr/, /pl/, /str/ and other combinations to afflict the learner. No wonder tongues get tangled! No wonder a profession has appeared to untangle them!

Finally, we have a few sounds that can only be made on the wing—with the mouth in motion. These are called the *glide* sounds. For example, to produce the /w/ as in *we* /wi/ you must form your tongue and lips for the vowel *oo* /u/ and then shift or glide into the vowel *ee* /i/, the distinctive sound of /w/ being made during the transition, during the shift. Another glide sound is represented by the letter Y in our usual alphabet, but the phonetic symbol for it is /j/. Like the /w/, the Y or /j/ sound is made by moving away from the tongue position for one vowel into the contour of another, but in making this glide the initial positon is that of the vowel *ee* /i/. The child must learn that you don't utter the vowel *ee* aloud as you start the word *you* /ju/; instead you merely form it in your mouth and the glide sound begins as you shift away from it into the *oo* /u/. (Alternately, say *ee* and then *oo* swiftly and repeatedly and you will hear yourself saying the glide sound Y or /j/ in the word *you*.)

So there you have most of the forty-five or more sounds of our English language; sounds that you have mastered in just a few years and that your own infants someday will have to master too. Knowing that any prospective student of speech pathology will have to take courses in phonetics, we have presented just the bare bones of the information he will need if he is to prepare himself to work successfully with persons who cannot utter these sounds correctly. Indeed, anyone who tries to help a child with an articulatory problem should have at least this basic knowledge, but our major point is that we should not be surprised, given the complexity of own speech, to find so many persons with defective articulation. Instead, we should be amazed to find so few.

Going still higher in the speech chain, we come to the structure of the ear. Its importance to speech is obvious. Deaf babies will babble for a time but because they cannot hear that babbling or the speech of others their speech and language are bound to be impaired. In a later chapter we shall present the basic information about hearing and its disorders. Here we wish merely to remind all those who may deal with persons who have a communicative problem that auditory acuity and auditory perceptual problems may be responsible for their deviant speech, or for their inadequate language, or for their learning disabilities.

We were once asked by a teacher of the emotionally disturbed to observe the speech of one of his pupils. "Frank gives me more trouble than all the others combined," he said. "He's always negative; won't follow directions; will not cooperate with the other children in any of our projects. All he does is raise hell. His speech isn't bad for I can usually understand him and the other children do not even seem to notice his mispronunciations. Perhaps he's just oversensitive about the way he talks. Anyway, he's such a problem that we're considering having him placed in the State Hospital School though I don't really think he belongs there." We found that Frank's speech had the kinds of errors characteristic of a conductive hearing loss. Referral to an otologist resulted in the removal of heavy wax deposits in both ear canals and once the boy could hear again his behavior changed so dramatically he was able to return to a regular classroom.

Students who investigate the field of speech pathology soon find
nervous system. Crucially responsible for the reception, perception,
organization, and transmission of messages, it is easy to understand
that injuries or malfunctionings of this system may be reflected in
speech and language problems. Let us give just a few illustrations.

When the maturation of the central nervous system is delayed
the child will be slow to talk. Later in this text we will discuss a disorder due to brain damage called apraxia in which the client cannot
voluntarily lift the end of his tongue to produce a /t/ or /l/ sound
even though he might be able to move its tip perfectly in licking a
bit of peanut butter from the same contact in the mouth. We have
also had to work with persons with only half a functional tongue in
whom the paralysis was caused by peripheral nerve damage and
we've taught them to make their sounds adequately anyway. Again,
certain voice disorders occur when one of the vocal folds is similarly
paralyzed. In aphasia we deal with the result of brain injury and in
the speech of certain cerebral-palsied persons we find the coordination difficulties produced by inadequate integration of the motor impulses controlled by the cerebrum and cerebellum. These few illustrations present only a tiny sample of the problems in speech pathology
that are due to neuropathology. Those who specialize in this field
will need to explore this area intensively.

Language

Students who investigate the field of speech pathology soon find
themselves confronting the nature of language itself and being surprised by how little they know about it despite having spent many
years in reading, writing, and speaking. The Book of Genesis in the
Old Testament tells how the ancient Babylonians began to erect the
Tower of Babel with its top in the Heavens as a challenge to God.
Whereupon "He confused the language" of the workers so they could
no longer understand each other and the result was that the tower
was never finished. Those of us who have tried to teach children
whose language is "confused" or stroke patients with aphasia to read
or write or speak again, can easily appreciate the havoc so wrought.

There are literally thousands of languages being spoken at this
moment on our planet and only a handful of us can understand more
than one of them. These languages differ widely one from another.
The Hottentot's click language and the Chinese tonal language or that
polyglot monstrosity called English would seem to have very little in
common, yet they do. All languages share three characteristics: (1) a

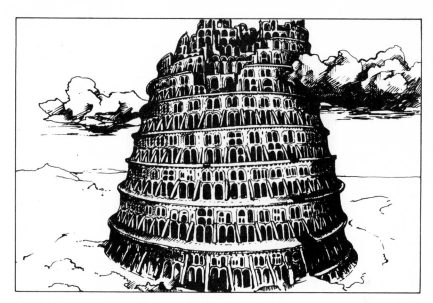

Figure 9 The unfinished Tower of Babel. (Based on the famous painting by Peter Breugel, the Elder.)

limited (finite) set of different sounds or phonemes; (2) a vocabulary or *lexicon* of meaningful combinations of these phonemes into units called *morphemes;* and (3) a set of rules for linking these units together. Every child must acquire this threefold repertoire and do so at the same time he is learning hundreds of other new coordinations, exploring the territory of his new world and testing the limits of his freedom. It is probably good that the student who feels overloaded by the unreasonable demands of his professors has forgotten the incredible amount he had to learn before he was four years old.

Phonology   In our presentation of the speech mechanism we briefly described the speech sounds of phonemes of our English language that comprise its *phonology.* As we noted, they fall into natural groupings according to how they are produced and where. Table II will summarize and review this information about the phonology of our language. Of course, you probably knew all this phonology long ago, or rather your lungs, larynx, velum, tongue, and lips did, and long before you could even read.

The linguist's term for a distinctive speech sound is the *phoneme* and the concept is important in speech pathology. You perhaps may be surprised to learn that the phoneme /s/ is not really a single sound but a family of sounds. However, if you listen carefully to the

TABLE II   *Classification of the Consonant Sounds*

	Nasals	Glides	Lateral	Fricatives	Affricates	Plosives
Bilabials	m	w hw				p b
Labiodentals				f v		
Dentals				θ ð		
Alveolar	ṇ		l	s z r	tʃ dʒ	t d
Palatal		j (l)		ʃ ʒ		
Velar	ŋ					k g
Glottal				h	ʔ	

s sounds in the words *see* and *sue* you will notice that the latter /s/ is much lower in pitch than the former. They are not at all the same sound but they are similar enough to be perceived as being identical. Moreover, there are no two words in English which have different meanings just because the two /s/'s differ in pitch. The pitch differences of these two /s/ sounds make no difference in meaning. To give another example, the /t/ in the word *take* is aspirated; it is released with audible airflow. On the other hand, in the word *stake* we do not hear that tiny rush of aspiration on the /t/ yet both /t/'s belong to the same sound family, to the phoneme /t/. Variant members of a phonemic family are called *allophones*.

And what has an allophone to do with speech pathology? Let us give just one example. A child with a lateral lisp produces a very low-pitched slushy sibilant for the standard /s/ phoneme and usually he is completely unaware of his error. Why? Because he perceives his defective sibilant as one of the *permissible* allophones or variants of the phoneme /s/. If he says *soup* using this laterally emitted allophone it still means *soup* to him and nothing else. His trouble lies in the fact that this particular variant is not permissible; it lies outside the boundaries of the phonemic family of /s/. This difference, of course, is what we must teach him. In other words, many articulation errors are not substitutions of one phoneme for another, but rather, they are the impermissible allophones we call *distortion errors*. They are hard to eliminate because to the child they make no differences in meaning. When such a child is corrected, he often says, "But I did say soup," using his slushy /s/. In the development of speech, then, the child must not only learn to produce all the standard phonemes of our language but also to recognize which allophones of those phonemes are acceptable and which are not.

But how does the child acquire the more than forty phonemes he needs to speak English? The basic process seems to be one of discrimination and experimentation. Through matching his own production with the models provided by other speakers, he comes to recognize that each of these forty phonemes consists of its own unique bundle of *distinctive features.* Any sound that does not have all of the set of distinctive features possessed by a particular standard phoneme is perceived as being a different phoneme or as an unacceptable distortion. The /s/ in *Sue* and the /z/ in *zoo* have several features in common since their manner and place of articulation are identical, but they are different phonemes because the /z/ is voiced and the /s/ is not. Voicing, then, is a distinctive feature of the /z/ in our language. The child gradually comes to recognize or has to be taught that all of the distinctive features belonging to a given phoneme must be present if he is to speak that sound correctly. Much of the work of the speech specialist consists of helping children with articulation disorders to recognize the distinctive features of the sounds that are incorrectly produced.

Semantics   It takes more than a collection of phonemes to make a language. Only when those phonemes are combined into meaningful units does one have the vocabulary he needs if he is to communicate. The linguist's term for the *smallest* meaningful unit of a language is *morpheme. Baby* is a morpheme but the word *baby's* consists of two morphemes, the first referring to the infant while the second, the *'s,* adds a second meaning, that of possessiveness. (The term morpheme, then, is not just a synonym for "word.") The phrase, "The baby's bottle", consists of only three words, but there are four morphemes in it. When a morpheme can exist by itself and still be meaningful (as baby or bottle can) it is called a *free morpheme.* The word *boys* has both, the first meaningful unit referring to a young male and the second, the /s/, referring to plurality. Therefore a child who says, "I *see* two duck" probably does not have an articulatory problem but a language problem. He does not know how to add the morphemes of plurality.

By the time the normal baby is a year old he has a production vocabulary of perhaps two to ten words and a recognition vocabulary of many more. You will probably have to work with some children who have fewer. For as long as he lives that baby will be adding to his collection of these meaningful units, but always *his* recognition vocabulary will be far greater than the one he uses in communication. Some highly educated adults can understand more than 100,000 words but they certainly don't use that many because if they did their listeners wouldn't be able to comprehend what they were saying.

Syntax   To speak a language you need more than phonemes and morphemes. You must also know how to combine these into phrases and sentences. In speech pathology we often meet children who have difficulty doing this. Perhaps they still speak in "one word sentences" at the age of four. Or perhaps they arrange the many words they do have in improper sequences. Also, some of your future clients may have failed to learn the grammatical rules they must follow in sending their messages and so they will need language training. Let us see how one child learned his language.

We persuaded a parent to write down all the utterances spoken by a young child which had the words "Daddy", "go", or "lake" in them sequentially over the period between fourteen months and four years of age. The list is not complete for there were also other transitional forms used but unrecorded, yet they illustrate how one child mastered his syntax. At fourteen months the boy was using several one-word sentences with intonations and gestures to indicate his meaning. Most of them were declaratives or commands. Among them were "Daddy", "Tommy" (his name), and "lake" (Tommy loved to splash in it and to go to it as often as he could.) Here are some sequential samples of his speech. Note how his mastery of the language evolved.

"Lake! Lake! Tommy Lake!" (One word sentence; two word sentence)

"Pity (pretty) lake" (while splashing in it). (Noun phrase)

"Tommy lake! Daddy lake!" (An imperative. He demanded to go.)

"Tommy go lake! Daddy go lake!"

"Tommy go lake and Daddy go lake!" (Note conjunction linking the two kernel sentences.)

"Tommy and Daddy go lake now!" (A better way, though shorter.)

"Tommy and Daddy go car and go to lake now!" (Note the first use of preposition.)

"Tommy go in lake now and go in, Daddy too!"

"Tommy and Daddy go in the car and go to lake." (Note the *"the"*)

"Me and Daddy go to the lake in car, now!" (Note personal pronoun and use of prepositional phrases.)

"Daddy, Tommy want to go to lake in the car now." (Two rules are still not applied.)

"Daddy no go lake now? Tommy wanna go in car and go to lake too." (Note length of utterance.)

"You going lake, Daddy? I wanna go."

"Why you no take me the lake, Daddy? I want to go to the lake."

"Mommy, why won't Daddy take me to the lake? I want to go fimmin (swimming)."

Some of the children with whom you'll work may fail to develop the different ways of expressing meanings that Tommy discovered. A few may never get past the early noun-phrase or verb-phrase level. Some may never learn the rules that govern personal pronoun usage or negatives or questioning. Some develop odd, inappropriate rules of their own. The student of speech pathology needs to know something about syntax. So does any teacher who must help a child with language problems.

The person with dysphasia often has difficulties with syntax, as well as with word finding. Trying to say "I now have to go to the bathroom" he might struggle and gesture and begin and hesitate before uttering "I . . . uh . . . bath . . . no . . . uh . . . go . . . now. "The rules for ordering the words of his message have escaped him and are lost momentarily, and without having these rules available he is helpless.

Any attempt to describe the syntax of our language in any detail would be inappropriate since this is an introductory text in speech pathology. Nevertheless, we can outline some of the rules for joining words together which must be mastered. First of all, we must be able

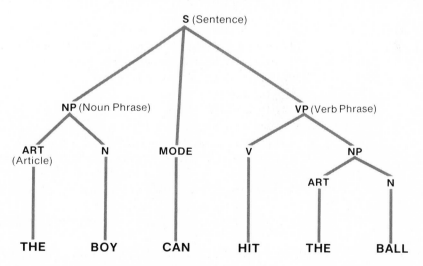

Figure 10   Tree diagram of a sentence.

to understand and produce noun phrases and word phrases, and then to link them together. "The boy" is a noun phrase consisting of the *determiner* "the" and the noun "boy." "Can hit" is a verb phrase, with "hit" as the verb and "can" as its auxiliary. The sentence "The boy can hit the ball" adds another noun phrase. The diagram of this typical sentence (Figure 10) may be thought of as the skeleton model for thousands of the sentences each of us will generate every year. Hidden in the linking of these words are eight rules, one of them being that a determiner must precede the noun (*the* must precede *boy*) and another that an auxiliary must precede the verb. "Boy the hit can ball the" breaks these rules and produces something that isn't English. A baby then must master something besides these words; he must find out not only how they must be combined but also how they shouldn't be linked together.

Of course, the illustration we have provided falls far short of portraying the whole picture of language structure. We do not speak only in such simple declarative sentences. Though thousands of sentences can be formulated in which different words can be placed in the slots of our diagram to say many different things, we need more complicated patterns to express other meanings. Expansion, coordination, subordination require much more elaborate diagrams.

For example, the child, in learning a language, must also master some transformational rules. "The ball is being hit by the boy" is an example of the application of a passive transformation. "Can the boy hit the ball?" is a rearrangement of the words and phrases so that they pose a question. (As any parent of a two-year-old child knows well, these interrogative transformations are mastered early.) These two examples of transformations show that there must be different rules governing the order of the words of a declarative or interrogatory utterance, as well as an active or passive one. The language learner will have to know these rules even if he cannot verbalize them. Again, all we provide here is the briefest of glimpses of the nature of the transformations in syntax. Not only the position of the words is changed; new words may have to be inserted or embedded in the new sentence structure. Modifying phrases or qualifying clauses which have their own rules may be necessary to express the altered meaning. Those who work with children who show language delay must be able to analyze their speech linguistically.

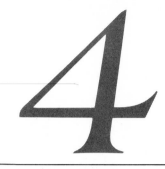

DEVELOPMENT
OF
SPEECH
AND
LANGUAGE

Projects [3]

1. Draw outlines of the head similar to that in Figure 8 and indicate the contact position of the tongue and palate for the following sounds: /t/, /d/, and /k/; /g/; and /l/ /ŋ/. (See C. Van Riper and D. Smith, *"Introduction to General American Phonetics,"* New York: Harper & Row, 1977 (3rd ed.), or almost any other phonetics text.)
2. Draw, and then label, the basic structures of the hearing mechanism. (See W. R. Zemlin, *Speech and Hearing Science,* Englewood Cliffs, N.J.: Prentice-Hall, Inc., 1968, p. 366, or almost any other text on speech science or audiology.)
3. Get some modeling clay and pipe-cleaners and create a model of the larynx showing the thyroid, cricoid, and arytenoid cartilages, the epiglottis, and the true and false vocal folds. (For information, see D.R. Boone, *The Voice and Voice Therapy,* Englewood Cliffs, N.J.: Prentice-Hall, Inc., 1971, pp. 25–32.)
4. Draw and label the main structures of the brain to show their involvement in speech production or reception.
5. Draw the upper surface of the mouth of a person with a cleft of the soft and hard palate. (See L. E. Travis (ed.) *Handbook of Speech Pathology and Audiology,* Englewood Cliffs, N.J.: Prentice-Hall, Inc., 1971, p. 769ff, or any other book on the cleft palate.
6. Make another set of key words for the phonetic alphabet.
7. Read pages 1163–68 in L. E. Travis (ed.) *Handbook of Speech Pathology and Audiology* and draw a tree diagram for the sentence "The astronauts photographed the moon."
8. Read P. Denes and E. Pinsen, *The Speech Chain,* Baltimore: Waverly Press, 1969.
9. Write the author a note in the phonetic alphabet telling him what you think of this book. The address is Speech Clinic, Western Michigan University, Kalamazoo, Mich. 49001.

[3] *Author's note:* We have deliberately chosen to use projects rather than a bibliography at the end of this chapter because most students gain a better knowledge of the speech mechanism, the phonetic alphabet, and simple language structure by doing them rather than by reading about these topics.

Since many of the disorders of speech have their onset early in life and reflect delays in maturation or acquisition of basic skills or competencies, we should understand something about how speech and language develop normally in the child. We begin our account from the moment of birth, trace the course of development through the stage of reflexive cooing and crying sounds, then through the period of babbling, and finally, into the acquisition of full-fledged language. To check the validity of this information you should have a baby of your own immediately.

There seems to be evidence that even before that baby emerges, it will show some responsiveness to sound, its heartbeat showing changes when the mother begins to speak. Researchers have shown that by placing a buzzing doorbell against the mother's stomach, they could cause an increase in the movements of the fetus. Even more incredible, Ostwald 1960 provided some shaky evidence that a few infants have actually vocalized while still in the uterus. All three of this author's babies, fortunately, were mercifully silent during the pre-natal months, but they more than made up for it thereafter. So will yours!

Many linguists, doubtless because their field is focused on language rather than on speech, have shown only minor interest in the output of the baby's mouth prior to the emergence of the first meaningful words. Their point of view is expressed by Carroll: "Despite the fact that the phonetic diversity noted during the period of babbling increases considerably, these phenomena have little relevance for the development of true language. It is as if the child starts learning language afresh when he begins to utter meaningful speech."[1] The

[1] J. B. Carroll, "Language Development." in A. Bar-Adon, and W. Leopold (eds.) *Child Language: A Book of Readings* (Englewood Cliffs, N. J.: Prentice-Hall, 1971), p. 201.

linguists point out that the sounds of crying, comfort, and babbling are not phonemic which, of course, is true. These early utterances are sounds (*phones*), not phonemes, and often they lack any precise identity because their boundaries are difficult to determine and their variability is great. Moreover, though the baby may repeatedly utter a few clearly defined sounds in the syllables of his babbling, some of them drop out of his utterances and seem to have to be relearned once he begins to string words together in his true language.

Nevertheless, during the period of pre-language, the child does build the foundation for the true speech which is still to come. In the very early reflexive sounds of crying and comfort-cooing, we certainly find him practicing the basic synergies of respiration and phonation. In his babbling we see him exploring articulation. As Fry says, "The learning that takes place on the motor side at this stage [babbling] is absolutely basic to the acquisition of speech."[2]

Reflexive Utterance.   The two main types of nonpurposeful reflexive utterances
Crying Sounds   your very young baby will produce are the crying and comfort sounds. Even the father of your baby will recognize the difference between them, though he may not be able to distinguish between the wail due to hunger or the howl caused by an open safety-pin. For the first month you both should expect more crying than whimpering, and more whimpering than comfort sounds. Hopefully, the ratio will change as the diapers go by. If you listen carefully to the crying, you'll probably be able to detect vowel-like sounds resembling the /æ/, /ɛ/, and /aɪ/ of our language but they will be nasalized. And if your imagination is good enough, you may hear a few sounds that crudely resemble the consonants /g/, /k/, or /n/, but since these sounds are reflexive they should not be viewed as the true ancestors of the phonemes your baby will eventually master. If the crying sounds like any contribution at all to the mastery of speech (which you may doubt at midnight) that contribution lies in the practicing of essential motor coordinations and the establishment of the necessary feedback loops between the larynx and the mouth and ear.

Comfort Sounds   These reflexive utterances are difficult to describe in words. Gurgles and sighs, grunts and little wisps of sound, you will probably lump them together under the category of "cooing." They

---

[2] D. B. Fry, "The Development of the Phonological System in the Normal and the Deaf Child," in F. Smith and A. Miller (eds.) *The Genesis of Language* (Cambridge, Mass: M.I.T. Press, 1966), p. 189.

mainly appear during or just after feeding, or diaper filling, or some other form of relief from distress. Again, if you listen carefully, the front vowels and back consonants will seem to predominate but they are not nasalized as in crying. Misery seems to want to come out of the nose, comfort from the mouth.

Over and over again in taking the case histories of children with very severe articulation disorders or speech delay we have found parents telling us that these children cried much more than their other babies. If we were to hazard a guess as to the significance of these reports it would be that the feedback loops between the ear and the vocalizing mechanism became loaded with the static of pain or unpleasantness. In contrast, when the ear of the baby hears the sound of his own voice in the context of pleasurable sensations, that baby may be more likely to experiment with his utterances, and so achieve better speech sooner. Anyway, of one thing we're sure. You'll enjoy those comfort sounds more than his crying. Crying may build parental character but the comfort sounds engender love. You'll need both.

Babbling Emerging from the stage of reflexive vocalizations is the appearance of babbling, a universal phenomenon found in all human infants. It is characterized by the chaining and linking of sounds together on one exhalation. We hear syllables of all types, the CV (consonant vowel as in "ba") which is most common, with the VC (vowel followed by a consonant, as in "ab") and the VCV ("aba") being found less frequently. These strings of syllables have no more semantic meaning than did the comfort sounds, though their component sounds are perhaps more similar to our standard phonemes. The baby just seems to be playing with his tongue, lips, and larynx in much the same fashion that he plays with his fingers or toes. A good share of this vocal play is carried on when the child is alone, and it disappears when someone attracts his attention. One of our children played with her babbling each morning after awakening, usually beginning with a whispered "eenuh" and repeating it with increasing effort until she spoke the syllable aloud, whereupon she would laugh and chortle as she said it over and over. The moment she heard a noise in the parent's bedroom this babbling would cease and crying would begin.

Parents who joyfully rush in and ruin this speech rehearsal are failing to appreciate its significance in the learning of speech. The child must simultaneously feel and hear the sound repeatedly if it is ever to emerge as an identity. Imitation is essentially a device to perpetuate a stimulus, and babbling is self-imitation of the purest vari-

ety. When the babbling period is interrupted or delayed through illness, the appearance of true speech is often similarly retarded. Deaf
babies begin to babble at a normal time but since they cannot hear
the sounds they produce, they probably lose interest and hence have
much less true vocal play than the hearing child. Mirrors suspended
above the cribs of deaf babies have increased the babbling through
visual self-stimulation.

And what are the contributions of babbling to the acquisition of
true speech? As we have mentioned earlier, many linguists would
say they are few. Certainly the vowel-like and consonant-like sounds
are not phonemic, but in babbling we often hear the repetition of intonation and stress patterns so similar to the patterning of adult sentences that many parents swear their baby is talking to himself or
trying to tell them something. Some of the strings of syllables have
the intonational patterns of command; others, of declaration or questioning; most are just randomly varied in pitch and stress. During
this babbling period we find sounds from many languages other than
English (even the tongue clicks of Hottentots) occurring in the free
speech flow. Interestingly, Weir[3] reports that the babbling of Chinese
children shows some of the pitch characteristics of the tonal Mandarin
language. The baby doesn't know, of course, what he is going to become or that soon he will have to learn how to make a variety of
sounds, combine them into syllables, and produce phrases and sentences with different intonation patterns. But in his babbling he almost acts as though he did know.

Socialized Babbling   About the fifth or sixth month, when the infant can sit up,
fixate an object with its eyes, grab an object to put into its
mouth, or hoist its hind end up to crawl, some of the babbling appears to have an instrumental function. He *seems* to use it to get attention, to support rejection, to express a demand. He babbles more
in a social context. Sometimes he even seems to listen and certainly
he is aware of the speech of others.

A bit later the child begins to use his vocalization for getting attention, supporting rejection, and expressing demands. Frequently he
will look at an object and cry at the same time. He voices his eager-
ness and protest. He is using his primitive speech both to express
himself and to modify the behavior of others. This stage is also

[3] Ruth Weir, "Some Questions on the Child's Learning of Morphology," in F.
Smith and G. Miller (eds.) *The Genesis of Language* (Cambridge, Mass: M.I.T. Press,
1966), p. 156.

marked by the appearance of syllable repetition, or the doubling of sounds, in his vocal play. He singles out a certain double syllable such as *da-da* and frequently practices it to the exclusion of all other combinations. Sometimes a single combination will be practiced for several weeks at a time, though it is more usual to find the child changing to something new every few days and reviewing some of his former vocal achievements at odd intervals. True disyllables *(ba-da)* come relatively late in the first year, and the infant rejects them when the parent attempts to use them as stimulation.

At this time the child will often "answer back." Make a noise and he makes a noise. The two noises are usually dissimilar, but it is obvious that he is responding. In his vocal play, most of the vowels are still the ones made in the front or middle of the mouth, but a few *oo* and *oh* sounds (which are back vowels) can be detected. There are also more consonants to be heard, the /**d**/, /**t**/, /**n**/, and /**l**/ having appeared; but it's still hard to separate them out of the flow of unsorted utterance unless you have long, sharp ears. Some private babbling continues throughout these months, but now the child seems to take more pleasure in public practice. He's listening to himself but also listening to you. He is talking to himself but also sometimes to you. This is *socialized vocalization.*

We must not conclude this section without pointing out some implications which babbling and vocal play have for speech therapy. Svend Smith, a Danish speech therapist, has devised a set of rhythms based on the bongo drum chants of South African natives, and he has his patients utter strange and unfamiliar cries in unison with the rhythmic beat. We too have used his methods, and often find that children and even adults can follow our own chanting as it progresses from these strange cries into standard sounds of English. We find that they can make sounds which previously they were unable to produce. Often we use the baby's comfort sounds or the repeated syllables of vocal play in these chants. The rhythm helps to create the freedom to try new sounds. Some children become so tense when attempting a sound which they have never successfully produced, that they cannot possibly find the new coordinations. Babbling and vocal play can free them from this tension. To vary our production of sound, we must feel some of the same freedom that the baby experiences when babbling or doing vocal play. In this regard, it is interesting to note that in England and elsewhere on the continent, a speech therapy session often begins with a period of relaxation. We know of no better way to relax than by free babbling, especially when the pathologist is babbling freely too. Perhaps we are returning to an earlier period when learning to speak was fun.

Inflected Vocal Play   Although some squeals and changes in pitch and loudness have previously occurred in the babbling, it is not until about the eighth month that inflection or intonational changes become prominent. It is then that the vocal play takes on the tonal characteristics of adult speech. We now find the baby using inflections that sound like questions, commands, surprise, ponderous statements of fact, all in a delightful gibberish that has no meaning. We hear not only the inflections and sounds of English but those of the Oriental languages as well. No baby can be sure he will end up speaking English.[4] So he practices a bit of Chinese now and then. We have tried hard to imitate some of these sounds and inflections and have failed. The baby can often duplicate whole strings of these strange beads of sounds.

The private babbling and social vocal play continue strongly during this period from eight months to a year. The repertoire of sounds increases. There is a marked gain in back vowels and front consonants. Crying time diminishes, though few fathers would believe it. They begin to get interested in their sons and daughters about this stage, however. The infant is becoming human. He'll bang a cup; he'll smile back at the old man. He'll reach out to be picked up. He begins to understand what "No!" means. But most important of all, he begins to *sound* as though he is talking.

We have previously spoken of various stages of development, but it should be made very clear that, although most children go through these stages in the order given, the activity in any one stage does not cease as soon as the characteristics of the next stage appear. Grunts and wails, babbling, socialized vocalization, and inflection practice all begin at about the times stated, but they continue throughout the entire period of speech development.

It is during this period that the baby begins to use more of the back vowels (u, ʊ, o, ɔ) in his babbling. According to Irwin and Curry, 92 percent of all vowels uttered by babies are the front vowels as compared to the 49 percent figure for adult speech.[5] They say, "It is evident that a fundamental process of development in early speech

---

[4] We use the word "inflection" in its traditional sense to denote pitch changes. In linguistics "inflection" refers to certain kinds of word endings such as the *s* of plurals or the *ing* ending of verbs.

[5] O. C. Irwin and T. Curry, "Vowel Elements in the Crying of Infants Under Ten Days of Age," *Child Development,* XII (1941), 99–109.

consists of the mastery of the back vowels." It is interesting that when we work with adult articulation cases, we prefer syllables such as *see* and *ray* and *lee* to those involving the back vowels like *soo* and *low*. Front vowels seem to be more easily mastered.

The baby, through his vocal gymnastics, gradually masters the coordinations necessary to meaningful speech. But it must be emphasized that when he is repeating *da-da* and *ma-ma* at this stage, he is not designating his parents. His arm movements have much more meaning than those of his mouth. It is during these months that the ratio of babbling to crying greatly increases. Comprehension of parental gestures shows marked growth. The child now responds to the parent's stimulation, not automatically, but with more discrimination. His imitation is more hesitant, but it also seems more purposive. It begins to resemble the parent's utterance. If the father interrupts the child's chain of *papapapapapapapapa* by saying *papa*, the child is less likely than before to say *wah* or *gu* and more likely to whisper *puh* or repeat the two syllables *puhpuh*. During this period, simple musical tones, songs, or lullabies are especially good stimulation. The parent should observe the child's inflections and rhythms and attempt to duplicate them. This is the material that should be used for stimulation at this period, not a long harangue on why mother loves her little token of heaven.

This period, too, has a message for those who wish to help the child with abnormal speech. We see that new sounds are not acquired solely in meaningful words; they appear singly, or doubly in syllables, and nonsense syllables as well. We note that they occur in the context of pleasurable contacts with others who share them. They are to be played with, not demanded. We have known many children who could make a perfectly good *r* sound in isolated words like *church*, yet who failed to say this sound when it occurred on a falling inflection as in the word *father*. Speech therapy should not be done in monotonous drill. The baby tells us that the way to acquire new sounds is to use them expressively and socially.

At any rate, in this socialized babbling or vocal play of the baby we find the basic pattern of communication, of sending and receiving, although it is only sounds, not meaningful messages, that are being batted back and forth.

By the eighth month inflections are very prominent and the prosodic features or melody of his gibberish make the give and take of a "conversation" with the baby a delightful experience. Social reinforcers such as a parental smile or gesture or touch or spoken word increase the frequency of his vocal behaviors. You will imitate him more than he will you, but you'll note that his repertoire of sounds is growing rapidly with a marked gain in back vowels and front consonants. It is about time for him to say his first meaningful words.

The First Words

When you have that first baby someone is sure to present you with a "Baby Book" in which you are to record a host of its accomplishments. One of them will surely be a section of "First Words." We have examined many such books without much profit from their perusal. (One mother claimed that her child's first word was "Kalamazoo" spoken at the age of seven months while babbling. It was probably just a sneeze.) The linguistic literature and our own observations of our own children and grandchildren have been more illuminating than these baby books.

Reviewing a large number of studies, Darley and Winitz (1961) cast some doubt on the usual parental reports concerning the time when the first words were spoken, though the age usually claimed was about one year. They found, as we have, that the criteria for those first words showed wide differences from parent to parent. Also, they pointed out "the inadequacy of parental records, the fallibility of parents' memory, parents' 'wishful hearing', 'optimism', 'pride', among other weaknesses." The dates of average onset of these first words vary from about nine to eighteen months for normal children. A few of them begin to speak much later and when they do, they may speak in multiple-word sentences, thereby showing once again that comprehension precedes performance.

Words are acquired (comprehended) before they are used, and long before the first one pops out the child has shown by his behavior that he understand the gestures, intonations, and meanings of some of the parent's speech. Since parents at this time tend to speak to their children in single words or short phrases and sentences when really trying to communicate with them (rather than adoring them, which produces a host of multi-word nonsense) it is not surprising that the first meaningful utterances of babies are single words.

These words are often not usually monosyllabic but duplicative. The child prefers "Dada" to "Dad" and "Mama" to "Mom" or "Ma", thus showing, perhaps, the influence of his previous babbling. The labial and dental sounds are most prominent in the first words of babies of all races but others may also occur. The author's son's first word was "aga" meaning "all gone" in the contexts of no more milk in his cup or the turning off of a light. As Carroll (1971) writes: "The

utterances learned in the period between 12–18 months are particularly likely to be learned as whole units even when, from the adult
point of view, they are composed of several words and their pronunciation is extremely imprecise. This is also the period of the 'one-
word sentence' when a single word or word-like utterance can stand
for a multiplicity of meanings.''[6]

The first words then are sentence words and you will soon hear
the same utterance spoken at one time with the intonation and stress
of a declarative statement, or at another as a command, or even as a
question. Often an appropriate gesture will accompany the utterance.
Even though only one morpheme is used, the tone of the voice and
the gesture show the other parts of the implicit sentence. When one
of our daughters heard the sound of the car in the garage, she said,
''Dadda?'' with an upward inflection and looked toward the door
through which he usually entered. Then when he came in, she held
up her arms to be picked up and imperiously demanded, ''Dadda!,
Dadda!'' with the appropriate inflection and stress of command.
These were sentences even though only single words were spoken.

How are the first words acquired? This question looks in-
nocently simple but it has troubled many students of language and
still has no universally accepted answer. Since you may have to teach
a non-verbal child to talk someday, your own or somebody else's,
you should be interested in the various explanations.

Learning Theory: Advocates of operant conditioning believe that whenever a
Operant   parent smiles, cuddles, or responds favorably to a child's vo-
Conditioning   calization, that vocalization or something like it will tend to
increase in frequency. If that vocalization has some similarity
to the intonation or phonemic patterns of adult language it will get
more reinforcement immediately, and then with each closer approximation the parent will tend to show more approval. Children echo or
imitate the word of the mother, saying something like *milk* when she
says it, and lo, there is the bottle and the mother's smile. When the
word is emitted and then rewarded, the probability that it will be uttered again in future but similar situations is thereby increased. The
development of syntax is explained by some theorists in terms of the
chaining of operants, each word of a phrase or sentence carrying a
cue which evokes the next one or next group of words. This sim-

[6] John B. Carroll, ''Language Development'' in A. Bar-Adon and W. F. Leopold,
eds. *Child Language: A Book of Readings.* Englewood Cliffs, N.J.: Prentice-Hall, Inc.,
1971. p. 447

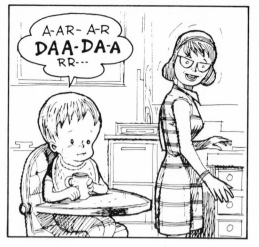
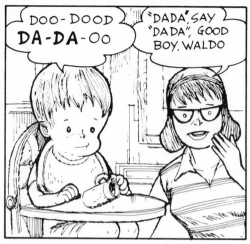
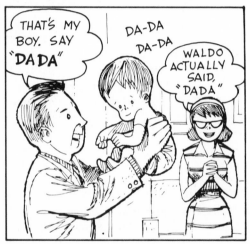
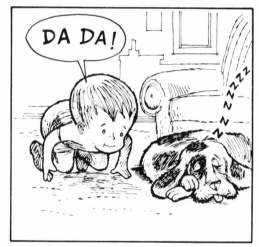
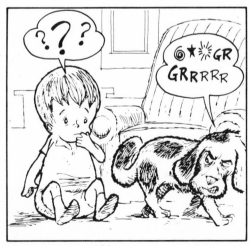

Figure 11 The first word. (From *Child Psychology*, Wallace A. Kennedy, Englewood Cliffs, N.J.: Prentice-Hall, Inc., 1971, p. 293.)

plistic account does not do justice to the operant learning explanation, but it describes its major features.[7]

The Autism Theory   Experiments in teaching birds to talk led O. H. Mowrer, a famous American psychologist, to formulate what is known as the autism theory of speech acquisition.[8] He found that his birds would reproduce human words only if these words were spoken by the trainer while the birds were being fondled or fed. After this had happened often enough, the word itself could apparently produce pleasurable feelings in the bird. Since myna birds and parakeets produce a lot of variable sounds, it is almost inevitable that a few of these sounds might resemble the human word that produced such pleasant feelings. Thus when the bird hears itself making these similar sounds it feels again the pleasantness of fondling and being fed. So it repeats them, and the closer the bird's chirp-word comes to resemble the human word, the more pleasant the bird feels. By properly rewarding these progressive approximations, we can facilitate the process. However, finally the bird will find that "Polly-wants-a-cracker" or "To-hell-with-Iowa"[9] is pleasant enough to be self-rewarding. The word "autism" refers to the self-rewarding aspect of the process. At any rate, these phrases seem to sound almost as good to the bird as a piece of suet tastes.

When this theory is applied to the child's learning of his first words, it seems to make a lot of sense. Certainly, the mother says "Mama" or "baby" a thousand times while feeding, bathing, or fondling the child. Also it is certain that the baby will find *mama mama* or *bubbababeeba* sometime in his babbling and vocal play. If these utterances flood him with pleasant feelings, he will repeat them more often than syllables such as "gugg" which have no special pleasant memories attached to them. It is also true that the closer the child comes to the standard words, the more reward he will get from the mother. There still remains the problem of giving meaning to utterance, and this is explained in terms of the context. "Mama" is used when the mama is present; "baby" is used when he sees him-

---

[7] For a more thorough presentation of the learning theory explanations of language learning, see Orlando Taylor and David Swinney, "The Onset of Language" in J. V. Irwin and M. Marge (eds.) *Principles of Childhood Language Disabilities* (Englewood Cliffs, N. J.: Prentice-Hall, 1972), pp. 53–62.

[8] O. H. Mowrer, "On the Psychology of 'Talking Birds'—A Contribution to Language and Personality Theory," in *Learning Theory and Personality Dynamics* (New York: The Ronald Press Company, 1950).

[9] One of the author's graduate students taught a parakeet to say this most reprehensible phrase, knowing well that the author had received his doctorate at that excellent institution. The author is presently engaged in teaching the bird to stutter when it says it, having found it impossible to extinguish the phrase, or, for that matter, the bird.

self in the mirror or plays with his body. This theory raises some objections, but it seems to be the best explanation we have yet been able to formulate.

Nativistic Theory   Another explanation states that the child has an inborn capacity for language learning which is mobilized when he discovers that the parent's noises have meaning and a structure which somehow fit those innate patterns. Just as Helen Keller, deaf and blind, suddenly discovered that water had a name when the word was traced upon her hand by her teacher, so little children discover that things and experiences and people have words (names) for them, that there are different classes of words, and that words can be arranged sequentially according to certain basic rules to represent other meanings. Even as the child organizes his visual perceptions to recognize the bottle from which he drinks his milk, so he is programmed to organize his auditory perceptions of language. Born in all human beings is a basic competence or propensity for language learning and the parent's speech merely triggers that latent capacity. Adherents of this theory insist that the other theories cannot account for the child's surprisingly rapid acquisition of the complexities of language nor for his ability to generate novel phrases and sentences (and even new words such as "bringed" for "brought") that he has never heard before.

Behavioral psychologists (Premack and Premack, 1972), however, have been able to teach chimpanzees to communicate with them and with each other using a non-vocal language involving gestures with symbols on them, blocks, and push buttons. Through a sign language, these chimps can learn to communicate. Perhaps as primates they too share the universal language competence the linguists have claimed for humans alone. Though the chimps must be taught this sign language and not merely be exposed to it or encouraged to use it, as human infants are, this does not mean that the achievement is any less impressive or troublesome to linguists of the Chomsky (1968) school. In summary, all we can say is that we still are not sure how the baby manages to say his first real words. But he does! He does!

Learning to Talk   At about eighteen months of age many children begin to join
in Sentences   words together, and this is probably the most important discovery the child will ever make—even were he to become the first man to walk on Mars. Indeed, it is probably the most important one the human species has achieved, for it enabled this two-legged

race of mammals to exploit the immense potentials of symbolization. Were we restricted to one-word utterances, we would be woefully handicapped.

How, then, does the child learn to join words together and to do so correctly? Some workers, such as Braine (1963), have suggested that they come to recognize that there are two different kinds of words, *open class* words and *pivot* words. Open-class words are similar to those the child has already been using in his one-word utterances. They are content words; they refer to things or activities; they are labels and can stand alone. *Milk, cup, car, Jimmy, shoe, drink, go* are all samples of open-class words. Pivot words are handles. By themselves they cannot constitute a sentence. They can modify (*"more* milk") or locate (*"that* cup") and do other things, but they need another word (an open-class word) before they make sense. Linguists such as Braine believe that when a child learns to join the two kinds of words together the first primitive sentences are formed.

Other linguists, however, (Slobin, 1971 and Brown, 1973) reject the pivot grammar approach, mainly because it ignores the semantic or meaningful aspect of language. Instead, they claim that the child begins to join words together when he recognizes the need for modifiers, for ways of expressing subject-predicate, action-object, possessor-possessed, and other relationships. They feel that the pivot grammar explanation of how a child learns to combine words is too simplistic, preferring an explanation which shows how the four basic kinds of one-word utterances (declarative, imperative, negative, and interrogative) are expanded in the interest of meaningfulness. Table III (taken from Wood, 1976) provides an illustration of this point of view. Neither explanation is completely satisfactory and so we shall describe how one real child, our grandson, Jimmy, learned to speak in sentences.

For the first six months of his second year we heard only one-word utterances, but they were accompanied by intonations and gestures which supplemented their meaningfulness. Thus "bye-bye"

*TABLE III   Development of Sentence Structure**

Sentence Type	Sequential Stages in Sentence Formulations		
Declarative	"Big boat."	"That big boat."	"That's a big boat."
Negative	"No play."	"I no play."	"I won't play."
Interrogative	"See toy?"	"Momm, see toy?"	"Did you see the toy?"
Imperative	"No touch!"	"You no touch!"	"Don't touch it."

*Barbara Wood, *Children and Communication* Englewood Cliffs, N.J.: Prentice-Hall, 1976. p. 137.

might be uttered as a question or as a command or merely as a comment on the fact that he was already in the car. He also had two negatives, "uh-uh" and occasionally "No!". "Ah-gah" (for "all gone") seemed to be a single sentence-like word and was used interrogatively, imperatively, and declaratively depending on the situation. Jimmy had achieved a vocabulary of about 32 words at eighteen months. Most of these, such as *milk, cup, car, plane, shoe,* were what Braine would call open-class words, but the boy also had some modifiers which could be termed members of the pivot class, words like *here, more, big,* and *that.* At any rate, by one year and ten months he had learned to combine these into two-word utterances which again were used with the appropriate intonations of command, questioning, commenting, and so forth. Many of these were novel combinations which certainly he had never heard before such as "bye-bye bed." He would say "more milk" which certainly had been modeled for him, but he also said "more shoe" when he wanted the other one put on, and this too could not have been learned by any sort of imitation.

Within a month Jimmy showed clearly that he had discovered how noun phrases and verb phrases could be constructed: "my cup," "that shoe," "that car," "big milk." In naming pictures he would use the article "a" or the demonstrative "that" before each of them. No longer would he merely say "cow" or "house." It was always "a cow" or "that house." If we forgot to put in the prefatory word, he would become enraged and say, "No, no! 'a' cow," and correct us. He wasn't going to have his newly learned rule violated. If we said "big cow," that was all right, but no more single words for him! Something similar also occurred with verbs, though this came later. Verb phrases consist of the combination of an antecedent verb with a noun or noun phrase. Jimmy's first one was "bang cup," but within a week he was saying not only "pay pono" (play piano) and "wah miuk" (want milk) but also "weed a booh" (read a book) and, showing us that he could do so, "frow duh bih bah" (throw the big ball), thus combining the verb with a noun phrase.

For almost two months, Jimmy stayed at this level of speaking in noun phrases and verb phrases, making many gains in vocabulary and practicing many different applications of the rules he had discovered. The noun phrases were then expanded: "Daddy big shoe." Verbs were followed by noun phrases as well as single nouns. He would say such things as "Jimmy want big ball' and even "Doggie eat Jimmy toast," thus indicating some sense of the possessive. Some of these verb phrases soon showed expansion by linking adverbs or prepositional phrases with the verb: "Fall down," "Go now in big car." It was fascinating to see him experimenting with these noun and verb phrase combinations. That he was not merely repeating phrases that he had heard his parents use, but actually and deliberately linking the words together is shown by some of these utterances: "Here bye-bye" (I've got to go now), "Go Mummy bed," and "No that button." These were not imitations of parental speech. They were the result of his attempts to construct a grammar, to relate words appropriately and meaningfully.

Then one day we heard more true sentences. "Jimmy want coat." "Jimmy go car." "Big ball fall down." He had found a new way of combining. Noun phrases could be joined to verb phrases. Subjects could have predicates. He didn't know these terms, but he had the idea. Whee! When he said one of these new combinations, he would run around in circles, shriek with pleasure, and collapse on the floor in ecstasy.[10]

For some time Jimmy seemed to be practicing these simple sentence combinations. Then we heard him restructuring them and adding the appropriate intonations of pitch and stress. "Jimmy want cookie!" (command); "Where Daddy go?" (interrogative); "Jimmy no go bed" (negation); "Jimmy big boy" (declarative). Soon he was no longer having to add two simple sentences together as in "Jimmy go car and Mummy go car" but was saying, "Jimmy and Mummy go in car now." Shortly thereafter, he was using more of what is called *embedding,* attaching a clause or phrase to the basic subject-predicate pattern. Instead of saying "Daddy go car?" he said, "I think Daddy go car?"

Next the boy showed a growing mastery in the use of prepositional phrases: ("Jimmy go to store" instead of "Jimmy go store"), then possessives, plurals, past tenses, passive voice, and other constructions appeared until by age four he was speaking very much like an adult. When you have that baby of yours, watch for these aspects of language growth. You will be amazed to watch the unfolding of the potential he seems to possess for becoming human. Besides, your enjoyment of his language development may help you bear all the other responsibilities with which his birth has bedeviled you.

Phonological Development

Thus far we have been tracing the way the child acquires the use of syntax, his grammar. Now let us see how he learns his phonology, how he comes to master the sounds (phonemes) of his language.

[10] So did his grandfather.

Phonemic Occasionally we meet a proud mother who insists that her
Acquisition child pronounced sounds like an adult from the very first, but
and Mastery we have never observed such a paragon personally. Certain
sounds appear before others in the child's early words, the
/m/, /b/, /w/, /d/, /n/, and /t/ consonants being those most often
used. Most of the vowels of these early words are produced fairly accurately from the first, though the /ɔ/ as in *ought,* the /ɛ/ as in *met,*
and the /ʊ/ as in *cook* seem to cause some difficulty.

The mere presence of a standard phoneme in a word or two obviously is not the same as its mastery. Ordinarily, we feel that a child
has really mastered a phoneme when he consistently uses it correctly
in the initial, medial, or final positions of all the words which require
it. We have little research on the age of the first appearance (acquisition) of phonemes. Instead, we have tables of mastery, such as those
shown in Figure 12.

An inspection of this figure reveals that the sounds first mastered are mainly the labials, nasals, stop consonants, and glides with
the fricatives, affricates, and the /r/ appearing after the fourth year.
We should also add that the consonant blends (such as /fl/, /str/,
/gr/) often are in error even later. Various explanations have been offered for this sequence of development. One is that the earliest
sounds to be acquired are those that involve the easiest coordinations. The /p/, /b/, and /m/, for example, are less complex motorically
than the fricatives, affricates, or the /r/ sounds, and they are also
more visible. Another explanation is based on the distinctive feature
concept, the belief being that the child masters the discriminations in
the following order: voicing, nasality, stridency, continuancy, and
place of articulation.

Mastering the standard phonemes of our language is not an
easy task for the child. "Goggy" does not sound much different from
"doggy" in the ears of a two- or three-year-old. One plosive seems
similar to another; one fricative resembles several others, especially
when the sounds are hidden in the flow of continuous parental
speech. How then does the child ever master the discriminations he
needs? In part, he learns what he needs to know through parental
correction. ("Don't say 'thoup.' Say 'soup'; "That's 'soup,' not
'thoup'." This is a crude way of presenting contrasting pairs, the
non-word and the real word.) And, of course, he never hears his parents using "rings" except in the context of fingers, whereas "wings"
are what birds fly with. Unfortunately, not all the words in English
have such contrasting pairs. If they did we suspect that we would
have far fewer children with articulation errors. If the name for spin-
ach were "tandy," no child would use that expression for "candy"
more than once or twice.

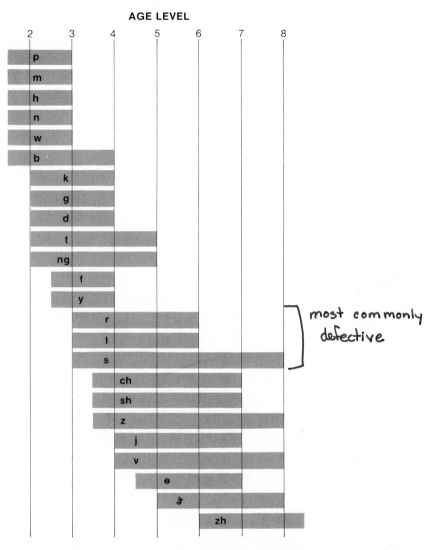

AGE LEVEL

most commonly defective

Figure 12 Average age estimates and upper age limits of customary consonant production. The solid bar corresponding to each sound starts at the median age of customary articulation; it stops at an age level at which 90% of all children are customarily producing the sound. (From Templin, 1957; Wellman et al, 1931.)

In the mastery of a new phoneme, we often find the child going through a series of approximations before the standard sound is produced. "Choo-choo" for *train* may be uttered with the two vowels alone, as *oo-oo* /u u/, then change to /tutu/, then shift to /tsu tsu/, before many months later it appears as "choo-choo" /tʃutʃu/. The substitutions reflect the use of easier and earlier sounds for those that are acquired later, and they are usually similar in that they possess some, if not all, of the distinctive features of the correct phoneme. Thus, we have never heard a normal child substitute a back plosive such as /k/ for the /m/ sound when he tries to say *milk.* If the standard sound is voiced, the child's substitution tends to be voiced. If it is a glide, the error will rarely be a stop consonant. He may say "wummy" for "yummy" but he won't say "dummy or chummy". Why does a child say "tandy" for "candy" rather than "sandy", "mandy", "randy", or "bandy"? As Menyuk (1968) explains it, the /t/ substitution used by the child has all the distinctive features possessed by the first sound of *candy* (/k/), all except one, the place of articulation. Both the /t/ and the /k/ are unvoiced, and stop plosives, and they are not nasal. They both involve the touching of the tongue to the roof of the mouth. It is the spot being touched which differs, the /t/ being in front and the /k/ in the back of the mouth. In terms of their distinctive features they differ in only one. Were a child to use an /m/, or /r/, or /b/ for the /k/ sound in *candy* the substitution would be much more unlike the standard sound. That is, more than one distinctive feature would differ. The child may not be able to hit the target phoneme's bulls-eye at first but he tries to come as close as he can; he does not fling out any old sound at random.

Finally, we should remember that progress in articulatory mastery is gradual. Even after the child has demonstrated that he is able to use the standard phoneme in some words, other words will still contain its usual error. Newly acquired phonemes seem very fragile. Under excitement, the child may return to the older forms and say "goggy" long after he has demonstrated that he can say "doggie". In certain phonetic contexts the new sound will tend to disappear. One child who had learned to say perfectly the word "fish" (instead of his earlier "fiss") could not say "Fish swim in water" for over a year because the /s/ in swim influenced the final sound of *fish* and turned it into another /s/ (assimilation). But eventually the child will master the phonemes he needs or have to have the help of a speech pathologist.

Semantic   Although there is much we still do not know about how a
Development child acquires the meanings of the words he hears and uses,
it seems evident that in early years the developmental process involves both extension and contraction. One of the author's children's very first words was "pih" for *pig,* probably because she enjoyed the animal's feeding times on our farm. She would say the word and point to the pigs, big ones, little ones, alike. But, through extension of the meaning inherent in the words, she also called all other animals "pih" too: dogs, horses, cows, and even her father

when he crawled on all fours under the fence. But then differentiation (contraction) appeared as she watched the cows being milked. She tried "pih-mik" (pig-milk?) a few times, then accepted our "moo-cow" by using her already acquired word for milk (mik) instead of our "moo" to produce "mik-kau". She never used "pih" for cow again, and very soon thereafter began eagerly to learn the names for other animals.

We also know little of the internal dictionaries being developed by the child. There seems to be some evidence that the early entries may be filed not as words but as phrases, *cup* meaning *something to drink from* or *ball* as *throw ball*. We do know that these internal dictionaries grow swiftly in volume. According to M. E. Smith (1926) a child of three years is already using 896 different words; at four years, 1540, at five, 2971, figures which are probably very conservative. Comprehension dictionaries are doubtless much more extensive. Like adults, children know many more words than they use in communicating.

Children also seem to learn the meanings of new words in a sequential fashion. First they learn those that refer to objects, events, or actions; next they seem to acquire the adjectives and adverbs that modify the words they've already acquired: ("*Big* dog", "Go *fast*"); then they master a set of terms that describe spatial and then temporal relationships, as shown in Figure 13.

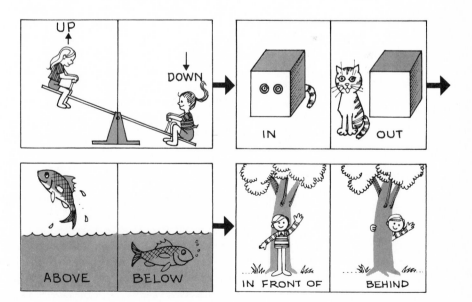

Figure 13   Developmental sequence of terms related to space.

We do not wish to imply that semantics is confined solely to vo-cabulary acquisition for, of course, it is the ways in which words are combined that enable us to communicate our meanings. Never-theless, any child who lacks the words he needs is very handicapped for he has to *have* them before he can string them together. We see this handicap vividly in stroke patients with aphasia who often have tremendous difficulty in word finding. As one of our clients told us, "I have lost my voc . . . my vocab . . . my, oh dear, my alphabet". And then he cried with frustration, knowing well that "alphabet" was not the word he needed.

Most parents are eager enough to help the child to get his first twenty or thirty new words. Some parents are even too ambitious at first; they try to teach such words as "Dorothy" or "Samantha." But their teaching urge soon subsides. The child seems to be picking up a few words as he needs them. Why not let him continue to grow at his own pace? Our answer does not deny the function of maturation in vocabulary growth. We merely say that parents should give a little common-sense help at moments when a child needs a new word, a label for a new experience. When parents notice a child hesitating or correcting himself when faced with a new experience, they should become verbal dictionaries, providing *not only the needed new word, but a definition in terms of the child's own vocabulary.* For example:

> John was pointing to something on the shelf he wanted. "Johnny want . . . um . . . Johnny want pretty pretty ball . . . Johnny wanta pretty . . . um . . ." The object was a round glass vase with a square opening on top. I immediately took it down and said, "No ball, Johnny. Vase! Vase!" I put my finger into the opening and let him imitate me. Then we got a flower and he put it in the opening after I had filled it partially with water. I said, "Vase is a flower cup. Flower cup, vase! See pretty vase! (I prolonged the *v* sound slightly.) Flower drink water in vase, in pretty vase. Johnny, say 'Vase!'" (He obeyed without hesita-tion or error.) Each day that week, I asked him to put a new flower in the vase, and by the end of that time he was using the word with assurance. I've found one thing though; you must speak rather slowly when teaching a new word. Use plenty of pauses and patience.

Besides this type of spontaneous vocabulary teaching, it is pos-sible to play little games at home in which the child imitates an older child or parent as they "touch and say" different objects. Children invent these games for themselves.

"March and Say" was a favorite game of twins whom we observed. One would pick up a toy telephone, run to the door of the playroom, and ask his mother, "What dat?" "Telephone," she would answer, and then both twins would hold the object and march around the room chanting "tepoʊn tepoʊn" until it ended in a fight for possession. Then the dominant twin would pick up another object, ask its name, and march and chant its name over and over.

In all of these naming games, the child should always point to, feel, or sense the object referred to as vividly as possible. The mere sight or sound of the object is not enough for early vocabulary acquisition. It is also wise to avoid cognate terms. One of our children for years called the cap on a bottle a "hat" because of early confusion.

Scrapbooks are better than the ordinary run of children's books for vocabulary teaching because pictures of objects closer to the child's experience may be pasted in. The ordinary "Alphabet Book" is a monstrosity so far as the teaching of talking is concerned. Nursery rhymes are almost as bad. Let the child listen to "Goosey Goosey Gander, whither dost thou wander" if he enjoys the rhymes, but do not encourage him to say the rhymes. The teaching of talking should be confined to meaningful speech, not gibberish. The three-year-old child has enough of a burden without trying to make sense of nonsense. When using the pictures in the scrapbooks, it is wise to do more than ask the child to name them. When pointing to a ball, the parents should say, "What's that!" "Ball." "Johnny throw ball. Bounce, bounce, bounce" (gestures). Build up associations in terms of the functions of the objects. Teach phrases as well as single words. "Cookie" can always be taught as "eat cookie." This policy may also help the child to remember to keep it out of his hair.

References

BRAINE, M. "The Ontogeny of English Phrase Structure." *Language,* XXXIX (1963), 1–13.
BROWN, R. W. *A First Language: The Early Stages.* Cambridge, Mass.: Harvard University Press, 1973.
———, *Psycholinguistics, Selected Papers.* New York: Free Press, 1972.
BULLOWA, J. M. L., G. JONES, and A. DUCKERT. "The Acquisition of a Word." *Language and Speech,* VII (1964), 107–11.
CARROLL, JOHN B. "Language Development." in A Bar-Adon and W. F. Leopold eds., *Child Language: A Book of Readings.* Englewood Cliffs, N.J.: Prentice-Hall, Inc., 1971, 200–11.
CAZDEN, C. B. "The Psychology of Language." in L. E. Travis, ed., *Handbook*

of Speech Pathology and Audiology (Englewood Cliffs, N.J.: Prentice-Hall, Inc., 1972).

CHOMSKY, NOAM. *Language and Mind.* New York: Harcourt, Brace, Jovanovich, 1968.

CURRY, F. K., "Speech Maturation." in A.S.H.A. Report No. 7. *Orofacial Function: Clinical Research in Dentistry and Speech Pathology,* 1972.

DARLEY, FREDERICK and HARRIS WINITZ. "Age of First Word: Review of Research." *Journal of Speech and Hearing Disorders,* XXVI (1961) 272–90.

DUNN, L., K. HORTON, and J. SMITH. *Peabody Language Development Kits.* Circle Pines, Minn.: American Guidance Service Inc., 1968.

FLEMING, J. D. "The State of the Apes." *Psychology Today,* VII (1974), 31–46.

FODOR, J. and J. KATZ. *The Structure of Language: Readings in the Philosophy of Language.* Englewood Cliffs, N.J.: Prentice-Hall, Inc., 1965.

FRY, D. B. "The Development of the Phonological System in the Normal and the Deaf Child." in F. Smith and A. Miller, eds., *The Genesis of Language.* Cambridge, Mass.: M.I.T. Press, 1966.

IRWIN, J. V. and M. MARGE, (eds.), *Principles of Childhood Language Disabilities.* Englewood Cliffs, N.J.: Prentice-Hall, Inc., 1972.

IRWIN, O. C. and T. CURRY. "Vowel Elements in the Crying of Infants Under Ten Days of Age." *Child Development,* XII (1941), 99–109.

McNEILL, D. *The Acquisition of Language.* New York: Harper & Row, 1970.

MENYUK, P. *The Acquisition and Development of Language.* Englewood Cliffs, N.J.: Prentice-Hall, Inc., 1971.

———, "The Role of Distinctive Features in Children's Acquisition of Phonology." *Journal of Speech and Hearing Research,* XI (1968), 844–60.

MOWRER, O. H. "On the Psychology of 'Talking Birds'— A Contribution to Language and Personality Theory." *Learning Theory and Personality Dynamics.* New York: The Ronald Press Co., 1950.

OSWALD, P. F. "The Sounds of Human Behavior," *Logos,* III (1960), 6–27.

PREMACK, A. J. and D. PREMACK. "Teaching Language to an Ape." *Scientific American,* CCVXXVII (1972), 92–9.

PREMACK, D. "The Education of Sarah." *Psychology Today,* IV (1970), 55–8.

SANDER, E. K. "When Are Speech Sounds Learned?" *Journal of Speech and Hearing Disorders,* XXXVII (1972), 54–63.

SLOBIN, D. *Psycholinguistics.* Glenview, Ill.: Scott-Foresman Co., 1971.

SMITH, F. and G. A. MILLER, (eds), *The Genesis of Language.* Cambridge, Mass.: M.I.T. Press, 1966.

SMITH, MADORA E. "An Investigation of the Sentences and Extent of Vocabulary in Young Children." *University Iowa Studies Child Welfare,* 1926, v. 3.

SWEENEY, SHEILA. "The Importance of Imitation in the Early Stages of Speech Acquisition." *Journal of Speech and Hearing Disorders,* XXXVIII (1973), 490–94.

TAYLOR, ORLANDO and DAVID SWINNEY. "The Onset of Language." in J. V. Irwin and M. Marge, (eds), *Principles of Childhood Language Disabilities,* Englewood Cliffs, N.J.: Prentice-Hall, Inc., 1972, 53–62.

TRANTHAM, C. R. and J. K. PEDERSEN. *Normal Language Development.* Baltimore: Williams and Wilkins Company, 1976.

WEIR, R. "Some Questions on the Child's Learning of Morphology." in F. Smith and G. Miller, (eds), *The Genesis of Language.* Cambridge, Mass.: M.I.T. Press, 1966.

WOOD, B. S. *Children and Communication.* Englewood Cliffs, N.J.: Prentice-Hall, Inc., 1976.

5

DEVELOPMENT LANGUAGE PROBLEMS

While the material on the development of speech and language is still fresh we go directly to a consideration of language disability. Children with such disabilities are often thought to be simply delayed in the acquisition of language, but studies (Leonard, 1972) have shown that some of them use *deviant* grammatical structures rather than more infantile patterns. One of our own young clients, five years old, never used any verb without adding the suffix *-ing* to it, an error that rarely is found in the speech of very young normal children. Sometimes he would say "Kitty be crying" or "Andy wanting no go to sleep now." We cannot assume, therefore, that a child with a language disability is fixated at an earlier level; he may instead have strayed from the normal path. So we shall use the term *language disability* because it can include both language delay and language deviancy.

However we label the problem, language disability is a common and difficult problem not only for the speech pathologist but for all workers in the field of special education. You will be sure to confront them at some time in your career. We are not even sure how many children are language handicapped, but careful estimates (Marge, 1972) show that the number of them in this country alone is larger than most of us would suspect, as demonstrated in Table IV.

The threefold classification used in the table is a crude one but it does give some idea of the problems you may encounter. Some children fail to acquire any usable language at all; they may be mute or echolalic or have at best a primitive and inadequate gesture language. Most of the profoundly mentally retarded belong in this category but some emotionally disturbed or congenitally deaf children may also show little or no language. The second and largest class includes those who are delayed or deviant in language acquisition. They have some language but it is so deviant or infantile and in-

114

TABLE IV   *Number of Persons with Language Disabilities**

	Ages 4–17 Type of Language Disability	Current Prevalence	Incidence (%)
I.	Failure to acquire any language		
	A. Age 4	22,854	0.6
	B. Ages 4–17	44,745	0.08
II.	Delayed language acquisition	3,467,784	6.2
III.	Acquired language disability	139,830	0.25

*From John V. Irwin and Michael Marge, *Principles of Childhood Language Disabilities,* Englewood Cliffs, N.J.: Prentice-Hall, Inc., (1972), page 91.

adequate in its structure that they are truly handicapped in communication. Some of these children are also mentally retarded or hard of hearing or emotionally disturbed, but others are not, though they may possess other learning disabilities, problems in motor coordination, hyperactivity, or environmental deprivation. Finally, in the third group, we find children who once had possessed adequate hearing but who have lost it, and children with aphasia or neurological impairments resulting from illness or trauma. Sooner or later you will meet some of these children professionally, and hopefully you will try to help some of them acquire their human birthright, the ability to use language effectively.

Non-Verbal Children   Since statistics alone, however, do not describe the human problems hidden therein, let us present a handful of word pictures of some children of the first type.

Dick is a post-encephalitic child with no motor or hearing defect. He was first seen at 4.8 years of age. An occasional grunt, used indiscriminately, comprised his total verbal output. No imitative oral responses could be elicited. Communicative contact was pointedly evaded, and he was extremely hyperactive. Gestures were infrequently used to indicate what he wanted. The prognosis made by physicians was that he would never develop the use of speech. At 6.8 years he was imitating sounds and producing word approximations. Spontaneous speech was limited to one-word sentences, but symbol meaning was clear only when the subject was known to the listener. Responsiveness and contact were improving. At 8.2 years he was able to

* a brain disease involving an alteration in the brain structure.

imitate most of the consonant sounds; spontaneous speech was frequently understandable, although still limited in output. Phrases and sentences such as "open the door," "your green car," "boy drink milk," objects and picture-naming, and ready responses to greetings were indicative of a much improved communication adjustment. (Schlanger, 1959, p. 358)

Here is another child, one who could only grunt and gesture:

Don was five years old, physically normal, and his parents were completely convinced of his intelligence. His hearing was good and so were his coordinations. He seemed to comprehend speech very well and could follow directions with ease. Possibly because of an early isolation on a farm with few playmates, he had few friends and preferred to play alone. He was well behaved, and his lack of speech and of interest in socialization seemed to be his only real difference. His parents had become quite anxious about his delay in learning to talk but seemed to love him. He was an only child. With this brief introduction, let us give you the observer's report. The observer watched the child and his parents through a one-way mirror and heard him over a hidden intercommunication system.

Father told Don to take off his hat and to hang them on the rack. Boy did this without hesitation, then returned to the play table and looked at toys. Father told him to help himself. He worked the little pump, and when the little ball came out of the spout he smiled, looked at the father and said, "uhn, uhn, uhn, uhn" and pointed to the ball. Father told Don to put ball back into upper hole of pump. Don did, then pumped handle, but ball was stuck. Looked at father who was not paying attention. Took pump to father and said, "oo." Father shook pump and ball came out. Don put ball back and shook pump. Ball did not come out so he put it down and put his thumb in his mouth. Father withdrew it without comment. Don said, "no," and put thumb back in mouth. Father said, "Cut it out, you hear me?" Don obeyed but held thumb in other hand. Father opened picture-book and said, "See cow? Say cow." Don looked but did not respond. Father said, "Say cow. Try it anyway." Don said, "uhn."

This was typical of the entire half-hour of observation. The only recognizable word was "No." The boy used monosyllables to get attention and then conveyed his meaning with gestures. If he could not make himself understood, he just gave up, waited quietly, or turned to something else.

Blake describes two seven-year-old boys, Jim and Ted, neither of whom had usable speech. We will use them here to show the marked variability in these problems of delayed language. Ted had been diagnosed as having been brain damaged; Jim had congenital heart disease. They differed markedly in personality, Ted being extremely hyperactive and aggressive, while Jim was shy and well controlled.

> At the beginning of therapy they both seemed to comprehend some spoken language fairly well, as demonstrated by the ability to follow simple instructions, understand simple gestures, play with and relate to objects, and by their response to other informal tests. Neither had adequate voicing in his attempted vocalizations. Ted's vocal quality was hoarse and extremely breathy, whereas Jim's vocalization attempts were whispered. Neither child was classified as verbal. Ted's main attempt at vocalization at the beginning of therapy was a rhythmical oronasal production of "k-k-k, k-k-k, k-k-k." He did attempt an approximation of *mama* which was vocalized as [a-a], with no attempt at labial (lip) closure or valving at the lips for the [m]. The word *daddy* was also approximated as [æ-i]. The words *yes* and *no* were vocalized as [hʌ] with the appropriate head gesture for each. This was the observable extent of Ted's intelligible vocabulary.
>
> Jim's mother described him as a child who seemed to understand what was said to him but who made very little or no attempt to verbalize on his own. His only intelligible vocabulary approximation was observed (and confirmed by his mother) to be a whispered production of "mama." (Blake, 1969, p. 364)

These two boys might appear to the casual observer as being hopelessly lost. We know that once the most favorable age of readiness for the acquisition of language has been passed—it is usually felt to be during the second to fifth years—the prognosis is poor. Nevertheless, Blake's experience and that of many of us who have worked intensively with these children may provide hope. Here is what he reports:

> Both Ted and Jim have developed functional speech far beyond the expectations of their parents and the clinician. Their vocabu-

laries are continuing to grow, and they use sentences with as many as seven or eight words now. They use functional speech in appropriate context and show promise of developing more complex speech and language skills. After one year of therapy, which has included two 30-minute sessions of language stimulation per week, Ted and Jim speak in sentences with an average length of four words [pp. 368–69].

Not all of these children are so restricted in their verbal utterance. Some of them vocalize almost constantly, but speak a gibberish which no one can understand. It resembles the jargon which many young normal children use. The utterances are full of inflections and are accompanied by gestures so that one almost believes that they are truly trying to communicate, but we have analyzed many of their vocalizations and have been unable to find any consistency which might indicate a self-language.

One of the children whom we examined vocalized every minute of her stay with us. She was a restless, wandering child whose attention constantly shifted. As she picked up one toy, threw it down, ran to the window, tapped at the pane, shook her skirt, sucked her thumb, laughed at her reflection in the mirror, and performed a hundred other consecutive activities, she accompanied each with a constant flow of unintelligible jabber. By using a hidden microphone, we were able to record some samples of her speech. The speech sample together with the object of her attention ran like this:

"Yugga boo booda . . . iganna min . . ." [jʌgə bu budə igæ nə min]. Picked up the toy automobile and threw it down. "Annakuh innuhpohee . . . tseeguh . . . tseekuh . . ." [ænakə inəpohi tsigʌ tsikə]. Looked out window and tapped at pane.

The Language Deviant Child Much more frequently found than any of the kinds of problems we have described are those in which the children do have some useful language and can communicate to some extent, but where it is clear that marked emotional problems or linguistic deficits are present. Wood describes a hyperactive and possibly schizophrenic boy named Paul with various difficulties.

Paul had developed speech, but failed to communicate ideas through speech. He usually talked at inappropriate times and on inappropriate subjects. He might begin with a specific idea, which he apparently wished to discuss, but his speech would wander away from the subject and he would include things which had occurred in the past, or objects which he had seen in his surroundings, or people's names which he seemed to remember suddenly. His conversation sounded something like this: "I saw a dog—ah—the chalk mama put to the desk—ah—on the picture pinned there—have you seen the car? My name is Paul. I am eight years old. Goodbye. (Wood, 1964, p. 109)

Although this speech indicates some comprehension of the rules of the language, yet in the sentence "the chalk mama put *to* the desk," we note just one small indication of deficit. In the following description, we find the telegrammic speech of early language development. Many of the function words are absent. The British girl who spoke this passage was eight years old. Hers was a disorder of language, not of speech.

I went to Reading. See, see bus. Long time. Went swimming. Mummy. Me. And the black man by. Mummy job. Down a stream. Quiet. Married. Long way. Very long way. Church. When I went there, fell I did. And I went soon, soon. Know her, she bride. Went to Reading, bus. Went to seaside. Not. Only next. Next. See the bridge. Way to holidays. (Renfrew, 1959, p. 35)

Many children with delayed language are not so impaired, but the flavor of the telegram with its omitted words is always present. The syntax is limited. Some of these children have not mastered the use of question words, the appropriate pronouns, plurals, or the use of verb tense. Others can use noun or verb phrases, but fail to combine them into subject-predicate sentences. Here is a sample of the speech of a five-year-old boy who was denied entrance into kindergarten because of his language deficiency:

Me Go. [Pause.] Outdoor. Mama in car now. Firsty [thirsty]. Dink Tommy cup. No dink now. Go Mama now. Tommy bed. [Was he trying to tell us he was tired?] Car. Car now. Dink mama car now. [He wanted to go home.]

Jenifer, a girl the same age as Tommy, spoke much better, but she too showed language difficulties. She was telling us what she was doing with our playhouse:

Here the kitchen and stove is there and Jenny cook stove eggs for breakfast. Um and Jenny go sleep here by bed. See! Oooh, bathtub. Soap no um in in a bathtub? [Questioning inflection.] You get soap for wash feet? Me like bathtub. Spash [splash] on water all over.

The examples we have given, of course, are those of children whose language ability is very poor.

Finally, let us present a group of school children who are not as profoundly handicapped yet still have language problems.

Five-year-old Gary with normal hearing caught the teacher's attention, and pointing to his mouth said, "Another one coming in back a tooth." Teacher looked in his mouth expecting to find a missing tooth. Instead, a six-year molar was just appearing through the gum.

John, age four, with hearing impairment, put his ideas in improper sequence when asked what he did after school. His answer, "Buy toys and go store."

Matthew, age five, with hearing impairment, was asked to tell what he remembered of the Thanksgiving party. His reply, "Teacher sit in the chair watching the children. The children all eating dinner. The children sitting down in the chair. Some of the children didn't ate all their supper. And the children went to get a drink of water in the cup and they was all quiet. And they came back in the room. Then they ate, and then they went back home. That sure is a long story."

A group of six-year-old children without hearing impairment were drinking their milk. John finished, looked up, and noticed Kerry had also finished. Instead of saying "We tied," John commented: "Me him beat together." (Bangs, 1968, p. 13)

Children Who Have Had Language But Lost It   You will also encounter some children with language disabilities who have suffered brain injuries due to trauma or illness, and others with a history of acquired rather than congenital deafness or severe hearing loss. Some of these have retained only the rudiments of their former language; other demonstrate their problem only in the use of occasional odd locutions. The range of language impairment in these clients is very great and it is difficult to present any representative or typical examples.

Deterrents to Language Acquisition

For many years writers on the subject of language disability have begun their discussion with a list of assumed causes for failure to acquire language mastery. In so doing, they follow the medical model which, for these and other speech disorders, may not be at all appropriate. Deviant language is not a disease. While it is clearly evident, as we have seen, that failure to master our language is often found in the seriously mentally retarded, the congenitally deaf, the brain injured, or in some children with severe emotional problems, we cannot be sure that these conditions *cause* the language problem in the same sense that one of the venereal diseases is caused by gonococcus. Rather it would seem wiser to view the relationship as deterrent or obstacle-creating. Severe hearing loss makes communication difficult rather than enjoyable, and it prevents a child from perceiving the models he needs to do the learning he must do. Mental retardation makes it hard for a child to recognize or recall meanings and relationships and both, of course, are vital to language learning. The emotionally disturbed child may reject the models or the interactions involved; the brain damaged child may find it hard to concentrate his attention on language stimuli or to see their patterning. Any one of these children, because of the way he was labeled or treated, may simply have learned not to learn. Tragically, all of them have been deprived in some way from having the crucial experiences for acquiring language which most children get over and over again. As Menyuk says, "The application of a diagnostic label such as deaf, aphasic, mentally retarded, etc., does not guarantee that we have isolated the factors which have determined the child's lack of 'linguistic behavior' ". (Menyuk, 1969, p. 13) Whatever may be the conditions that have deterred or prevented language learning, the job of the clinician is to help the child master the language code, both in comprehension and in output.

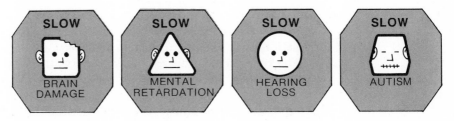

Figure 14 Some deterrents to language acquisition.

Sensory Deprivation   Output must always follow input in the development of language. If a child cannot hear the words and sentences of his parents and playmates, or hears them distortedly and faintly, he will have a very hard time in acquiring his word tools and in deciphering the rules of the linguistic code that makes speech possible. Even adults who learned speech early and have used it adequately all their lives begin to find a decay in the precision and intelligibility of their utterance when they become deafened. Consonants become fuzzy, the vowels distorted. We need a monitoring ear to speak a language without abnormality. One can readily see how difficult it must be for the child who does not hear well. The sounds of speech may be faint or missing or unintelligible. It would be like learning to speak Chinese with your fingers in your ears. You might give up; you might even manage to learn a little, but it wouldn't be very good Chinese. Children who are born deaf seldom, if ever, acquire a normal voice or natural speech sounds despite the best of teaching. Some of them can master enough intelligible speech to get along.

However, not all children who have impaired hearing are deaf; some may merely have hearing losses. By hearing loss we mean that some usable hearing still exists. The person can hear certain sounds at a certain loudness level. He may hear some of what you say. He may be able to hear sounds which are low in pitch yet fail to hear the high-frequency sounds. He may be able to hear pretty well by bone conduction, although when sounds come through the air they seem muffled and distorted.

There are two major kinds of hearing losses: conductive and perceptive (or sensori-neural.) By the first, the conductive, we mean that the loss is caused by some defect in the outer or middle ear. There may be wax in the ear canal; there may be fixation of one of the tiny bone transmitters in the middle ear behind the eardrum. There are many possible reasons for conductive loss, but the important thing to remember is that the lower and middle frequency tones are usually heard as being more muffled or fainter than they should be. Children with conductive loss usually learn to speak, though a little retardation may occur. They often, however, show many severe articulation errors of substitution and omission.

The other type of hearing loss is perceptive. It may be due to an injured or malfunctioning cochlea in the inner ear, or to a damaged acoustic nerve, or to injury to the brain itself. Of the two types of hearing loss, this is usually the more serious for speech learning or maintenance, because it introduces distortion as well as muffling of sound. The reason for this is that the hearing loss is not equal for different frequencies of sound. Most children with perceptive loss have a harder time hearing the high-pitched sounds than they do those lower in pitch. Sounds such as /s/, /θ/, /f/, /tʃ/ and /t/ are some of the high-frequency sounds. If you had a perceptive loss, these would be faint or unheard at the same time that the vowels and the /m/, /n/, and a few other consonants would be quite loud enough. If you could not hear the announcer on the television because you had such a perceptive loss, turning up the volume wouldn't help you much because the low sounds would seem to be blasted out so much louder proportionally. The tiny high-pitched overtones would still be lost. A person with a high-frequency loss can never hear normal speech as it really is. What he is able to hear will be a distorted fac-simile. Engineers have invented filters to cut out all the high-frequency sounds of speech. When we listen to recordings played through such filters, we are lucky to understand barely forty percent of what we hear, and even then we have to guess.

But even more important is the difficulty that children with auditory disorders experience in figuring out the structure of lan-guage itself. The child with normal hearing is provided with a wealth of speech samples from which he can find the combination rules that are acceptable; the deaf child is impoverished. However, even when taught very carefully in a highly favorable environment, the pro-foundly deaf child seldom seems able to overcome completely the handicap of his sensory deprivation. He is usually four or five years behind his hearing peers, even in the activity of silent reading. His written language is not only sparse but is characterized by many er-rors which show that he has not mastered the rules of the language, as evidence by some sentences spoken by a boy who was about to graduate from high school and who had been deaf from birth:

> Which best game you played? Are you brave or coward? He hit you like bee's sting. Want to play bridge game? Don't park be-tween this signs. Joe can one blow lick anybody. As well as I better leave now although there aren't any space left.

Deprived of the auditory experience of his own speech attempts and those of others, many children who do not hear often lose heart and make little effort to communicate except on the most primitive levels. Why try to talk when other people do not seem to understand? Why try to understand when others present only the picture of silent, moving lips? Confused and frustrated, they often retreat into a re-stricted, isolated as well as silent world. Finally, because these chil-dren have been severely limited in language growth and have had to rely primarily upon visual and tactual concepts, they tend to have great difficulty with abstractions. Their concepts tend to deal with the concrete. They have trouble with most relationships that cannot be seen or felt, and language involves many of these.

Neurological Dysfunctions and Deficits Anyone who has ever viewed the impact of brain damage on an adult who has long been able to comprehend and speak normally and then suddenly becomes aphasic will have no trouble understanding that children who suffer such damage may also have difficulty in mastering the complexities of language.

Some children get off to a bad start on the road of life by having birth injuries. Others start well but fall victim to severe illnesses or accidents along the way. When the brain is damaged by any of these traumata, there is always the possibility of speech delay. If the central nervous system is damaged, we may find a general mental deficiency causing delay in most functions, but, in other instances, we may find instead the awkward coordinations of cerebral palsy or the inability to use meaningful symbols as in aphasia. In other injuries, a central hearing loss may be the result. There are also some less conspicuous aftermaths of brain damage—hyperactivity, irritability, inability to tolerate stress, perceptual difficulties—all of which may make it difficult for the child to learn to talk. To learn to speak, we must hear; we must be able to coordinate our muscles; we must be able to handle symbols; we must have good auditory perception. Brain injury can affect any or all of these items.

Dysarthria This term refers to distorted speech caused by injuries of the central nervous system which make the coordinations needed for speech very difficult. Tongues may be clumsy; the lips may flutter tremulously, the jaw may fail to move on time or move sidewise; the larynx may be wrenched out of place; the chest may be expanding as in inhalation at the very time the child is trying to talk. The degree of involvement may be either widespread or almost hidden to all but the expert eye. We have worked with individuals whose only dysarthria was in the utterance of the tongue-tip sounds. Some cerebral palsied individuals find the task of coordination so difficult they never learn to speak.

Aphasia The term aphasia refers to the loss of speech, and so it may seem appropriate to use it in children who have never developed speech. Some speech pathologists prefer to use the term "developmental aphasia" instead. As we have seen in Chapter 2, aphasia refers to disorders of symbolization, to disorders of language rather than speech. It may include disabilities in reading, writing, gesturing, calculating, drawing, as well as in speaking. The basic problem revolves about the use of symbols. So far as speech is concerned, these children find difficulty in formulating their thoughts in words, in expressing them verbally, or in comprehending what others are saying. It's hard for them to send messages or, less frequently, to receive them. Formulating, expressing, comprehending, these are the functions which trouble the person who is aphasic. Some aphasic children have more difficulty with visual symbols; others, more trouble with symbols involving sounds. Some who cannot read (alexia) can write or copy the symbols they see on the printed page. Others can read but cannot write (agraphia). There are many varied disabilities lumped under the name of aphasia, but we hope that we have made our point—that aphasia refers to the difficulty in using symbols meaningfully; it is a disorder due to brain damage.

There is no doubt that aphasia can occur in children who have had speech and then lost it as a result of brain injury. We have worked with many such children. Here is one.

> Walter had been speaking very well, indeed much better than most children his age, when the automobile accident occurred on his fifth birthday. Thrown from the wrecked car, his head had struck a concrete abutment, and he was unconscious for over a week. When he was able to leave the hospital, he was almost mute although occasionally a snatch of jargon would pass his lips. He had difficulty recognizing his parents and sister but a gleam of recognition came when the family dog nuzzled him once they were home. His first word was "Tiber" which he used for the dog's name (which was Tiger). Even his gestures were confused at first. He shook his head sideways for yes and vertically for no. He had forgotten how to cut with the scissors or to hold a crayon. Emotionally, he now appeared very unstable. He cried a lot and had uncontrollable outbursts of temper. It was difficult for him to follow directions or to remember. Occasionally he would come out with swear words his parents had never heard him speak. Gradually the speech returned, aided by our patient tutoring and the parent counseling that was so necessary. At the present time, four years later, he is speaking very well but has a marked reading, writing, and spelling disability.

There exists some argument among certain speech pathologists concerning the concept of congenital or developmental aphasia. These terms refer to disabilities in the *learning* of symbols or language as contrasted with the *loss* of ability previously learned which is what we find in true aphasia. Our own position, based upon our clinical experience, is that such congenital or developmental aphasias do exist. These aphasic children present different problems than those whose delay in speech is functional or due to mental retardation or hearing loss, although they may not become apparent until after some speaking has been learned. They may have gaps in their comprehension, intermittently appearing almost deaf; they may show inabilities in finding or uttering words which they have often used before. They confuse opposites, saying *hot* for *cold;* they use associated words instead of the ones they should use. One of our cases who could always name a chair when he saw its picture, could not say anything but "sit" when he desired to talk about it.

> You want to sit down in that little chair?
> Yes . . . No-no-no! Me want baby sit. . . .
> You want the little chair?
> No, no, no, no. Me no, no. Want baby bear, no big man sit, sit down.

We gave him the big chair that he wanted and noted the repeated perseverations, the confusions of opposites, the use of the rhyming word *bear* for *chair* and, once more, the use of the action verb *sit* for the noun *chair.* We do not find this sort of thing when we teach the nonbrain-damaged child to talk.

Wood has a good passage which testifies to this confusion:

> If one word were selected to describe children with aphasia that word would be *confused.* Dennis was a good example of this particular kind of confusion. He was unable to follow simple commands or directions, unable to match colors, unable to assemble puzzles or form boards adequately, unable to sort objects into common groups, and generally unable to perform adequately on any task which required organization. Dennis was distractable on many occasions, particularly when unpredicted movements or light changes occurred. On rare occasions he seemed to respond to sounds in his environment, but these responses were inconsistent and infrequent. Either his expression was one of questioning, with furrowed brows and an intense look, or, completely to the contrary, his expression might be totally blank, as if a veil had dropped between him and all that surrounded him. He had periodic temper tantrums, frequently unrelated to any of the activities which were going on about

him at the time. His temper tantrums and emotional outbursts seemed to be related to his inability to communicate and to his general disorganization. He gave the impression that he knew what he wanted to do and what he wanted to say, but that he was at a total loss to find his way out of the communicative maze he was in, all of which increased his confusion and disorganization. (Wood, 1964, pp. 112–13)

When we examine these children we find a wide range of behaviors and deficits. Dennis, in the passage above, is far from typical. We tried to find from our own case records an example which would be more representative, but we could not. The variation is just too great. Wood's impressions of Dennis are used primarily because they show clearly how hard it would be for a confused and disorganized child to learn his language. Or perhaps "unorganized" would be a better adjective since, to a large degree, it is through our ability to use language that we organize the reality about us.

The Minimally Brain-Damaged Child   There are some children who have no history of cerebral injury nor any discernible neurologic signs that indicate brain pathology and yet who show many of the same behaviors and difficulties in acquiring language which the aphasic children demonstrate. No truly satisfactory term for them has yet been accepted, but generally, they are classified as "brain-injured," "perceptually handicapped," "minimally brain-damaged" children. The diagnosis is based upon an analysis of the child's behavior rather than upon electroencephalographic examination or any of the other methods used by neurologists to reveal true impairment. These children do not seem to have hearing losses; they are not mentally retarded; they do not resemble the emotionally disturbed. Their labeling and their diagnosis is therefore based upon inference and presumption; but since these children exist and present real problems to parents and teachers, some term to classify them had to be found.

This is the general picture they present: (1) They clearly have an inadequate ability to regulate or control themselves, as shown by hyperactivity, great distractability, perseveration, violent shifts in emotionality, incoordination, and impulsivity. (2) They show an inadequacy in being able to integrate sensory information as demonstrated by perceptual difficulties involving awareness, discrimination, figure-ground relationships, sequencing, retention and recall, and many other similar deficits. They also show difficulties in forming concepts, in categorizing and classifying, in handling abstractions. (3)

They have disturbed self-concepts and disturbances in laterality and in self-identification. They have small tolerance for frustration, little sense of past or future. They are often controlling, negativistic, and very hard to live with, for they do not perceive the needs of others. They do not relate well.

Not all these children fail to acquire language, but it should be obvious from their characteristics that they do so with difficulty; and some of those who do learn to speak continue to show marked disability later on when faced with the other language skills of reading and writing. There are also some whose lack of self-control, inability to integrate, or inadequate sense of self are just too overwhelming to enable them to learn the language system. Perhaps the many frustrations experienced by an intelligent brain-damaged child who tries to live meaningfully in a world full of words often make him seem hyperactive and excessively irritable. In working with these children you often have to do speech therapy on the wing. They are squirrelly, on the move constantly. It's hard for them to sit still, to concentrate, to be patient. Their frustration tolerance may be abnormally low, but we suspect it is only that they are overloaded with frustration. Occasionally they may go berserk, and show what in the adult aphasic is termed the "catastrophic response." One such boy, who had been working at his table quietly, suddenly began to scream, ran around wildly, tearing his clothes and shuddering. It was not a seizure. We held him firmly but soothingly for a while until he calmed; then he went back to his work. If these children find it harder to inhibit emotional displays than the normal child, we must understand and help.

Can they be taught to talk? Or read or write, or understand speech? We feel that the answer is yes, although we have had enough failures with some children to say the word hesitantly. It's so hard to get through to a child who cannot talk, who sometimes cannot understand. Somehow it's harder for a clinician to remember his successes than given failures. Perhaps the best way to put it is to say that many of these children can be taught to talk and do all the other things if given the proper help at the proper time.

Emotional Problems All of us have difficulty putting our deepest emotions into words, and perhaps only the poet manages to do so. Some unfortunate children experience almost constant storms of emotion, and it is easy to understand why they would have trouble learning to talk. When we speak we enter into a relationship with our listener; if most of our unpleasant emotions center in that listener, we find it hard to talk to him. Emotionally disturbed children cannot find the words to express the surges of unpleasantness that flood their beings. Perhaps their private world of protective fantasy has few words in it. When there are no words for communicating the incommunicable and when one fears or hates his listeners, why try to speak the unspeakable?

The range of problems encountered in this category is wide. In it we find children who are psychotic or autistic at one extreme, and children who are emotionally immature or negative at the other. They do not learn to talk because, perhaps, they fear the communicative relationships which speaking demands or because their flood of inner emotional static prevents them from hearing the models they need. Some of these children live in a world of their own. Others find their *lack* of speech a powerful tool for controlling others. There are children who find the awaiting world of adult life too unpleasant a prospect after they hear their parents screaming at each other, and so they prefer to remain infants all their days. What better way than to refuse to talk? Why should a child wish to put something into his mouth if it is unpleasant or painful? Why should a child speak if speaking puts him in contact with someone he fears or hates? Speaking is revealing; there are children who cannot bear the exposure.

Childhood   The child with this type of mental illness may show normal
Schizophrenia   language development until the ages of two or three and probably does not belong in the category of delayed language. However, he is truly delayed in using the language competence he has achieved to communicate and relate to others. When overheard, the verbalizations are bizarre. Here is one sample:

> Big train . . . under bed . . . [screams]. . . . I eat um up . . . and go toidy [toilet] . . . hurt hurt . . . [screams] . . . choo-choo-choo-choo . . . was dirty . . . I big house . . . green house and red and black and blue and . . . Mama, you go bed now.

All of this speech was uttered while playing with a truck on the floor. These children live in a private world, one often full of terrors perhaps, but yet better than the intolerable world of reality.

Rubin, Bar, and Dwyer give this account of another case:

> An older girl, with excellent language but poor articulation, which she wasn't interested in modifying, was preoccupied by birds. The clinician here had not only to restrict the topic to

feathered creatures but to enter actively into the girl's fantasies about birds before she cooperated eagerly with his attempts to improve her articulation.

This concentration upon certain restricted language themes is characteristic of this population when they do talk to other people. (Rubin, Bar, and Dwyer, 1967, p. 245)

Some of them show very little verbal output. They are so mute that they often are thought to be deaf. Their refusal to speak is compulsive rather than voluntary. In the histories of some of our cases of delayed speech we find that at one time they had begun to talk not only in single words but also in kernel sentences. Then something happened, a shock, an accident, a frightening experience, a separation from the mother, a stay at the hospital—and the child stopped talking.

Austra was a Latvian girl of seven who had experienced many of the terrors of displacement and bombing raids. She came to us two years after her father had finally managed to get to the safety of the United States. Her mother and brother and two sisters had been killed. Austra seemed to comprehend everything we said to her and her performance on the Wechsler Intelligence Test was superior but she talked only in grunts and gestures. The father told us that she had spoken very well until the age of three. She seemed to be a very happy child. Her father put the matter succinctly: "Austra has forgotten, but her mouth remembers." It took a lot of doing, but Austra learned to talk and graduated from college.

Autism The schizophrenic child often talks more to himself than to other people, but will communicate with them at times, though his speech often reflects his obsessions. The autistic child—a very strange child—resists verbal interaction with others. He won't answer questions and he rarely asks one. If he does reply to a demand it is a perfunctory reply, often an exact but monotonous repetition of what was said to him, and often it appears three or four minutes afterward. Although, according to Rimland (1964), whose work is the classic on the subject, about half of all autistic children are mutes and remain so all their lives, we personally have been able to evoke considerable speech from some of them. It is strange speech, full of exotic words at times, or unusual metaphors, sometimes interspersed with odd snatches of singing. But what strikes the observer especially is that the speech sounds dead, lifeless. There is no emotion or inflection in it. Here is a picture of one who spoke very little until treated:

> Kipper's parents' complaints were that "he can't pay attention," has "no speech," shows "inconsistent hearing" and "other unusual behavior." In particular, his unusual behavior consisted of periods of "finger flicking" (strumming the index or small fingers of his left hand with the index finger or four fingers of his right hand), and periods of sitting very still and "staring off at something."
>
> He was essentially unresponsive and inactive during our initial evaluation. He sat where placed without moving. He showed no response to his name. When eye contact could be achieved, his face remained expressionless ("mask-like"), giving the impression of a "blank stare." He was heard to utter only a few random sounds. When tickled he made only a slight flinching movement. As far as could be determined, he showed no response to auditory stimuli or social reinforcers. (Schell, Stark, and Giddon, 1968, p. 43)

The autistic child is a strange child, and he is sometimes very intelligent. It almost seems as though he is too hypersensitive to be able to bear the barrage of stimulation in which our children must live. Alexander Pope once wrote of the sensitive soul who "dies of a rose in aromatic pain." Autistic children are threatened by too much noise (and even a little noise is too much), too much color, too much movement, too many people—and sometimes even one parent is too much. They build walls around themselves, barriers to stimulation. Some of them do not seem to hear because they refuse to listen. Some of them sing the same little nameless tune over and over again to mask out the sounds and speech that can overwhelm them. Certain autistic youngsters concentrate on puzzles or mathematic manipulations to keep the world's fingers out of their lives. They may rock back and forth interminably to keep everything the same. Some of them do not talk at all or talk to themselves in a strange tongue. Other autistic children will talk a little, and even answer questions, but always in a detached and perfunctory fashion with a minimum of meaning and little feeling. They are strange children, not of this world. We have worked successfully with a few of them and have failed with more than a few. They require time and devotion which few of us can afford.

Negativism   Our culture demands much of its young. At the very time that the child is learning to talk, a hundred other demands are put upon him. He must learn how to eat at the table, how to control his bowels, how to be quiet, how to pick up his toys, how to behave himself. And this is the age at which we find out that we are *selves*, not objects, and that we are important in our own right. This is the "bullheaded" obstinate age, when the child learns how to say that favorite word of his parents: "No!" There are children who fiercely resist the constant pressure to conform, who fight a gallant but losing battle against incredible odds. And there are a few children who actually win, by discovering the one way they can refuse and get away with it. They refuse to talk.

You can't *make* a child talk. The tenacity with which some children resist their parents' efforts to eliminate thumb-sucking is minor compared to that shown by some children who triumph by not speaking. It's a tough problem to handle, once it seems to be focused on speech alone. First, we must convince the parents and associates of the child to stop making the usual demands that he say this and say that, and inhibit their complaining expressions of anxiety. We must remove the rewards which negativism brings. Here is one brief account of a child who had but one word in his vocabulary.

> The teacher said to the child in a rather peremptory tone, "Johnny, you go down to the drugstore this very minute and get yourself an ice-cream cone!" The child answered "No" and the teacher asked another child, who accepted and returned to eat the ice-cream cone under Johnny's regretful nose. Such a program soon brought a discriminatory answer to requests and commands, and when reward for positive response was added, together with humorous attitudes toward the negativism, the child's whole attitude changed, and his speech soon became normal.

Many of these children profit from a change in environment—placement in a nursery school—where they can learn from other children that speaking can be more pleasant than refusing to speak.

If we are to summarize these observations about the role of emotional disorders in the delay of language and speech, we would say first of all that most unpleasant emotionality involves human relationships. Communication also involves these relationships and it therefore is dependent upon them. If the very young child is immersed in negative emotion, he will have little inclination to learn language. If he is older when reality becomes unbearable to him, he will not use language enough to realize its fullest potentials.

Experience Some children are born into homes where conditions are un-
Deprivation favorable to speech development. There are silent homes
where the parents rarely talk to each other. There are homes
so confused with the noise and distraction of other children that the
harried mother has no time to create the relationship out of which
speech comes. Sick children are slow to talk, and there are sick
homes too. Some children hear little but angry speech. One of our
cases, who had lived with his grandmother, stopped talking when he
was returned to his real parents, who were deaf-mutes. Often we
have seen speech decay and disappear when an orphan child was
shuffled from one foster home to another. When two languages are
spoken in a home, one by the older children and the other by the
parents, some children get too confused to talk.

If a child is to talk there must be some identification with the
parent. We knew one little girl whose mother was a drunkard with
whom no child could identify as she staggered around the house,
dirty, cursing, and in half collapse. We have worked with children
too hungry, too weak or tired to talk, and had to take care of these
basic needs before they had a chance to learn. The county sheriff
once brought us three almost-wild children from a hut in a swamp
only a few miles from Kalamazoo. The father was a feeble-minded
junk scavenger who fed them when he could. The mother had abandoned them. The tale is too incredible to put in a textbook, but these
three nonspeaking children in the observation room were animal
children. Yes, there are environmental conditions which prevent
speech development.

Most of the research has clearly demonstrated that some children from the lower socioeconomic classes are delayed in language
skills. As Bereiter and Engelmann (1966) show in their review, pre-
school-aged children from this sort of environment are deficient in
vocabulary, sentence length, and complexity of grammatical structure.
In such life situations, there is often crowding, competing noise, and
little time for a parent to give the sort of language stimulation that fa-
cilitates learning.

It should be made clear, however, that a gross injustice has been
done to such ethnic groups as the black American, the Spanish-
speaking American, and American Indian minorities by stating that
they are linguistically delayed merely because they do not follow the
grammatical standards of upper- or middle-class American usage.
These children usually possess a competence in their own variant of
English which is quite as adequate as that of their other classmates,
even though they may speak differently. For example, as Baratz has
pointed out, the sentence spoken by a Negro child, "They don't have
none" instead of "They don't have any" does not reflect linguistic in-

competence but the standard usage of his community. When such a child says, "He there" instead of "He is there," he is not violating the rules of the language spoken by his associates.

Diagnosing the Since this is an introductory text we shall not treat diagnosis
Language Problem in any detail. What the language clinician probably does at first is to collect a corpus or sample of the child's utterances which is representative of his problem. If the child is mute and completely non-verbal she tries to learn his gesture language, if any, or to scrutinize his vocalizations for any intonations that might indicate meanings. She hunts for any evidence of comprehension of the speech of others. If the child has only a few words, she tries to ascertain whether they are true one-word declarative, imperative, or interrogative sentences, or merely stereotyped meaningless parroting of adult utterances and used only for display. If the child has progressed further and is combining words into real phrases and sentences, the clinician records and categorizes these to determine what the child has mastered and what he has not. Then she assembles the latter findings into a sequential hierarchy of targets for her training.

The clinician also has some tests that she can use to assess both comprehension and performance of language in a child who has sufficient language for analysis. Two of those currently in use are the Northwestern Syntax Screening Test (Lee, 1971) and the Carrow Elicited Language Inventory (Carrow, 1973). Developmental language testing is in its infancy and there are many unstandardized or questionably valid and unreliable tests being used for lack of any better ones.[1]

In addition to these analytical language tests,[2] the clinician will also try to determine such contributing deterrents to language acquisition as hearing loss (audiometric testing), deficits in reception, organizing and processing of information (Illinois Test of Psycholinguistic Abilities, the ITPA), inadequate intelligence (Bender Gestalt for Children), or certain tests of motor coordination. Also, she usually will gather case history material through parental interviews and scrutinize medical or school achievement records. This very cursory

[1] Some tests or procedures for assessing language development require special training in linguistics for their interpretation. Among these are the *Linguistic Analysis of Speech Samples* (LASS; Engler, Hanna, and Longhurst, 1973) and the *Indiana Scale of Language Development* (ISLA; Dever and Bauman, 1971).

[2] One of the most useful references dealing with the diagnosis of language disabilities is *Language Disorders of Children* (Berry, 1969). In it the student will find not only a thorough discussion of assessment procedures, but also five detailed case presentations showing both diagnosis and training.

review is far from comprehensive, but it indicates the complexity of the factors that may play a part in language disability. Nevertheless, once the language clinician has achieved a preliminary understanding of the general outline of the presented problem, she begins her language training.

Language Training

"The task of the clinician faced with teaching language skills to a deviant child is enormous. Considering the infinite number of utterances a child could produce, it is clear that the clinician must call upon some basic rules to teach in order to insure only that a mildly language-deviant child produces most of his utterances in a normal manner." (Leonard, 1973, p. 182) If this quotation from Leonard is as valid as most language clinicians would agree, one can imagine the greater challenge presented by children with greater language disabilities. Unfortunately, there are many of them who may be placed in your professional hands, and so you'd better know what to do and how to begin.

The Sequencing of Language Training Most clinicians make some attempt to follow what they believe to be the normal course of language development in their language training even though the research on this topic leaves much to be desired. First they seek to elicit vocalization as a response to stimulation if this is not shown by the child. Then they try to get him to acquire a few sentence-like words. These should be chosen with some care so that they can be easily combined with other words to make noun and verb phrases, can be used with intonations and gestures, may be truly useful in the child's communication, and finally, are not too difficult to say. A corpus of such words may be found in the reference by Holland (1975). Once the child has acquired these "sentence words" the clinician stimulates him with simple noun phrases and word phrases, and tries to get the child to say them in meaningful context.

Next the language clinician tries to get him to expand these and other sentence-like single words into noun phrases and verb phrases with their modifiers. Following this, the clinician helps the child to generate simple sentences of various types by combining the noun and verb phrases to reflect the subject-predicate or designative or actor-action relationships.

Once these simple sentences have been acquired, the clinician then seeks to have the child combine, expand, or modify these sentences through the use of conjunctions, prepositional or adverbial words, and phrases. She then might work on the transformations and the changes in word order that express questions, negatives, and commands. Or she might instead set up as the training targets those constructions which reflect pluralization, amount, time, place, verb tense, and so on until most of the complex structures of adult speech have been mastered. In the later stages of training the appropriate priorities are difficult to determine and most clinicians "teach to the deficits," selecting as their targets those grammatical structures which seem most needed or are most easily taught.[3] What then, is the best way for training these children who have language disabilities? Not all language clinicians agree as to what the proper strategy should be. Some insist that the best way lies through operant conditioning; others feel that a cognitive approach stressing the perception of concepts and relationships is preferable. Currently, most language clinicians seem to be basing their training methods on the principles of transformational (generative) grammar.

The Linguistic Approach: Discovering the Hidden Rules of the Language
Speech pathologists, or language clinicians, whose basic orientation is linguistic, view their essential role as being that of a provider of simplified language models so that the child may discover the basic patterns and rules which seem to have escaped him. These workers insist that the goal is not to have the child, through imitation, simply repeat the clinician's modeling of phrases and sentences of increasing complexity. Instead, they desire that he discover how words and phrases can and must be joined together to express meanings. As Laura Lee (1969) puts it, "The clinician's task is to unravel the linguistic complexity for the child, to help him recognize the information bearing kernel sentences, and to build up a slow but meaningful set of transformational operations which he can use both receptively and expressively." (p. 273)

Modeling
If you were to overhear a speech pathologist of this persuasion talking to a severely language-deviant child as they played with dolls or doll furniture, you might hear her using only noun phrases in her commentary (if this is the structure she wanted

[3] For more detailed information on the developmental order in teaching syntactic structures, see Norma S. Rees, "Bases of Decision in Language Training," *Journal of Speech and Hearing Disorders*, XXXVII (1972) 283–304; and Laura L. Lee and Susan M. Cantner, "Developmental Sentence Scoring: A Clinical Procedure for Estimating Syntactic Development in Children's Spontaneous Speech," *Journal of Speech and Hearing Disorders*, XXXVI (1971), 315–40.

the child to discover): "Dollie . . . big dollie . . . more dollie"; "Mama dollie" . . . "baby dollie" . . . or, many weeks later on, using simple subject-predicate models such as "Dollie jump" . . . "Dollie sleep" . . . or, in later sessions, using such transformations as the negative "Dollie no eat" . . . or the interrogative "Where Dollie?" . . . "Where bed?" . . ., or even exploring the possessive, "Where Dollie's bed?" What this clinician is using here is not the itsy-cooing kind of baby talk with which some silly persons bedevil their babies or their poodles, but a carefully programmed kind of simplified language stimulation so formulated that the child has a very favorable opportunity to discover how words can be joined together to code or decode meanings. By using these models at the very instant that the child is perceiving or experiencing what is being referred to (about that dolly), the child learns how to comprehend language structure and how to use it. Moreover, the clinician often finds that, once he has been exposed to the models sufficiently, the child spontaneously begins to use the simplified models without being asked to imitate them, and to use them in generating untaught phrases or sentences of his own. Occasionally, some prompting must be done and there must always be some kind of reinforcement for accomplishment or progress.

Expansions   When the child shows (by the new phrases or sentences he formulates by himself) that he has mastered the target constructions, the clinician moves onward to more complex ones, usually those characteristic of the next step in normal language development. Thus, if the child has moved from the one word sentence stage to the mastery of noun phrases and verb phrases including modifiers, she may next elect to stimulate him with her self-talk commentary on what he is doing, perceiving, or feeling at the moment with new target sentences. Or she may use what are called *expansions,* echoing his utterances but providing a model of a more highly developed construction. Thus if the child says, "Timmy go in doggie house" the clinician might say "Timmy go in doggy's house", if there were two houses, one for dolls and one for dogs (and if Timmy is at the stage for acquiring the rules governing possessives). In these "expansions" the clinician repeats what the child has said, but in a changed form, the change reflecting a more advanced construction.

Extensions   This term refers to the procedure whereby the clinician or parent responds to an utterance of a child, not merely by expanding it into a more mature construction by filling in the words he has omitted or misused, but by adding other phrases or sentences which make his meaning clearer. For example, if the child says, "Johnny bye-bye", the expansions might be "Johnny go bye-bye" or "Johnny wants to go bye-bye". But if instead the clinician or parent says, "Johnny wants to go bye-bye in the car. Johnny likes to ride in the car" they are using extensions, providing not just revisions of his simple utterance but models of how his meaning might be even better expressed. Parents tend to do this anyway but often they use far too complicated utterances. The idea is to show the child that there are other more meaningful ways of saying what he might say. It is semantic training.

Correction   Probably the most frequently used technique for helping a child learn the rules of the language is simple correction. All parents use it—and often abuse it. It can certainly be overdone. We have known children to stop talking altogether after being corrected too much, especially when the correction model is accompanied by parental irritation. "Oh, stop talking like a baby. Don't say, Timmy, see one, two, three car! People don't talk that way. They say, Timmy sees three cars. That's how they say it. Now say it right!" And then, if the boy says, "Timmy see three car," the parent might say, "No! Three cars. CARSZZ! Lord, won't you ever be able to talk right?" Sometimes it's hard to be a little child trying to learn his language.

The Modeling of   A much better way is to have the clinician or parent herself
Self-Correction   provide models of self-correction. For example, suppose the child needs to discover how past tenses are coded in our language. When describing what happened when the toy dog drank some play milk before hiding under the dollhouse bed and the boy had said, "doggie drink milk and hide bed" the clinician might say, "The dog drink the milk . . . No, I mean, the dog drinked his milk and hide under bed." She is not too worried about the improper use of the -ed ending here for the past tense of the verb. He can learn "drank" later. And she will feel good when he says "goed" for "went" so long as he is saying "banged" or "showed" or "tickled" to demonstrate that he is beginning to catch on the way some verbs must be changed to indicate the past tense. The important thing is that he has seen that big people can correct themselves too, that there is a right way and a wrong way to say what he means.

Let us give another example. Suppose the child is having a hard time with his plurals. Instead of correcting him everytime he says "chair" for "chairs" or "spoon" for "spoons," the clinician might deliberately insert the singular in her own speech and then calmly correct it with the plural form before continuing. She is thereby helping him discover the rule for the plural, and she won't be upset if the boy says "deers" for "deer" or "sheeps" for "sheep." Always, the clinician seeks evidence that the child is finding the rules he needs, not merely mimicking her.

Thus, if an older child is having trouble with prepositional phrases and never seems, for instance, to use the words "over" or "under", the clinician and child may do a lot of crawling over and under the tables in the therapy room or putting things under or over others as she verbalizes the shared experiences, expanding on his inadequate utterances such as "Go table" by saying "Go *under* table," or perhaps using his inadequate phrases or sentences before correcting them; "Put dollie chair, no, no, I mean 'put the dollie *under* the chair.'" Or the clinician may even ask him to say it correctly, "Timmy, say: 'put dollie *under* the chair.'" Again, if the child's pronouns are all askew,[4] we show him the differences between the correct and incorrect usages by making his error first and then correcting it. Thus the clinician might say, "Me go outdoors now. . . . No, *I* go outdoors now" before indeed doing so. You might possibly feel that the clinician should never use models which are linguistically defective even though they are simplified. Should the clinician ever speak "childrenese?" The answer seems to be yes since research shows clearly that simplified models as compared to standard ones were much more effective in language training.

> Just last week we were working with a little boy who was thoroughly confused by plurals and possessives. So we emptied out his pockets and our own into a pile and said, "That's your . . . and that's *mines* . . . No, I mean that's *mine*. And that's yours, and that's mine. Yeah." Before the end of the session, the boy had recognized not only the difference between *yours* and *mine* but also that even while plural objects were designated, we did not add the *s* to *mine*. By demonstrating and self-correcting our own errors, we helped him recognize the correct usage as we took turns identifying the objects on the floor. And he also incidentally learned some new words. In all of this interaction we never once corrected the child's usage; we merely corrected our own deliberate errors.

With an older child, we may work more directly, confronting him with his mistakes and providing the standard usage mold as soon as the error occurs. We play "Catch me!" games in which we deliberately make the mistakes, and they are his usual mistakes

---

[4] It must be hard to learn these pronouns, to comprehend that when I say *I* it means *you* to you, and when I say *you* it means *I* to you.

which he is to identify in order to get rewards. By "catching" these mistakes and having to show why they were mistakes and what the correct forms would be, most of these children learn the rules of the language very swiftly. They need help and they need careful teaching, but it is surprising how quickly they get the insights they need once the language task is simplified. Also, it has seemed to us that often the child seems to have already acquired the necessary linguistic competence, but has not been able to convert it into performance until we provide this focused sort of language stimulation:

> We were helping a four-year-old child who, among other problems, had shown great difficulty in getting his past tenses straightened out. After some prompting and error recognition activities which he enjoyed hugely, we were trying to get him to discriminate between "growed" and "grew." Suddenly, he grinned at us and said, "I growed-grew, knowed-knew that all the time. I knew it but now I got it." Unfortunately, the English language has many traps for the unwary, and we had to straighten out some tangles when he overgeneralized and told us how he "shew" his mother how well he could ride his tricycle. In Chaucer's time, he would have been correct.

As we have said before, some speech pathologists who use the generative grammar approach that we have been describing tend to downplay imitation, drill, or requesting the child to repeat sentences spoken by the clinician. They don't want a simple parroting of their stimulus phrases or sentences. They want the child to be able to generate phrases and sentences of his own which are coded appropriately, and used meaningfully. Often an observer might hear very little speech being produced by a child during a therapy session, the clinician concentrating rather upon understanding and comprehension. For example, the clinician might be commanding, "Put car *in* bed," showing the child what he should do, or telling him instead to "Put car *under* bed," or finding picture cards which show not only "the toy car in a bed," but also a "bed in a car" to test his comprehension. Concepts are provided before they are coded.

Having the Parents Help A child who is severely deficient in language will require much help at home as well as in the therapy room and so the parents must be brought into the program. We have found it wise to let them observe our sessions for a period of time before asking them to join us in helping the child acquire language. And we rarely try to acquaint them with linguistic theory. Instead, we ask them to stop asking the child questions and to stop drilling him on trying to get him to repeat the inappropriate things they usually demand that he imitate. We train them to use what we call "self-talk" and "parallel talk" for these are techniques which they readily understand and will use.

Self-Talk By self-talk we mean that the parents should talk aloud to themselves so the child can overhear them verbalizing very simply what they are seeing, hearing, doing, or feeling.

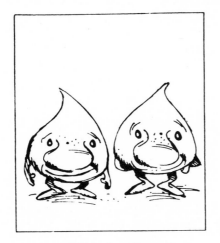 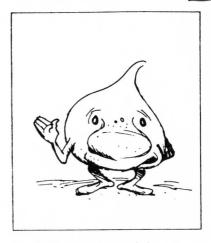

"This is a Boop."   "Here are two of them"

"There are two . . . ?"

Figure 15 Testing the child's comprehension of pluralization. (Modified from J. Berko, *The Child's Learning of English Morphology*, 1958.)

Here are some samples of a mother's self-talk:

Where cup? Oh, I see cup. Cup on table. Here cup. . . . Milk in cup. . . . Mummy drink milk. . . . Johnny want cup? . . . OK . . . Johnny drink. . . . Milk all gone. . . . Give Mummy cup. . . . Mummy wash cup. . . . Here water. . . . Here soap. . . . Give cup bath. . . . All clean. . . . Where towel? Here towel. . . . Wipe, wipe. . . . Give Johnny cup. . . . Put on table. . . . Johnny good boy.

This child was only making a few vowels, grunts, and gestures at the time but he was alert and interested. Note the mother's simple speech, within reach of the child's ability. Note the commentary accompanying what she did or saw. Note the recall and prediction. Here there is no demand for display speech. Here is self-talk used as verbalized thinking. It wasn't long before the boy was talking to himself too. Mothers and clinicians must learn to talk this way for the time being, to build the bridge between where the child is and where he should be in language usage. He cannot jump the chasm. As he begins to talk, they can gradually increase the complexity of their models. With some children who are speaking only in grunts or gestures, we would begin therapy by doing our own self-talk in a similar fashion, then progress to single-word utterances, then to short phrases, and finally to sentences which gradually increase in complexity and completeness. We have to begin where the child is. We must join him before we can lead him.

A surprising bit of behavior comes when we get to the early sentence stage. If we occasionally fumble a bit, leave a self-talk sentence hanging uncompleted in mid-air, omit a key word, the child will often say if for us. When this occurs it is unwise to make much of an issue of the achievement. Just feel good and use the technique more often. If we put words in his ears he will find them in his mouth.

We have found that most parents cannot do much better than this in modeling what the child must learn. Though occasionally the language clinician may ask her to try to use the constructions she is concentrating on in therapy, the mother usually forgets or finds the restrictions on her output too onerous. Usually, if you ask the parent just to say what she says to the child in very short simple phrases and sentences, the models she provides come pretty close to being those taught by the clinician.

Parallel Talking   If the clinician will show her, the mother can also learn to use what is called parallel talking. This technique does not require the child to say anything, thus freeing him from the usual bombardment of parental commands to "Say this" and "Say that." And it relieves some of the mother's anxiety. She must have something to do to help her child, something not too difficult to understand or carry out.

In parallel talking, the mother verbalizes not her own thoughts but those of the child. She tells him what he is doing, what he is feeling. If he appears to be predicting that Jack will jump out of his box, she might say, "Jack pop out, pretty soon." If he is about to turn off the light, she says, "Light go away now." If he is remembering

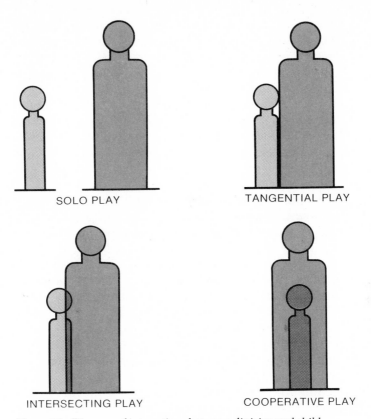

Figure 16 Diagram of interactions between clinician and child.

where she hid the cookie, she says, "Cookie in bag." As he bounces, she tells him what he is doing. When he tumbles from the chair, she says, "Johnny fall down. Ow, ow. Hurt foot. Ow!" Emotions can be expressed in self-talk and parallel talk too.

This parallel talking is fascinating stuff. Ideally, we should say the necessary word or phrase or sentence at the very instant that the child should be needing it. Practically, we seldom get the timing so precise. It is a skill which develops with use. We have known mothers to become wonderfully adept after a little practice. It requires careful study of the child and a lot of guessing, imagination, and the ability to identify with the youngster. Every speech clinician should learn the art, for it is very useful in treating the adult aphasic as well as the child who cannot talk. Training in empathy is vitally important in speech pathology.

We have spoken earlier of the importance of speech as a magical tool for controlling others. Nowhere do we see this so clearly as in delayed speech. As soon as we possibly can, we teach this function.

We have used puppets, dolls, even ourself as our victims. We command these beings. We tell them to fall down, to cry, to clap hands, and they must obey! The child watches us and sees the power of speech. Soon he is commanding too. Our knees still creak from a session with a little boy who insisted that we get "Unduh taybo!" thirty-seven times by actual count. This spontaneously achieved command had been preceded by much self-talk on our part, commanding first a puppet and then ourself to follow orders.[5]

We also use self-talk to set models for egocentric speech, for the expression of the self. Yesterday, with the same little boy, we crouched on the floor and said, "I'm little. . . . I baby. . . ." Then we got up on all fours, and said, "I kitty . . . meow!" Then we stood up and said proudly, "I big man . . . big as a house." The boy liked the display and gestured that he wanted us to do it again. We looked puzzled, paused a bit, then said, "More! . . . You want more?" He grunted. So we did it again and again, and soon he was imitating first our postures and our animal noises, and finally a little of our speech. He climbed aboard the table, stuck out his chest and arms and crowed, "Man . . . bih MAN!" This was the beginning of speech as the display of the self.

We teach speech as communication a little later. Often it begins to come in by itself, once speech as thought and speech as social control are activated. Usually, we combine it with command at first. "Mummy blow bubble. . . . Big Bubble . . . Oh, oh . . . No more bubble. . . . All gone. . . . Go ask sister for soap. . . . Sssssssssoap. . . ." If he's interested enough he might just possibly do it.

Direct Language Teaching   Not all language clinicians are content merely to stimulate the child with simple models of the constructions he needs and to wait until he discovers and begins to use them. Feeling that his chances of discovering them are better when they appear in his own speech productions rather than in the expansions or models which they present, they train the child deliberately to imitate their utterances. Thus, if the child is having difficulty in using the perpendicular pronoun "I" in contrast to the word "me" in discovering the variant forms of the subject versus object relationship, they would try to get the child (repeating after the clinician) to say such sentences as "I hit dolly" as he does so; or to say "Dolly hit me," in unison when this is acted out. Also, many clinicians, as we have said

[5] A psychological rationale for commentary and command in self-talk in terms of "tacts" and "mands" may be found in the book *Verbal Behavior* by B. F. Skinner (Englewood Cliffs, N.J.: Prentice-Hall, Inc., 1957).

before, resort to direct correction. When the child says, "Me go car" they respond by saying "*I* go car" and then insist that the child repeat what they have said. This procedure probably reflects the kind of parent-child interaction which has failed in the past to help him discover the difference between the two pronouns, but when the clinician repeatedly focuses on the problem and reinforces the correct one, it often does facilitate the discovery that must be achieved.

Although each child's language problem is unique, it is possible to work with small groups of children with language disabilities, as the text *Interactive Language Development Teaching* (Lee, Koenigsknecht, and Mulhern, 1975) demonstrates. These clinicians, using a story telling technique with the children in a group, have developed a comprehensive set of lessons organized according to a developmental sequence. They *teach* the grammatical constructions the children need using a variety of methods; they don't merely stimulate or model and wait for the child to discover the rules. This is their rationale:

> "Normally developing children are capable of generalizing grammatical rules from the conversational speech of parents, but clinical children have shown reduced ability for the self-discovery of grammatical rules. A structured interchange between clinician and child helps to highlight the grammatical problems the child is encountering. The clinician needs to reformulate, remodel, correct or expand a child's utterances in an effort to elicit more mature language from him. While parents may produce these corrections on expansions only occasionally, the clinician must do it constantly." (p. 8)

The Operant Conditioning Approach: Behavior Modification Procedures   You should know that there are many other speech pathologists who feel that the best way to help a child acquire language is through operant conditioning, and several studies have been reported in the literature wherein autistic or mentally-retarded children have made considerable gains in language through careful programming and reinforcement. These workers believe that language is learned, not discovered, and that when a child has failed to master the proper linguistic codings for his thoughts, he can be taught (conditioned) to do so.

Suspecting that most of you have a basic knowledge of operant conditioning, we will only describe it briefly, then illustrate how it can be used in language teaching. The basic principle of operant conditioning is that most behaviors, including language behaviors, are affected by their consequences. Some consequences increase the probability that the behavior will reoccur in the future and are therefore termed reinforcing; others, called punishers, decrease that probability.

The operant language clinician's task, then, is to define the behaviors he wants the child to emit more frequently, to carefully devise a serial program of successive objectives, and to provide and contingently apply the reinforcements according to an appropriate schedule. The criteria of successful achievement at each step of the program must be met before the child goes to the next successive step. If the child cannot meet the criterion for a given step, the program is revised, or the reinforcements are increased, or help in the form of *"prompts"* is given until success is obtained. Sometimes, because the desired response is too complex or does not exist (even intermittently) in the child's repertoire, a program of successive approximations called *shaping* is used. In this shaping, the clinician at first reinforces a response which may have very little similarity to what must be learned. But as it occurs again and again, however, some variability is usually shown and when it appears the clinician contingently reinforces only those behaviors which increasingly resemble the target behavior.

Conditioning the   If the child has no verbal language at all the operant clinician
Non-Verbal Child   devises programs to establish imitative behaviors. For example, the child may be contingently reinforced first for looking at the clinician whenever the clinician makes a sound. When this behavior is being consistently shown (perhaps eighty percent of the time), the reinforcement is faded out for simply looking but it is given again when the child looks and also opens his mouth as the clinician makes a sound. If this is unsuccessful, the clinician may insert an additional smaller step of reinforcing the child when he imitates her head shaking or hand clapping. If she accomplishes this, the clinician may return to reinforcing the imitative mouth opening, or even use the prompt of opening the child's mouth with her hands as a response to her stimulation. Usually, the child will emit some sounds in the course of the interaction and through reinforcement, the rate of this imitative sound production can be greatly increased.[6]

Then the clinician may move on to establishing the imitation of a few target words (names of objects or pictures or activities). In order to prevent mere parroting at this step, the clinician may insert a

[6] A description of this shaping may be found in N. Kerr, L. Meyerson, and J. Michael, *A Procedure for Shaping Vocalizations in a Mute Child'* in L. Ullman and L. Krasner, (eds) *Case Studies in Behavior Modification* (New York: Holt, Rinehart, & Winston, 1965).

substep into the program wherein the child must imitate the clinician's pointing to the object or picture as it is being named by both. Then the clinician would probably point to the picture but provide the name herself only occasionally (thus fading out her prompting), and usually the child will finally be able without help to point and name often enough to get the reinforcement.

An Operant Program   Most of the children with whom the speech pathologist deals are not mute or completely non-verbal. There are some who have at least a few single words which they occasionally use with their gesture language at one time or another. The following table from *A Language Program for the Nonlanguage Child* (Gray and Ryan, 1973) presents an overall picture of the sequence of objectives:

TABLE V   *Language Curriculum**

A. CORE	21. Cumulative noun/pronoun/verb/ verbing
1. Identification of nouns	
2. Naming nouns	22. Singular and plural past tense (t and d)
3. In/on	
4. Is	C. OPTIONAL
5. Is verbing	23. Was/were
6. Is interrogative	24. Was/were interrogative
7. What is	25. What was/were
8. He/she/it	26. Does/do
9. I am	27. Did
10. Singular noun present tense	28. Do/does/did interrogative
11. Plural nouns present tense	29. What is/are doing
12. Cumulative plural/singular present tense	30. What do/does/did
	31. Negatives not
13. The	32. Conjunction and
B. SECONDARY	33. Infinitive to
14. Plural nouns are	34. Future tense to
15. Are interrogative	35. Future tense will
16. What are	36. Perfect tense has/have
17. You/they/we	37. Adjectives
18. Cumulative pronouns	38. Possessives
19. Cumulative is/are/am interrogative	39. This/that/a
20. Cumulative what is/are/am	40. Articulation

*From Burl Gray and Bruce Ryan, *A Language Program for the Nonlanguage Child'* (Champaign, Ill.: Research Press, 1973), p. 27. Used by permission of the authors.

For each of these objectives a detailed operant program was written with the stimuli, target responses, type of contingent reinforcement, schedules of reinforcement, and criteria of success being specified for each step. Let us look at only one of them (Number 4).

When teaching the child the use of "is" (Number 4) Gray and Ryan program 22 steps in sequence; the reinforcement consisted of redeemable tokens or verbal praise; the target responses were the use of "is" either alone or in a sentence consisting of a noun, plus *is*, plus an adjective (e.g., "The boy is old" or in later steps "The boy is in the car," etc.); the schedule of reinforcement varied from 100 percent (given for each correct response) in the early steps of this program to 10 percent in the later steps; the criterion of success was either ten or twenty successively correct responses before moving on to the next step. Pictures and the clinician's verbal model ("The girl is walking.") were the stimuli used to evoke the responses.

This program of 22 steps was further divided into five series with different target responses required for each. The last three of these steps employed questions, story-telling, and conversation to allow for transfer. After the child has completed the entire program, he is then tested to be sure that he has learned how to use the word "is" in all the specified contexts, and if he has done so, he would then begin the next program (No. 5 in the language curriculum), designed to teach him to combine the "is" with a verb ending in "ing". ("The boy is running.")

Despite the complexity and length of this language curriculum, Gray and Ryan admit that it does not teach all of the constructions a child really needs to speak our language correctly. Nor do they feel that it is necessary to do so. What they do try to establish is a "mini-language" which the child can use as a foundation for later acquisition on his own. Nor do they always follow the normal course of language development, preferring instead to teach what can be learned most easily and employing a logical rather than a strictly developmental sequence of steps.[7]

Lovass (1968) describes another operant program consisting of a sequence of steps. In Step One the child was reinforced for all vocalization. Then when he was making more vocalization about every five seconds and watching the clinician's mouth more than half of the time, Step Two of the program was begun. In this step, the clinician (or parent) said a word once every ten seconds, and the child got his reinforcement only if he made some kind of vocalization shortly afterward. When this behavior increased to a substantial level, then Step Three was introduced. In this step, the child only got the reinforcement

[7] Another comprehensive program which could be used either by the advocates of operant conditioning or by those of the discovery approach can be found in *Emerging Language* published in 1973 by John Hatten, Tracy Goman, and Carol Lent, *The Learning Business,* 30961 Agoura Road, Westlake Village, California.

when he was able to match the adult's utterance. This was usually fairly simple and consisted of isolated sounds or syllables which were easily seen and could be facilitated by manipulating the child's mouth; or they were sounds the child had uttered before. When this was accomplished, Step Four was initiated, and this was followed by other steps which introduced new sounds and words and phrases according to the basic methods of reinforcement used in Step Three. This account illustrates the practices used by most of those who have attempted to get a nonspeaking child to talk through operant conditioning, though, of course, different children require different programs.

They also require different reinforcers. Sloane, Johnson, and Harris (1968) describe some of these reinforcers as follows:

> A great variety of reinforcers were used, based upon what "worked." When a reinforcer no longer "worked," new ones were tried until something was found that seemed to exert control. Some children received one of their regular meals as a reinforcer; that is, the ordinary meal was delivered in small spoonfuls contingent upon appropriate responding. Other edible reinforcers used were candies (M & M's, Pez, Neccos), spoonfuls of sherbet or ice cream, small marshamllows, bits of graham cracker, milk, soda pop, water, pieces of dry cereal (especially sugar-coated cereals), and raisins. (p. 84)

Some children respond to less tangible rewards—to social reinforcers such as praise or a smile or approval. Some will work hard to get tokens such as poker chips, which can be exchanged for opportunities to escape or to play or to use preferred toys for a time. It is usually wise to pair the clinician's approval with a primary reinforcer such as the candy so that the smile or "good boy" may later become effective controls. It is also important that the scheduling of these reinforcements be shifted from a consistent schedule—a marshmallow everytime he responds appropriately—to an intermittent or partial reinforcement schedule as soon as this can be done, if rapid extinction is to be prevented.

Other Approaches   Although the discovery and operant conditioning approaches are probably those used most frequently at the present time, there are some others which should be described. The first of these might be called the *cognitive approach.* Its basic tenet is that the use of language is based upon thinking and that the focus of therapy should not be on verbal output, but on the underlying concepts which must be coded in language. These workers insist that thought and comprehension are basic and they stress acquisition of the meanings which underlie the grammatical structures the child must discover. Other cognitive workers concentrate on concept formation and development following the outlines laid down by Piaget or Vigotsky. The Montessori schools which feature graded activities involving perception as well as initiative and coordination have been very successful in teaching language to some intellectually deprived children or to some whose home environments have prevented normal development.

A more recent example of the cognitive approach is found in the tutorial system of training preschool children in abstract thinking. Rather than working on developing language structures in these socially disadvantaged children, the clinicians train them in selective attention, categories, imagery of future events, inner verbalization, cause and effect relationships, and many other such processes.

Still another strategy for helping the language impaired child might be called the *phonetic approach*. Based upon the assumption that a non-verbal child cannot produce words if he has not learned the sounds which comprise them, clinicians of this persuasion begin by teaching the child directly how to make the sounds and to combine them into words which can then be associated with their referrents. The Moto-kinesthetic method, representative of this approach, consists essentially of the manipulation, touching, stroking, or pressing of the child's face and body by the clinician in such ways as to provide tactual and kinesthetic cues for the sequence of sounds that compose the word. The clinician thus helps the child to locate the structures needed to produce the sound, indicates the direction of their movement, and gives some clues with respect to voicing, nasality, plosion, or continuousness. At the same time that the clinician is manipulating the child's oral structures, she is also clearly pronouncing the sounds of the word being produced.

We taught one nonspeaking child his first meaningful word "No!" by asking him if he wanted to stay on the table on which we had laid him, telling him that only if he said "No!" he could get down. We placed his fingers on our nose and lips as we slowly said the word. Then we took his forefinger, placed it alongside his own nose, and then shifted it and the thumb to round his lips. Next we showed him how we used these movements to form our own "No." Then, after asking him again if he wanted to stay on the table, we went through the same series of manipulations, he pronounced the word perfectly, and we let

him get down to play for a time. To make sure, we asked him if
he wanted to get back on the table, and it was interesting to
watch him touch his nose and round his lips again as he said
the word clearly. In that same session we also taught him "Yah"
and invested it also with meaning. Throughout the half-hour
period the boy would intermittently relapse into his usual jargon and gestures, but these we simply ignored. The boy's
mother, who had watched the proceedings, then took over and
successfully got both a meaningful "Yah" for a proffered bit of
candy and a meaningful "No" when she asked him if he
wanted to stay with us as she went home. For both words, the
boy used his fingers on his face to help him say them, but the
parent reported that within a week he was saying these words
appropriately and without the motokinesthetic gestures. What
was most important, the boy had learned that speech was a tool.

Not all clinicians who use the phonetic approach use the motokinesthetic method, but they all teach sounds and sound sequences
as a means for creating words. Auditory discrimination, imitation,
and much drill work are employed, and after words are acquired they
are associated with meanings. The child is then taught through imitation to use his new words in phrases and sentences of increasing
complexity.

Which Approach   Language therapy is still in its infancy. There are many prob-
Is best?   lems still to be resolved and so this question cannot be answered at the present time. Both the grammatical stimulation-
discovery approach and operant conditioning have been shown to
help some children acquire some language ability. Most of the speech
pathologists we know use both approaches, though they usually begin with the discovery approach first. Also, they use operant conditioning for special problems such as when teaching an older child to
stabilize the use of proper plurals or the past tense. Any teacher of
language-impaired children needs to know the rationale and application of both these approaches as well as the others. The child's
needs and difficulties and capacities must determine how he is to be
helped. As Marge (1972) states, "Unfortunately, there is no reported
evidence on the effectiveness of any approach in current use. The literature reveals discussions of individual cases of successful results
with language disabilities in children, but one finds it difficult to
generalize because of the multiplicity of factors which may individually or in combination lead to failure or success in managing language handicaps." (p. 308)

Children with language disabilities will have a rough time of it in school and out. Their parents will be ashamed of them and they will come to feel that way about themselves also. Not only speaking, but reading and writing skills, will be affected. If many people think they are mentally retarded (even if they aren't); they eventually may come to believe those others and respond accordingly. These children need understanding and expert help. We hope that you will see that they get it.

References

ADAMS, J. "Delayed Language Development." *Journal of Speech and Hearing Disorders,* XXXIV (1969), 169–71.

ADLER, S. *The Non-Verbal Child.* (2nd ed.) Springfield, Ill.: C. C. Thomas, 1975.

BANGS, T. E. *Language and Learning Disorders of the Pre-Academic Child.* Englewood Cliffs, N.J.: Prentice-Hall, Inc., 1968.

BAR-ADON, L. and W. F. LEOPOLD. (eds.) *Child Language: A Book of Readings.* Englewood Cliffs, N.J.: Prentice-Hall, Inc., 1971.

BARATZ, J. C. "Language and Cognitive Assessments of Negro Children: Assumptions and Research Needs." ASHA, XI (1969), 87–91.

BEREITER, C. and S. ENGELMANN. *Teaching Disadvantaged Children in the Pre-School.* Englewood Cliffs, N.J.: Prentice-Hall, Inc., 1966.

BERRY, M. F. *Language Disorders of Children.* Englewood Cliffs, N.J.: Prentice-Hall, Inc., 1969.

BLAKE, J. N. "A Therapeutic Construct for Two Seven-Year-Old Nonverbal Boys." *Journal of Speech and Hearing Disorders,* XXXIV (1969), 362–69.

CARROW, SISTER M. *Test for Auditory Comprehension of Language.* Austin, Texas: Educational Concepts, 1973.

CHAPPELL, G. E. "Childhood Verbal Apraxia and Its Treatment." *Journal of Speech and Hearing Disorders,* XXXVIII (1973), 362–68.

CHOMSKY, N. and M. HALLE. *The Sound Pattern of English.* New York: Harper & Row, 1968.

CRABTREE, M. *The Houston Test for Language Development.* Houston: Houston Tests Company, 1963.

—— and E. PETERSON. "The Speech Pathologist As a Resource Teacher for Language/Learning Disabilities." *Language, Speech, Hearing Services in the Schools,* V (1974), 194–97.

EGLAND, G. *Speech and Language Problems.* Englewood Cliffs, N.J.: Prentice-Hall, Inc., 1970.

FAY, W. "On the Echolalia of the Blind and of the Autistic Child." *Journal of Speech and Hearing Disorders,* XXXVIII (1973), 478–89.

GOLDMAN, R. and M. LYNCH. *Goldman-Lynch Sounds and Symbols Development Kit.* Circle Pines, Minn.: American Guidance Service, Inc., 1971.

GRAY, BURL and BRUCE RYAN. *A Language Program for a Nonlanguage Child.* Champaign, Ill.: Research Press, 1973.

—— and L. FYGETAKIS. "The Development of Language As a Function of Programmed Conditioning." *Behavior Research and Therapy,* VI (1968), 455–60.

HATTEN, J., T. GOMAN, and C. LENT. *Emerging Language.* Westlake Village, California: Learning Business, 1973.

HEGRENER, J. R., N. R. MARSHALL, and J. A. ARMAS. "Treatment As an Extension of Diagnostic Function: A Case Study." *Journal of Speech and Hearing Disorders,* XXXV (1970), 182–87.

HEWETT, P. M. "Teaching Speech to an Autistic Child Through Operant Conditioning." *American Journal of Orthopsychiatry,* XXXV (1965), 927–36.

HOLLAND, A. L. "Language Therapy for Children: Some Thoughts on Context and Content." *Journal of Speech and Hearing Disorders,* XL (1975), 514–23.

IRWIN, JOHN V. and MICHAEL MARGE. *Principles of Childhood Language Disabilities.* Englewood Cliffs, N.J.: Prentice-Hall, Inc., 1972.

JOHNSON, D. and H. MYKELBUST. *Learning Disabilities: Educational Principles and Practices.* New York: Grune and Stratton, 1967.

KERR, N., L. MEYERSON, and J. MICHAEL. "A Procedure for Shaping Vocalizations in a Mute Child." in L. Ullman and L. Krasner, (eds.) *Case Studies in Behavior Modification* (New York: Holt, Rinehart & Winston, 1965).

KIRK, S., J. McCARTHY, and W. KIRK. *The Illinois Test of Psycholinguistic Abilities* (Res. ed.) Urbana: University of Illinois Press, 1968.

LEE, L. L. "A Screening Test for Syntax Development." *Journal of Speech and Hearing Disorders,* XXXV (1970), 103–12.

—— "Linguistic Approaches to Developmental Language Disorders." *Folia Phoniatrica,* XXVI (1974), 33–67.

—— *The Northwestern Syntax Screening Test.* Evanston, Ill.: Northwestern University Press, 1969.

—— and S. CANTNER. "Developmental Sentence Scoring: A Clinical Procedure for Estimating Syntactic Development in Children's Spontaneous Speech." *Journal of Speech and Hearing Disorders,* XXXVI (1971), 315–40.

—— R. A. KOENIGSKNECHT, and S. MULHERN. *Interactive Language Development Teaching.* Evanston, Ill.: Northwestern University Press, 1975.

LEONARD, L. B. "Teaching By the Rules," *Journal of Speech Hearing Disorders,* XXXVIII (1973), 174–283.

—— "What is Deviant Language?" *Journal of Speech and Hearing Disorders,* XXXVII (1972), 427–46.

LENNENBERG, E. H. "Case Report. Understanding Language Without Ability to Speak." *Journal of Abnormal and Social Behavior,* LXV (1962), 419–25.

LEREA, L. *The Michigan Picture Language Inventory.* Ann Arbor: University of Michigan Press, 1958.

LILLYWHITE, H. S. and D. P. BRADLEY. *Communication Problems in Mental Retardation: Diagnosis and Management.* New York: Harper & Row, 1969.

LOVAAS, O. I. "A Program for the Establishment of Speech in Psychotic Children." Chapter 7 in H. N. Sloans and B. D. Macauley (eds.) *Operant Procedures in Remedial Speech and Language Training.* (Boston: Houghton-Mifflin Co., 1968).

—— L. Schreibman, and R. L. KOGEL. "A Behavior Modification Approach to the Treatment of Autistic Children." *Journal of Autism Childhood Schizophrenia,* IV (1974), 111–29.

McGRADY, H. J. "Language Pathology and Learning Disabilities." New York: Grune and Stratton, 1968, 199–233.

MECHAM, J. J., L. T. JEX, and J. D. JONES. *Utah Test of Language Development.* Salt Lake City, Utah: Woodruff, 1967.

MENYUK, P. *Sentences Children Use*. Cambridge, Mass.: M.I.T. Press, 1969.

MICHAEL, MARGE. "The General Problem of Language Disabilities in Children." in John Irwin and Michael Marge (eds.), *Principles of Childhood Language Disabilities*. (Englewood Cliffs, N.J.: Prentice-Hall, Inc., 1972).

REES, NORMA S. "Bases of Decision in Language Training." *Journal of Speech and Hearing Disorders*, XXXVII (1972), 283–304.

RENFREW, C. E. "Speech Problems of Backward Children." *Speech Pathology and Therapy*, II (1959), 35.

RIMLAND, B. *Infantile Autism*. Englewood Cliffs, N.J.: Prentice-Hall, Inc., 1964.

RUBEN, H., A. BAR, and J. H. DWYER. "An Experimental Speech and Language Program for Psychotic Children." *Journal of Speech and Hearing Disorders*, XXXII (1967), 242–48.

SCHELL, R., E. J. STARK, and J. J. GIDDON. "Development of Language Behavior in an Autistic Child." *Journal of Speech and Hearing Disorders*, XXXIII (1968), 42–7.

SCHLANGER, B. B. "A Longitudinal Study of Speech and Language Development of Brain-damaged Retarded Children." *Journal of Speech and Hearing Disorders*, XXIV (1959), 358–59.

SKINNER, B. F. *Verbal Behavior*. New York: Appleton-Century-Crofts, 1957.

SLOANE, H. N., M. K. JOHNSTON, and F. H. HARRIS. "Remedial Procedures for Teaching Verbal Behavior to Speech Deficient or Defective Young Children." Chapter 5 in H. N. Sloan and B. D. Macauley, (eds.), *Operant Procedures in Remedial Speech and Language Training*. (Boston: Houghton-Mifflin Co., 1968).

STUECHER, U. *Tommy: A Treatment Study of an Autistic Child*, Arlington, Va.: Council for Exceptional Children, 1972.

SULZBACHER, S. and J. A. COSTELLO. "A Behavior Strategy for Language Training of a Child with Autistic Behaviors." *Journal of Speech and Hearing Disorders*, XXXV (1970), 256–76.

TAYLOR, O. and D. SWINNEY. "The Onset of Language." in J. V. Irwin and M. Marge (eds.), *Principles of Childhood Language Disabilities*. (Englewood Cliffs, N.J.: Prentice-Hall, Inc., 1972), 53–62.

ULLMAN, L. and L. KRASNER. (eds.) *Case Studies in Behavior Modification*. New York: Holt, Rinehart & Winston, 1965.

WESSELL, M. H. "A Language Development Program for a Blind Language Disordered Preschool Girl." *Journal of Speech and Hearing Disorders*, XXXII (1967), 331–36.

WOOD, BARBARA. *Children and Communication*. Englewood Cliffs, N.J.: Prentice-Hall, Inc., 1976.

WOOD, N. *Delayed Speech and Language Development*. Englewood Cliffs, N.J.: Prentice-Hall, Inc., 1964.

WYATT, G. L. *Language Learning and Communication Disorders in Children*. New York: Free Press, 1969.

YOUNG, E. H. and S. STINCHFIELD-HAWK. *Moto-Kinesthetic Speech Training*. Stanford, Calif.: Stanford University Press, 1955.

YUDKOVITZ, E. and E. ROTTERSMAN. "Language Therapy in Childhood Schizophrenia: A Case Study of Monitoring and Feedback Approach." *Journal of Speech and Hearing Disorders*, XXXVIII (1973), 520–32.

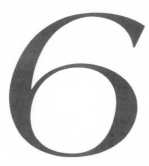

6

DISORDERS OF ARTICULATION

Of all the speech disorders, those of articulation are found most frequently. At least eighty percent of the case loads of those speech pathologists who work in the public schools is comprised of children who have not mastered the phonology of our language, children who erroneously substitute one phoneme for another, or omit or distort other sounds. They are handicapped because their speech deviates from the norms of our society, a society that depends upon effective communication and demands it.

Disorders of articulation vary widely in severity, from speech which is almost entirely unintelligible to a tiny transitional lisp in which a *th* /θ/ sound prefaces or follows the /s/ as in "sthoup" /sθup/ or "yeths" /jɛθs/. Generally, the more defective sounds that are exhibited by the client, the more severe will be the speech handicap. An articulatory error on a single sound can be quite noticeable, but when many standard sounds are defectively produced there is also a marked decrease in intelligibility and this compounds the problem greatly.

It is hard for most normal speakers to appreciate the distress of persons, especially adults, who cannot utter some of their speech sounds correctly. They are mocked and mimicked occasionally, especially by children who overhear them. Frequently they are misunderstood or asked to repeat over and over again what they have just said. Listeners respond with half-hidden amusement when the mistakes occur. Some of our clients have told us that they often encounter the common impression that any adult who cannot "talk right" tends to be assessed by prospective employers as being incompetent or immature or weak-willed. After all, even babies learn to talk correctly! But besides these adverse listener reactions, there is also a feeling of helplessness and inadequacy that appears when a person

156

tries repeatedly to say his sounds correctly and cannot. We vividly remember a sweet old lady who had spoken correctly all her life until being fitted with the dentures which resulted in a high-pitched, shrill whistle every time she produced an /s/ sound. Each session used up a half box of our tissues as she wept her way through therapy. The dentist had done his utmost to revise the dentures to eliminate the *strident lisp,* but it was not until we taught her to anchor her tongue tip against her lower teeth as she made her sibilant sounds that the piercing whistle disappeared and she was unafraid to go to the grocery store again.

Children, especially the younger ones, do not seem to be as sensitive, for our society tolerates more deviant sounds in a child than in an adult, unless there are just too many such errors for his age, or if he cannot be understood often enough. Indeed, one of the major problems in helping children with articulatory errors, as we shall see, is that they do not recognize their mistakes. Nevertheless, there are some children who have been hurt very deeply by their jeering playmates or by parents who have "corrected" them blunderingly or cruelly and then rejected them when the inevitable failures occurred.

Professional Therapy: Diagnosis A professional speech pathologist begins his work with a person with an articulatory problem in a systematic way. Perhaps the first thing he does, as the relationship is being established, is to make a preliminary analysis of the sounds which are omitted or deviantly produced. A bystander might fail to recognize that this is going on as the clinician skillfully evokes enough speech to enable her to get a pretty good idea of the person's articulatory disability. We have been amused at the amazement expressed by students in training when at the end of such a casually conducted exploratory session, the clinician was able to identify not only all the defective sounds but their consistent or inconsistent errors and many of the phonetic contexts in which the usually defective sound was uttered correctly. "How does she do it?", they ask us, and we answer by saying that as she was talking to the client her well-trained "phonetic ear" was probably scanning the client's speech against an internalized phonetic inventory of the common errors.

Nevertheless, no matter how skillfull or experienced she is, the clinician knows that such a first impression is bound to be inadequate, and so she administers more comprehensive and systematic tests as soon as she accepts the client for therapy. There are just too many sound combinations to assess through casual conversation alone, and a phoneme may be defective in one combination or phonetic context when it is correct in another. This is important information since if the client is already able to produce the standard sound in some word positions or contexts, these can be used in treatment.

Varieties of Articulation Tests[1]   Although some speech pathologists construct their own test materials, we now possess several widely used instruments for determining proficiency in articulation. Of these, the *Templin–Darley,* the *Laradon,* the *Photo–Articulation Test,* and the *Goldman–Fristoe* tests are probably most representative. All of them employ pictures of common objects to elicit spontaneous speech. (Those of the Photo–Articulation Test are actual color snapshots of the objects, while the stimulus materials in the other tests consist of line drawings in black and white or in color.) The *Goldman–Fristoe* also uses a film-strip test as a supplement. The pictures are chosen to test the accuracy of each of the English phonemes in the various positions within the word. In addition, most of these tests provide either sentences to be read or repeated or stories to be retold, and they include other materials that will elicit samples of consecutive speech. Test forms for recording whether the errors are substitutions, omissions, or distortions are also available.

Another articulation test instrument, the McDonald *Deep Test of Articulation,* has a different format in that the test pictures and stimulus materials are presented in pairs, the child being asked to link their names together without pausing. McDonald feels that a person tends to misarticulate certain sounds only in certain contexts, and that deep testing will reveal many instances in which a usually defective sound will be produced correctly. He therefore devised stimulus materials that would present any given sound so that it precedes or follows each of the other sounds. For example, if the clinician desired to know whether a child could say the *th* sound correctly in a certain phonetic context, he would ask him to "See if you can make a 'funny big word' out of these two little words," and then show the child the paired pictures of *teeth* and *sheep* so that he will say "tee*thsh*eep" and with *tub* to make "tee*tht*ub," and again and again with a large number of other words. McDonald insists that the accuracy with which a sound is articulated varies not only with the type of consonant produced but also with the kind of overlapping movements characteristic of ordinary utterance. He says that the basic acoustic

[1] Sources of these tests will be found in the bibliography at the end of this chapter.

and physiological unit of speech is not the isolated sound but the syllable, and the consistency of an articulatory error will vary according to its role in arresting or releasing that syllable. One of the disadvantages of such a deep test lies in its length. To test every speech sound in every phonemic context would take far too much time to be practical. Therefore McDonald advises that the clinician check the spontaneous speech in conversation or in memorized material to locate the obvious errors before doing the deep testing. Deep testing will then locate the combinations in which the usually defective sound might be produced correctly as well as incorrectly. He has also devised a shorter form that deep tests for only those sounds which are usually misarticulated.

Screening Tests   Most of these tests may also be used not only to determine articulation proficiency and type of error, but also as screening tests—i.e., to locate the children in a given school system who may need speech therapy. A screening test is used, as Winitz says, "to provide a comparison of a child's articulatory performance with that of his peers." In the public schools where large numbers of children enter the elementary grades each year, the speech clinician has found that she must screen the children to find those with speech problems. Most of those she does find have articulation errors and so, as quickly as possible, she examines them, not at this time to analyze the articulation problems presented, but merely to locate them. She must identify those children from the others with normal speech or other types of speech disorders. Analysis will come later.

Type of Error   These diagnostic tests usually consist of sets of pictures, words, nonsense syllables, or reading materials which can be used to elicit the speech samples to be analyzed for error. Both spontaneous and imitative responses may be demanded because if a child can match the clinician's model through imitation and thereby produce a correctly articulated sound or word which usually he misarticulates, the prognosis seems to be better than if the child does not seem to profit from such stimulation. The test items present each of the phonemes as it would occur in the initial (the beginning) position of words, as well as the medial and final positions. In most of these tests, there are sufficient items containing the phonemes most frequently misarticulated (the /s/, /l/, /r/, /θ/ and their blends) so that if the client happens to say a specific phoneme correctly on a given test word but makes errors when it occurs in others, this can be ascertained. It's good to know that he can say it right on the test word but we must also make sure that his mastery of the phoneme is complete. Almost anyone could administer these articulation tests but it takes training before one is able to identify the inconsistencies and recognize and record the kinds of errors that are shown.

Generally, the more defective phonemes shown by a client the more he will be handicapped, and so the speech pathologist's report of the diagnostic examination will always show how many there are and what they are. When a child shows that he has not mastered eight or nine of the phonemes of our language, the clinician knows that a lot of work is ahead. Nevertheless, she is also vitally interested in the kinds of errors that have been revealed by her testing for certain types of errors are more difficult to eradicate than others. The distorted sibilants of lateral lisping, for example, are usually more difficult to correct than the substitution of a *th* /θ/ for the /s/ in a child with an interdental lisp. The same holds true for the distorted /r/ and /l/ sounds which are usually difficult to remedy. A child who substitutes a /t/ for the /k/ should have less trouble conquering that error than one who replaces the /k/ with a little cough-like glottal fricative. It is necessary, therefore, to scrutinize and analyze the articulatory errors.

Error Analysis in Terms of Distinctive Features   When the child shows multiple articulatory errors, the speech pathologist is also interested in their patterning for he knows that many of them may reflect the child's failure to discern or produce certain of the distinctive features which characterize the phonemes he does not produce correctly. Pollack and Rees (1972, p. 453) describe the phonological analysis in terms of four questions: (1) Is a specific feature totally absent from the child's repertoire? (2) Does a feature appear in combination with one or more other features, but not in combination with a different feature or set of features? (3) Are all the features present, but inappropriately incorporated into the child's phonemic system depending upon positional variables within a morpheme or word? (4) Are all the features pertinent to a specific phoneme present in one phonetic context (independent of position within the morpheme or word) but absent in another?

Let us give just one example of the usefulness of this sort of analysis:

One of the children with whom we worked never uttered any of the following phonemes correctly /s/, /z/, /θ/, /ð/, /f/, and /v/. Instead, she used various stop plosives as their replacements or omitted them entirely. For the sibilants, she substituted a /t/ or /d/; for the labiodentals she used /p/ or /b/; for the affricates she substituted a /k/ or /g/. The distinctive feature which was missing in all these misarticulations was that of *stridency,* so instead of teaching one sound after another we concentrated on teaching the girl to hiss and whistle and buzz, then to recognize the stridency feature in our own speech as we prolonged these sounds when we talked with her. Then we asked her to imitate us and to talk as we did in this peculiar way. As soon as she could do so with some adequacy, we then concentrated first on the /f/ and /v/ sounds and next on the /s/ and /z/ until when she spoke carefully she could speak words containing these sounds without error. Progress was very rapid thereafter and we never did have to teach her how to make the other phonemes. Once she had gotten the idea that some sounds had to have the little noises of stridency in them if they were to be spoken correctly, she then could apply the principle to all other sounds that required this distinctive feature.

Kinetic Analysis   The speech pathologist also makes an analysis of the articulation errors themselves, a kinetic analysis. It is important to know which sounds are being misuttered, but we need also to know how they are being produced. The label "lisp" is a *phonetic* term; the modifying adjectives "lateral," "occluded," "interdental," or "nasal" are *kinetic* terms. They describe how the error is being made. They refer to the *manner of production.* The term "lalling" is such a kinetic or kinesiologic term. It refers to the type of speech produced when the individual characteristically makes most of his speech sounds without raising the tip of the tongue from the floor of the mouth. It tells us only that his tongue position is at fault. If you were told that a child was a *laller,* all you could guess about his actual speech would be that certain of the consonants which normally are made with an elevated tongue tip would be defective. You could be sure that the /r/ would be defective; the /l/ probably would be poor, and perhaps the /dʒ/ and /tʃ/ or even the /t/, /d/, and the sibilants. Those would be the probabilities, but you could not be certain. Only by analyzing the manner of error production could you know what the person is doing incorrectly.

Each of the speech sounds can be incorrectly produced in several ways. The most frequent error of such *stop-plosives* as *k* and *g* seems to be due to (1) the wrong location of the tongue contact. Other errors include (2) the wrong speed in forming the contacts; (3)

the wrong structures used in contacts; (4) the wrong force or tension of the contacts; (5) too short a duration of the contacts; (6) too slow a release from contacts; (7) the wrong mode or direction of release; (8) the wrong direction of the air stream; and finally, (9) sonancy errors in which voiced and unvoiced consonants are interchanged. Examples of these errors are now given for illustration:

1. The child who says "tandy" for "candy" is using a tongue-palatal contact, but it is too far forward.
2. A breathy k sound [xki] for [ki], results when the contact is formed so slowly that fricative noises are produced prior to the air puff.
3. A glottal catch or throat click [ʔæt] for [kæt] is often found in cleft-palate cases. They make a contact, but with the wrong structures.
4. Insufficient tension of the lips can result in the substitution of a sound similar to the Spanish v for the standard English b sound.
5. When the duration of the contact is too short, it often seems to be omitted entirely. Thus the final k in the word sick [sɪk] may be formed so briefly that acoustically it seems omitted [sɪ].
6. Too slow a release from the contact may give an aspirate quality to the utterance. "Kuheep the cuhandy" [kʰip ðə kʰændɪ] is an example of this.
7. The lowering of the tongue tip prior to recall of the tongue as a whole can produce such an error as "tsen" for "ten" [tsɛn] for [tɛn]. In this error the case is not inserting an s so much as releasing the tongue from its contact in a peculiar fashion.
8. Occasionally the direction of the air stream is reversed and the plosion occurs on inhalation. Try saying "sick" with the k sound produced during inhalation, and you will understand this error.
9. The person who says "back" for "bag" illustrates a sonancy error.

Most of the errors in making the *continuant* sounds are caused by: (1) use of the wrong channel for the air stream (using an unvoiced l for the s); (2) use of the wrong construction or constriction ("foop" for "soup"); (3) use of the wrong aperture (a lateral lisp); (4) use of the wrong direction of the air stream (nasal lisp, inhaled s); (5) too weak an air pressure (acoustically omitted s); (6) the presence of nonessential movements or contacts (t for s, occluded lisp); and (7) cognate errors (z for s, or vice versa).

Most of the errors in making the *glide* sounds are produced by combining the types of errors sketched above. They may be generally classed as movement errors. They include: (1) use of the wrong beginning position or contact ("yake" for "lake"); (2) use of the wrong ending position [fɪu] for [fɪr]; (3) use of the wrong transitional movement in terms of speed, strength, or direction [rweɪd] for [reɪd]; (4) the presence of nonessential contacts or positions [tjɛlou] for [jɛlou]; (5) cognate errors [wɛn] for [hwɛn].

It is necessary to analyze any given articulation error according to the above scheme so as to understand its nature. It is not sufficient merely to start teaching the correct sound. We must also break the old habit. Many of our most difficult articulatory cases will make rapid progress as soon as they understand clearly what they are doing wrong. Insight into error is fundamental to efficient speech correction.

To show you how we would record the results of a *kinetic* analysis, let us present the summary report of both the phonetic and kinetic procedures:

Client

Summary of errors:		Phonetic	Kinetic
k/g	(I.M.F)		Confusion of voiced and unvoiced
t/d	(I,M,F)		sounds; cognate or sonancy errors.
f/v	(I,M,F)		
s/z	(I,M,F)		Ditto: Vocal cords silent.
θð	(I,M,F)		″ ″ ″ ″
w/r	(I,M)		Uses lip glide instead of tongue glide.
−r	(F)		The *r* position was made but it was unvoiced.

This client mastered all of his errors at once except the w/r. He was taught the concept of cognates: that there are pairs of sounds, articulated in much the same way, but one is voiced or sonant while the other is unvoiced or surd. He learned that the /v/ was made by having his vocal cords vibrate as he made the lip-teeth position for an /f/. He found out that the /s/ was a whispered /z/. By feeling both his own and his clinician's throat as the pairs of sounds were produced, he learned to discriminate between them. By holding his fingers in his ears as he shifted from the prolonged /s/ to a prolonged /z/, he learned to recognize one sound from its twin.

Under What Conditions Do the Articulation Errors Occur? In studying any articulation case it is also necessary to discover the circumstances in which the errors occur. Some of our lispers have difficulty with their sibilants only when emotional. We worked with an exasperating case who never made an error when speaking at a normal rate of speed, but who became unintelligible when hurried. Some children can utter words perfectly when repeating from a model and yet substitute, omit, and distort their speech sounds in spontaneous speech. Some children who can produce every consonant correctly in isolation or in nonsense syllables will seem to be unable to use them in meaningful words. All of these observations point to the necessity for studying the articulation errors in terms of the type of communication being used. The importance of these factors in therapy is obvious. It would be silly to spend a lot of time drilling a child to produce the /r/ sound in nonsense syllables if he has always been able to do so. For these reasons, we examine each error in terms of the following: (1) type of communicative situation, (2) speed of utterance, (3) kind of communicative material, (4) discrimination ability. Here is a typical summary report:

> Our analysis of the conditions under which articulation errors occurred is as follows: Jackson substituted θ/s (I,M,F) and ð/z (I,M,F) consistently in swift, emotional speech, swift nonemotional speech, when carefully trying to speak correctly in oral reading, and when repeating single words after the examiner. One exception occurred: he said "six" correctly when repeating it carefully. He made the same errors on nonsense syllables when they were spoken at fast speeds, but had good final *s* sounds occasionally when the nonsense syllables were spoken slowly. He prolonged good isolated *z* sounds when prolonged with teeth closed. The *s* was only occasionally good in isolation, even with strong stimulation by examiner. He was always able to hear the error in another's speech but did not seem to be able to hear his own except on isolated words.

The only reason for such diagnostic procedures is that they may help us in therapy. In the above case, the therapy plan called for the teaching of the /z/ sound prior to the teaching of the *s*. A great deal of discrimination ear training was used. Recordings and auditory training units, which enabled Jackson to hear his own /z/ and /s/ at high amplification, were used. The /s/ sound was first taught by isolating it from the key word *six,* and no attempt was made to have oral reading or conversation employed in therapy until the new sounds were thoroughly habituated. The /s/ sound was used in the final position of nonsense syllables (*ees-oss-oos*) and in the final position of familiar words (*house, glass, ice*) before it was taught in the initial position (*see, sandwich, sick*). By analyzing the conditions under which errors occur, we are able to treat our cases much more efficiently.

Misarticulation: Its Causes

Although it is essential that the articulatory errors be identified if we can hold any hope for their correction, the speech pathologist also tries to determine why they exist, why this person failed to master his phonology. Therefore, in the diagnostic examination, he always tries to see if there are any perceptual, organic, or developmental factors still existing which he must take into account as he plans his therapy. Some of his exploration may require parental interviews; some of it involves the use of certain tests; all of it demands careful observation.

Hearing Loss As we found in our discussion of language disabilities, impaired hearing can create many difficulties and we certainly find this factor playing a part in the mastery of standard articulation. If a child cannot hear a sound with fidelity or if it is perceived distortedly, that sound will be difficult to produce correctly. While we shall consider this matter more fully in our chapter on hearing disorders, we should make clear at this point that some children have a loss of auditory acuity that affects the perception of all the phonemes, while others who can hear certain sounds very well may be unable to identify the characteristic features of other sounds. In high-frequency hearing loss, for example, the vowels and voiced sounds may be heard very clearly, whereas the high-pitched sibilants such as the /s/ may be heard so faintly as to be virtually non-existent to the child. Speaking loudly, or shouting at him will only amplify the sounds he can already hear and mask out those he hears weakly. Moreover, due to the hearing loss, even if he hears the sound, he may hear it so distortedly that it cannot serve as a model for correction.

Auditory Memory Span There are some few children who find it very difficult to remember sounds even when they can hear them. Sounds disappear very swiftly once they are spoken. In the swift rush of conversation the life of a given consonant is very brief—much shorter than a fruit fly's. Most of us find it easy to hold a familiar sound in memory, but have great difficulty in hanging onto one that is strange. It seems to fade so fast. We even find it difficult to repeat a snatch of our own free babbling or jargon after a short period of silence. Most children with articulation errors do not have defective auditory memory spans. They can hold a sound as well as we can. But there are others who have much difficulty. They may remember the meaning but not the characteristics of the sounds which have been spoken. Indeed, often they cannot even recall how they have uttered their own sounds. We can readily see how such a disability would make it difficult to correct articulatory errors. Fortunately, it is possible to improve this deficiency through training.

Phonetic Discrimination   As we said earlier, many children with misarticulations as such find it difficult to identify the sounds that give them trouble. Often they will say things like "But I did say tandy!" when corrected by their parents. Since this apparent inability to tell the error from the correct phoneme is bound to play an important part in the design of therapy, speech pathologists frequently administer tests of discrimination. You might even see them placing a little object (see Figure 17) on a child's tongue and then asking him to draw it or to pick out a picture that represents it. This is called a test of *oral stereognosis,* and it is used to determine whether or not a client has difficulty in discriminating the tactual and kinesthetic sensations that are important in the production of speech sounds. Locke (1969), for example, found that ten children with poor oral stereognosis were less able to learn new consonants than a matched group whose tongues could recognize the objects.

But most of the discrimination difficulties shown by persons with articulatory errors are auditory, not tactile or kinesthetic. If a child cannot tell the difference between a *th* /θ/ and an /s/, if in other words the /θ/ seems to him to be merely a nondistinctive variant or allophone of the /s/, then how could he be expected to say that sibilant without error? Much research has been conducted to determine whether or not the majority of children with misarticulations show such discrimination difficulties, and although there are some negative findings, most of the studies do seem to indicate that inadequate auditory discrimination ability is an important factor, especially with regard to the phonemes they cannot produce correctly (Powers, 1971). Speech pathologists, therefore, often include some testing of discrimination in their diagnostic examination.[2]

Tests of Phonetic Discrimination Ability   One of the problems in using these tests is that they may be based on the erroneous assumption that the child's main discrimination problem lies in being able to discern the differences between two sounds (such as the /t/ and /k/) *when they are presented in pairs by the clinician.* His big difficulty, however, often

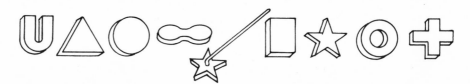

Figure 17   Some of the forms used in testing oral stereognosis.

[2] Three of the standardized tests being used widely at the present time are the Templin (1957), the Wepman (1958), and the Goldman-Fristoe-Woodcock (1969). (See references at end of chapter.)

seems to be in comparing *his own* sound with the standard sound. He may know very well that the /t/ and /k/ as produced by another speaker are different, but he may not recognize at all that the /t/ he used in the word "candy" is not the /k/ sound that others use in that word. Aungst and Frick (1974) and others have shown, for example, that many children who can easily distinguish between two sounds when they are produced by another speaker, have trouble doing it when they have to compare their own utterance with that of another. Most clinicians know this, and so they seek to determine the child's awareness not only of his own error but also his ability to distinguish it from the standard sound.

Stimulability   A clinician's diagnostic report on a client with an articulatory disability will also include an assessment of the person's ability to say the usually defective sound correctly when strongly stimulated. Beginners in speech pathology are often amazed to find that a child can sometimes produce the correct sound immediately if it is presented in isolation or in a nonsense syllable. Of course, this does not mean that he will also be able to say it in a word he has misarticulated thousands of times or that he can use it correctly in connected speech. However, if a child can make a certain phoneme correctly under strong auditory and visual stimulation it usually means that he will master it more easily than another phoneme which does not respond to such stimulation. Often, if six or seven phonemes are in error, the clinician elects to begin therapy with those he can imitate after strong stimulation.

Organic Factors   Most of the research (as reviewed by Winitz, 1969) seems to indicate that organic deviations of the tongue or other articulatory structures do not play an important part in the problems presented by most children with defective phonemes. Nevertheless, the speech pathologist finds some clients which seem to present an exception to this general rule. One of them was a child who had filled his mouth with lye, resulting in speech which was so slurred as to be almost unintelligible. His clinician noticed, however, that the child could elevate the middle and back of the scarred tongue to some degree. Accordingly, she formulated a therapy program in which the child was taught to speak with his teeth held together and to use the bulging middle of his tongue to produce pretty fair facsimiles of the front consonants. If you will try to talk with your teeth together and the tongue tip flat in the mouth you will see that it is possible to speak intelligibly this way if you speak very slowly and carefully, though some muffling occurs. Later therapy activities allowed the child to open his mouth more widely and took care of that problem.

In Figure 18 you will find another child, one with a frenum so short that he found difficulty in learning his /l/, /r/, and /s/ sounds since he was unable to raise the tip of his tongue. This so-called "tongue-tie" is rarely found to play a part in an articulatory problem, but when it does the speech pathologist, of course, notes it on his diagnostic report and refers the client to a physician for surgery or plans a program for teaching compensatory ways of producing the sounds which are made incorrectly.

Figure 19 shows another person, a girl with a different organic problem, a severe malocclusion, who presented several error sounds, notably distortions of the /s/, / z/, /r/, and /l/, along with some unseemly facial contortions as she vainly tried to compensate for her extreme overbite. Occasionally, speech pathologists have to work with clients who, because of cancer surgery, accident, or paralysis, have lost much of the tissue or use of their tongues. These are often diffi-

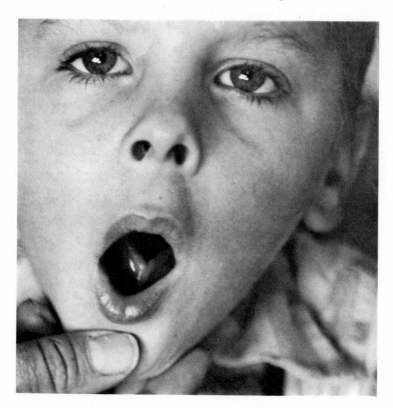

Figure 18 Tongue-tie.

cult clients to work with, but we have found that they can achieve good articulation when taught to compensate for their disabilities.

Motor
Incoordination
Difficulties

Since the speech pathologist knows that the production of certain phonemes requires the simultaneous and successive timing of many muscle contractions, he is always alert for any evidence of poor motor ability. Anyone who has observed the difficulty that children with cerebral palsy show in walking or writing will not be surprised to find that they also may have misarticulations. Motor coordination ability must also be assessed.

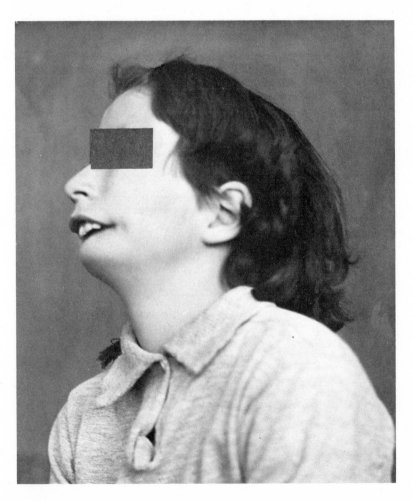

Figure 19   Malocclusion (overbite).

The articulatory disorders shown by most of our clients, however, represent a non-organic problem. Most of them have simply failed to master the phonology of our language. The technical term for their articulation problem is *dyslalia.* But when, as in cerebral palsy, brain damage creates a real motor disability, the problem is called *dysarthria.* The speech of a client with a partially paralyzed tongue is termed *dysarthric,* as is that of adults who formerly spoke normally before they contracted such diseases as multiple sclerosis or musculature dystrophy. It should be understood that these are etiological (causal) terms and that they do not describe different types of defective sounds. (The distorted /r/ and /l/ sounds of a person with dysarthria may sound little different from those of a person with severe dyslalia.) In many ways, both terms are unsatisfactory. Some so-called dyslalics show a certain clumsiness in coordinating their tongues, a minor motor disability confined primarily to speech rather than to gross motor coordinations, and yet they show no other neurological signs of brain or nerve damage.[3] Long ago, speech clinicians spent much of their time in administering tongue exercises to all children with articulatory problems of every kind; this is not our present practice. Winitz's (1969) summary of the research, for instance, indicates that motor disability is not a general characteristic of these clients. Nevertheless, most speech pathologists incorporate some assessment of this factor in their diagnostic examinations.

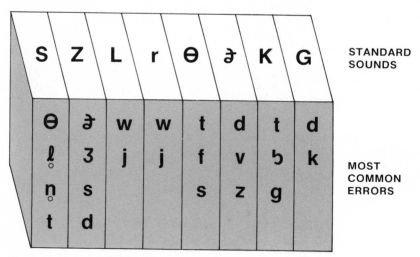

Figure 20   Common consonantal errors (most frequent substitutions).

[3] Muriel Morley, the British speech pathologist, in her book, *The Development and Disorders of Speech in Childhood* (Baltimore: Williams and Wilkins, 1972) has described some of these motor disorders under the headings of *developmental dysarthria* and *developmental dyspraxia.*

Predictive Tests   Since there are large numbers of children who seem to be able to master their defective sounds without therapy, it would be a waste of time to treat them. The problem is to know which ones they are. This is a problem frequently encountered by the public-school speech pathologist who often has case loads so large that she must always put certain children on waiting lists. Several attempts have therefore been made to determine whether or not articulation tests could be made prognostic, i.e., whether they could discover and identify those misarticulating children who will be able to master their standard sounds without therapy. The *Laradon Articulation Scale* yields a prognostic score, but to date no data are available to indicate its reliability or predictive validity. Since several studies had indicated that such a predictive test was possible, Van Riper and Erickson (1969) devised the *Predictive Screening Test of Articulation (PSTA)*, an instrument which, when applied to first-grade children with articulation errors, seems able to predict fairly well those children who will "outgrow" their misarticulations by the time they enter third grade.

Summarizing the   To illustrate how we bring all the test and interview data to-
Diagnostic   gether to give an overall picture of an articulation problem,
Examination   we provide the following illustrative report:

> *Case:* John Smith   *Age:* Ten   *Grade:* Fifth   *Referral:* Mrs. K. Jones
>
> *Informant:* Mother   *Examiner:* Madrid
>
> *Previous Therapy:* None   *Type of Disorder:* Articulation
>
> *Case History Data:* No foreign language background; parental speech and attitudes toward child, good. No evidence of imitation as a factor. Birth history normal. Developmental history: child experienced great difficulty in sucking; bottle fed with large opening in nipple required; digestive troubles during first two years of life; much crying, "little babbling." Normal physical development. Usual childhood diseases were mild. Cut tongue tip with paring knife at 22 months; no permanent injury or scar tissue; intelligence normal: Binet IQ at eight years was 108; good student and excellent reader (silently); well-adjusted child with no pronounced emotional conflicts or behavior problems; interests normal for his age; first words spoken at 13 months and was speaking in "long sentences" by his second birthday; parents tried to correct child by demanding he repeat his difficult words after them, but this method failed and no further attempts have been made except by the kindergarten

teacher, who also had no success. Child is aware of the fact that he does not talk correctly but is not too concerned. Some teasing to which he reacted by laughing and making his speech even worse.

Hearing: Audiometric examination reveals no hearing loss.

Organic Examination: No abnormalities. Palatal arch fairly high but with normal variation. No frenum interference.

Motor Coordinations: Large muscular coordinations adequate for his age norm. However, child seems unable to move tongue independently of jaw except at very slow speeds. Tongue thrust and strength seem normal. Tongue-curling and lifting are accomplished with great difficulty. Cannot sustain half-lifted tongue tip in a fixed position. It always returns to lower gum ridge, or teeth.

Perceptual Deficiencies: Auditory memory span normal; cannot discriminate *w* from *l* and made one error on *t* and *k;* cannot locate or recognize own errors in conversation or in single words; vocal phonics very poor: could integrate only two stimulus sounds (sh-oe); failed consistently in trying to integrate three sounds. Has little conception of words as sound sequences. Poor rhyming ability. Hears words as "chunks of sound."

Articulation Test Results: The *Templin-Darley Articulation Test* was first administered. Child cooperated fully. Of the screening test items, forty were produced correctly and ten defectively, thus showing that the child was performing at about the seven-year level at best. Three single sounds were misarticulated, the *k, g,* and *l.* Error types were as follows:

t/k   (I.M.F)   −k   (F)
d/g   (M.F)   −g   (F)
w/l   (I.M)   −l   (F)
o/l   (F)

All *l* blends (sl, pl, etc.) have the *l* omitted. All *kr* and *gr* blends defective. Occasionally defective *r* (I) distorted by lip protrusion.

Following stimulation, John could correctly articulate the *k* and *g* sounds in isolation and in nonsense syllables but not in blends of words. The final *l* was never uttered correctly, but stimulation produced it normally in consonant vowel (CV) syllables but not in words.

McDonald's *Deep Test of Articulation,* supplemented by other word combinations, was then given to John, using the cards for *k* and *l*. These sounds were correctly articulated in the following context: /uk/; /ok/; /nk/; and /tl/; /lt/ /nl/. We also discovered several key words in which the usually defective sound was employed correctly. They were "OK"; "Go"; and "li-" (Like).

Manner of Error Production: This case tends to anchor the tongue tip on the lower gum ridge and produces the acoustically correct *t, d,* and *n* as well as the defective sounds by raising the blade of the tongue instead of the tip.

Conditions Under Which Errors Occur: Case can produce the *k* in isolation [kə], but only with strong stimulation and at slow speeds. The *g* can be produced in isolation and in nonsense syllables in all positions by repeating after the examiner and without need for strong stimulation. Case also uses *g* occasionally in his conversation. Fails consistently if excited or hurried. Omissions of both these sounds in the final position are most prominent in swift conversation. Discrimination of correct versus incorrect sounds as made by examiner is good. Self-discrimination is poor. Child cannot produce or discriminate a good *l* sound even with strong stimulation. Error on this sound always occurs.

Intelligibility: Generally good. Occasionally when speaking swiftly or excitedly, some difficulty in understanding a word or two was experienced by examiner. Other children and his parents and teacher understood him readily.

Attitude Toward Prospective Therapy: Fifteen minutes of trial therapy were administered in which discrimination of /t/ from /k/ was attempted . Child seemed interested. Cooperative. Rapport easily established. Should be a good case if motivation can be achieved.

The Treatment of Articulatory Disorders

Once the speech pathologist has performed the diagnostic procedures described in the preceding section of this chapter, his next task is to design a tentative plan which takes into account the findings of that diagnosis. We use the word "tentative" because there will always be a need for revisions as the therapy proceeds. We remember vividly, and with some chagrin, one instance in which some new information suddenly caused us to work with a different client than the one we had examined. In taking the history we had asked the mother if the boy had any older or younger brothers or sisters with a similar speech problem and she had said no. What she had not told us was that he had an identical twin, the more dominant one of the pair, whose speech was almost unintelligible. So we worked only with that twin instead and the less dominant one, our original client, showed a swifter improvement than that achieved by the other. New information always comes in during the course of therapy and the clinician must always make adjustments to the treatment plan.

Designing the Therapy Program   Nevertheless, there are certain goals and subgoals which are to be found in all articulation therapy no matter how it is done or what strategies are used to enable it to be successful. (1) The client must become aware of the characteristics of the standard phonemes if they are to serve as the targets of treatment; (2) He must also come to recognize the characteristics of his misarticulations and how they differ from those target sounds; (3) He must discover how to produce the standard phonemes at will and be able to use them in isolation (/ssss/), in syllables (/sa/, /isi/, /os/), and in words and phrases or sentences. Finally, the client should be able to use the target sound in spontaneous speech of all kinds and under all conditions. This latter objective is usually included under the terms "transfer," "maintenance" or "carry-over."

There are differing points of view concerning the most appropriate way to structure the learning and unlearning process that takes place in articulation therapy. Our clients learn in different ways. For some, the cognitive kind of learning (in which the clinician structures the training so that vital insights can be achieved) seems most useful. Other clients learn the standard speech sounds more readily when the learning process is highly structured as when operant conditioning procedures are employed. Clinicians, as well as clients, show preferences for one or another of these approaches and so they design the kind of therapy which suits their own needs and competence. We suspect that most speech pathologists are as eclectic as this author and will use whatever learning strategy seems most promising in terms of the client's personality, motivation, perceptiveness, and response to different kinds of trial therapy. Moreover, it is possible to use different kinds of learning procedures at different phases of the treatment. Often, for example, in training a child to produce a phoneme which he has never made correctly, we have used the cognitive approach, then shifted to operant conditioning when we wished to strengthen the new sound or to extinguish the habitual errors which he no longer needs to make.

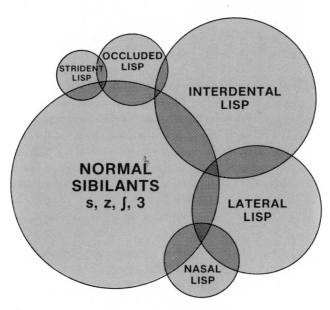

Figure 21   Types of sibilant errors. Where circles intersect, blends and distortions characteristic of the phonemes concerned are indicated.

The First Targets   If a client has only one misarticulated phoneme, it is, of course, the first target of therapy. However, most of our clients have more than one error, and so some decisions must be made. Few speech pathologists do what most parents do—try to correct all of the defective sounds at the same time. Instead, they decide to work on only one or a few of them with similar features (such as the cognates /s/ and /z/, or the /f/ and /v/ in which the manner of production is similar except for the feature of voicing.) Usually: (1) They select as the first targets those phonemes which occasionally in certain phonetic contexts (as revealed by deep testing) are already produced correctly; (2) Or they choose phonemes whose coordinations are relatively simple. (If a child has difficulty with the /r/, /l/, and /f/, they would begin with the /f/.); (3) Or they would choose the sound which responds most readily to strong stimulation. (If the child with /θ/ and /s/ errors can imitatively produce the /θ/ sound in isolation or a nonsense syllable but cannot make a good sibilant when imitating the clinician's /s/, that clinician would probably start therapy with the /θ/.); (4) Of a number of defective phonemes, those which are acquired earlier by normal children would be chosen over those that usually develop later (A misarticulated /k/ or /g/ sound would be worked with before an affricate such as the /dʒ/.) The clinician has to use her own judgment as to the importance of these features and at times disregard them altogether if other critical factors are present.

We worked with a little boy who had been teased unmercifully because he could not say his own name—Rodney. Though he had many other defective sounds which might have been easier to teach, which he could produce after stimulation, and use correctly in a few words, we chose instead to begin with the /r/. Once he had mastered it and was able to use it in his own name, the progress with all his other misarticulations was rapid. This illustrates again that motivation may be the most important factor of all in choosing the first target sounds.

The Operant Conditioning Approach   In the last few years many speech pathologists have begun to use operant conditioning procedures in their articulation therapy. Since we have presented the basic rationale for this approach in our chapter on language disorders, we shall not repeat this information here. However, we wish to emphasize that all of the goals and activities described in this chapter may be programmed according to the methodology of operant conditioning. Indeed, many of the commercially available operant programs for articulation disorders are based on some principles we have outlined.[4]

Were you to observe a speech pathologist using the operant approach in helping a child recognize the difference between the correct sound and its error, you might see him presenting paired sounds, syllables, or words and giving the child a marble for each time (or every three times) he correctly identifies that they are the same or different, and then later letting the child choose a small prize in exchange for those marbles. You would note that the speech pathologist has set up a hierarchy of discrimination tasks, beginning with the easy ones and then proceeding to those more difficult. He will establish baselines and then chart the child's progress as the criterion for each sub-

[4] Representative of these are the *Swirl Speech Articulation Kits for the /s/, /l/, /r/, and /θ/* (American Book Company, 300 Pike St., Cincinnati, Ohio); the *R-Kit for Articulation Therapy*, (Speech Systems, Albuquerque, New Mexico); the *S-Programmed Articulation Control Kit, rev. ed.* (Educational Psychological Research Associates, Palos Verdes Estates, California). There also are several texts containing operant programs for eliminating misarticulations. One of the most useful is R. D. Baker and Bruce P. Ryan, *Programmed Conditioning for Articulation* (Monterey, California: Monterey Learning Systems, 1971).

sequent step is successfully accomplished. At times, when the task seems too difficult (e.g., in identifying the clinician's deliberate errors in coversational speech), the program will be revised or *branched* with additional substeps until the child can again be successful and get his reinforcing tokens. Occasionally, the clinician will use *prompts* (helpful comments or suggestions) to keep the child progressing.

Speech clinicians have been using similar techniques for years but the program used by operant workers are much more systematized and objective. There is no doubt that such programs can help a client identify the distinctive features of the correct phoneme and to recognize his errors. However, in contrast to its use in facilitating discrimination, the application of operant conditioning methods in helping a person acquire a new sound initially has been less successful. Although some individuals are able to produce the correct sound as soon as they can tell the difference between it and its error, this is not usually the situation. Far too many persons just cannot discover by themselves the necessary coordinations that will produce it. If a lateral lisper, for example, never emits a normal sibilant, it is obvious that we have nothing that can be reinforced. Punishing such a person for his errors usually just makes the matter worse. In such a situation, programs are designed which involve what is called "shaping." A chain of target responses is set up, beginning with a sound the person can already produce, and then gradually progressing through a series of slight modifications which more and more resemble the standard sound. At each stage in the sequence, the patient is reinforced for successful production until that particular component sound in the chain is learned. Then this production is no longer reinforced and the client gets his reinforcement only when he varies his attempts enough to achieve the next transitional target sound. By working through this series of transitional sounds, the standard sound is finally acquired. We shall discuss and illustrate this shaping process later under the heading of "progressive approximation."

The Distinctive Some speech pathologists, however, set as their first targets
Feature Approach not the learning of the correct forms of one or two phonemes, but instead the discrimination and production of distinctive features. Linguistically oriented, these workers feel that the child either has not learned the rules that govern our phonology or has learned improper rules of his own. They, therefore, seek to help the child discover these rules, to recognize the distinctive features that he

omits or replaces with others. Weber (1970) illustrates this point of view:

(1) The main difference from traditional therapy was that an entire pattern was worked on by involving all the sounds in that particular category. In other words, the immediate goal was to correct a deviant pattern, not to correct one sound at a time. The child who had used stops for fricatives, was taught in one session to make /s/, /z/, /f/, /θ/; then in subsequent sessions these sounds were worked on as a group of sounds in order to teach and reinforce the common fricative element in each sound. (2) The second important difference stemmed from the use of contrasting sounds in the phonemic and auditory discrimination analyses. Therapy was based on pairing contrasting features. The child was taught not only to make voiceless fricatives but to contrast these sounds with the voiceless stops which he usually substituted for them. Throughout every stage of therapy the child was asked to make both the erred feature (e.g., voiceless stops) and the correct feature (the voiceless fricatives) one after the other.

The basic point of view of these linguistically-oriented clinicians is that the child does not need to learn how to make specific phonemes. Instead, they believe that once he is trained to discriminate and produce appropriately the distinctive features he needs in order to speak correctly, all the misarticulations containing these feature errors will tend to be discarded. As McReynolds and Bennett (1972) have stated and demonstrated: "If an error is a feature error, it should not be necessary to train the feature in all the phonemes in which it is relevant. The feature should generalize to other phonemes without specific training on each one."[5] (p. 264)

But just how does the clinician administer the distinctive feature approach? McReynolds and Bennett (1972) describe their procedures as follows: First the child was taught to produce the desired feature in the initial (the beginning) position of a nonsense syllable.

[5] More information on the distinctive feature approach to articulation therapy may be found in the following references: E. Pollack and N. Rees, "Disorders of Articulation: Some Clinical Applications of Distinctive Feature Theory," *Journal of Speech and Hearing Disorders*, XXXVII (1972), 451–62; J. L. Weber, "Patterning of Deviant Articulation Behavior," *Journal of Speech and Hearing Disorders*, XXXV (1970), 135–41; A. J. Compton, "Generative Studies of Children's Phonological Disorders," *Journal of Speech and Hearing Disorders*, XXXV (1970), 315–39. For some information concerning the limitations of this approach, see Harry Walsh, "On Certain Practical Inadequacies of Distinctive Feature Systems," *Journal of Speech and Hearing Disorders*, XXXIX (1974), 32–43.

In these syllables the feature was discriminated and then produced through imitation. Stridency, for example, was taught on the /s/ phoneme in these syllables, then generalized to other strident phonemes. Contrasts between strident and non-strident phonemes or productions of the same phoneme were made vivid by the clinician and taught to the child using the operant approach. Then the same procedure was used with the phoneme in the final position of nonsense syllables and words. This brief description probably does not do justice to the intensive therapy that was carried out, but it illustrates the basic methodology.

Traditional Therapy   Most speech pathologists do not confine themselves to either the operant or linguistic approaches we have described, although they may employ some of the procedures from each for special purposes in therapy. For example, they may use the distinctive feature approach when this seems appropriate to the discrimination difficulties of a child as he compares and contrasts the characteristics of the standard sound and its error. And again, they may use operant conditioning procedures only for strengthening and stabilizing a newly acquired standard phoneme. Or they may use neither.

The hallmark of traditional articulation therapy lies in its sequencing of activities for (1) identifying the standard sound, (2) discriminating it from its error through scanning and comparing, (3) varying and correcting the various productions of the sound until it is produced correctly, and finally, (4) strengthening and stabilizing it in all contexts and speaking situations. This process is usually carried out first for the standard sound in isolation, then in the syllable, then in a word, and finally in sentences. (See Figure 22.)

Operational Levels   The mastering of a new sound so that it can be used in all types of speaking may be viewed in terms of four successive levels: (1) the isolated sound level, (2) the sound in a syllable, (3) the sound in a word, and (4) the sound in a meaningful sentence. This is the staircase our patients must climb. Once they have reached the top step of this staircase they find a wide platform on which they must explore the communicative, thinking, social control, and egocentric functions of speaking, using the newly mastered sound in each.

With such a concept, it is possible for both clinician and client to know just where the latter is at each moment during therapy, and to know what has been achieved and what remains to be accomplished. There is no excuse for unplanned therapy, for random activity or busy-work when a child or adult is unable to talk as others do. The clinician has many responsibilities when working with an articulation case. She must establish a close relationship, provide many rewarding reinforcements, create situations in which learning can occur, and provide models not only of the correct utterance but also of scanning, comparing, varying, and correcting processes. But she has one other responsibility of paramount importance: She must know where the case is, where he has been, and where he has to go in therapy. And she must help the case to know too.

The Focus of Therapy   Since the essential error consists of a defective sound, it is upon this that we usually focus our therapy. Let us repeat: It is the *sound* which is in error. It is the misarticulated, nonstandard sound that spoils the syllable, spoils the word, spoils the sentence, and spoils whatever type of speech is being used. In whatever context it occurs, the acquisition and use of a standard sound must be our goal. The child's playmates say to him, "What's the matter with you? You talk funny. Say it this way!" and they provide him with an entire sentence to attempt. The child fails. Parents and teachers focus their therapy on the word level. "Don't say wabbit," they command. "Say rabbit!" The child fails again, or if, by chance, he does say it correctly, there is no transfer to any other /r/ word and there are thousands of /r/ words he must use. The speech clinician usually focuses her efforts on the sound first, and then on the syllable, for she knows that these are the foundation stones of standard speech. Once a lisper can make a good *s* in isolation, in various nonsense syllables, and has learned how to incorporate it in a few words, he has acquired the tools needed to conquer all *s* words. He need not learn each one individually.

As we have seen, some controversy exists as to whether the new sound should be taught in isolation, or in a syllable, or in meaningful sentences. Our own practice has been to begin with the level which seems most appropriate for the individual case. For example, if our client can make the correct sound at will in words and sentences but fails to do so consistently, we would probably begin at the sentence level. Thus we would even find the sort of treatment used by Marshall (1970) in treating an adult with an unrecognized and mildly inconsistent interdental lisp to be quite appropriate. What he did was merely to have the person talk spontaneously and to give him an electric shock every time he made an error. As the author states, "The patient understood the reasons for the use of punishment and was not overtly disturbed by the mild shocks administered during the

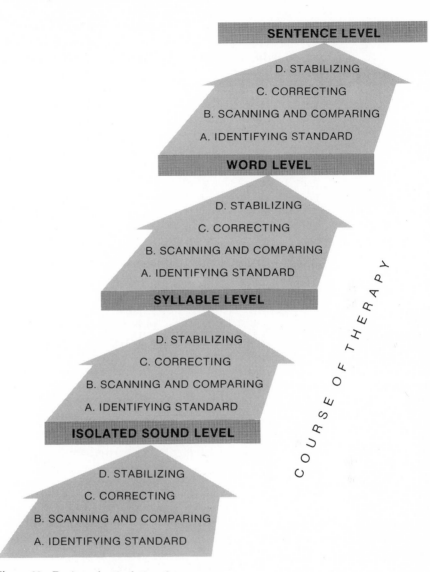

Figure 22 Design of articulation therapy.

conditioning segments of each therapy session." It is quite possible in such a case that the shock or the threat thereof served as an efficient alerting device as well as a punishment. But most of our clients do not present so easy a problem.

One of the reasons for the deep testing we described in the preceding section of this chapter is to identify those words (key words) in which the usually defective sound is used *correctly*. When there are a good many of these words, it is often possible to begin therapy by merely increasing their number and finding ways of implanting enough of them in the person's habitual speech until, through the process of generalization, the misarticulation disappears. Many normal children probably master their infantile misarticulations in this way. Again, if this testing reveals that a substantial number of certain syllables containing the sound in question are spoken correctly, we may begin immediately by working on syllables rather than isolated sounds. Some persons find it very difficult to break words into syllables or to recognize isolated sounds. With these we would probably begin at the word level. We also find persons with so many articulatory errors that their speech is almost unintelligible. It would be folly to begin treatment by concentrating on only one of so many defective sounds. Such persons need concrete evidence that they can indeed say something right, and they need it in a hurry. We would try to give them some intelligible words and phrases or sentences as soon as possible so that they can have some hope of being able to communicate. Nevertheless, most clinicians prefer to begin therapy by teaching most of their cases to produce the new sound in isolation. We feel that immediate and direct focusing upon the isolated sound or syllable has much to recommend it. It defines the target immediately. A new sound when mastered can spread very quickly to many syllables, many words, and not just those used in structured conversation. A child who learns to use the /th/ sound in "Thank you" in a pretended picnic in the therapy room may remember to say the phrase correctly when his father gives him a dime to spend; but he may have more trouble saying "birthday" or "think" or "bath" than those who have learned immediately to say "th." There are transfer problems in all types of articulation therapy.

Therapy at the Isolated Sound Level

All of the continuant sounds such as /s/, /l/, /r/, or /th/ can be produced in isolation since they are easily prolonged. Plosives such as /k/ and /g/ and affricates such as /ch/ can be uttered only syllabically; and so when we teach these in isolation, we begin usually by using the *schwa* (or neutral vowel), *uh*/ə/, or/ʌ/ to create syllables such as *kuh*, *guh*, and *chuh*. We work on only one or two target sounds at a time. When too many quail flush at once, most marksmen miss. We shoot better when we have our sights focused on a single target. Nevertheless, there are times when we do work with a group of sounds at once. If a child's multiple errors seem to be due to the fact that he has failed to distinguish between stops and fricatives, we would begin by helping him learn the contrasts between these features. Thus one of our children was almost unintelligible because (except for the nasals) the only consonants he used were the /p/ and /b/, the /t/ and /d/, and the /k/ and /g/. Instead of saying "We went swimming yesterday and I saw a fish," he said something like this: "Me met timmun tettaday and I taw a tit." With this boy we did not single out one sound as the nucleus of therapy. We began by teaching him to recognize the contrasts between sounds that "popped" and were made suddenly, and those that were prolonged. We showed him that he could prolong the /f/ and /sh/ and /v/ as he walked all the way across the room, but that this was impossible for the /t/, /d/, /p/, or /k/. We also rewarded strongly all words that he did say correctly.

Identifying the Characteristics of the Sound to be Taught   The task of learning to correct an articulation error is much more difficult than one might think. The stimulus sounds that a child must learn are very brief, and they vary with the phonetic context; different sense modalities are involved in the discrimination process. Their perception depends upon the sort of stimulation provided by others. Comparison of the standard sound with the error poses many problems. Many a child has persisted in his articulation errors simply because he has never really recognized the distinctive features of the standard sound. He has never heard it in isolation. At best the only help he has had is when others have said it to him, "Don't say fumb, say thumb!" The memory traces of sounds fade fast. Usually the sound he must learn has always been buried in the fast-flowing words, sentences, and communications of other people. The child, consumed by his need to listen for meanings, not for sounds, may hear the standard sounds flicker by, but he does not attend to them. Hidden as these sounds are in the fast torrent of speech, they have little stimulus value. Somehow we must make the characteristics of the sound vivid enough to be mastered. The task of the speech clinician is to aid the child to recognize the distinctive features of the correct sound and to know the contrasts between it and its error. We must help him know how it looks, and especially how it sounds. If the child already has some key words in which the usually misarticulated sound is spoken correctly, we can even help him pay attention to how it feels, and we can use tactile and kinesthetic cues to identify the target sound he has always been able to use correctly in these few words.

Discrimination of
the Target Sound
from Other Sounds

Here is an account of how a clinician tried to help a child who had a consistent interdental lisp to know the characteristics of the sibilants he had to learn:

Peter was a fast-talking child, and he talked freely and almost constantly. So far as I could tell, he was completely unaware of his consistent substitution of the voiced and unvoiced *th* for the /z/ and /s/ sounds. My first job was to get him to recognize these latter sounds as the ones he had to learn. Using a variety of activities in which he had to do something as soon as he heard me make an /s/ or /z/, I helped him to discriminate these from other sounds. For example, I covered him up with a towel which he could throw off; and he could "scare" me whenever he heard me make one of these sounds as I pronounced a series of isolated sounds, syllables, words, or finally, when I spoke to him in sentences. He missed some of these at first, but he learned rapidly. Next, I taught him to tell when the *s* sound occurred at the beginning or at the end of a syllable, first using nonsense syllables, then monosyllabic words, then longer words. I would pronounce a series of these, and it was his task to shout "Head" or "Tail," depending upon whether the /s/ occurred at the beginning or the end; and if he got the discrimination right, both of us would have to waggle our heads or tails. He enjoyed seeing me do this and learned swiftly when he made a misjudgment and I didn't do what he expected. When he got so he could locate these sounds in my speech pretty well, I then spent some time in showing him just what the /s/ sound looked like—that my teeth were together and my lips retracted—and also that in it there was a high-pitched hiss. By pantomiming isolated sounds, syllables, and words, some of which contained the /s/ sound and some did not, I taught him this visual discrimination. Then I put big paper sacks over our heads and repeatedly said the name of an object in the room which began with the /s/ sound, but he was not to throw off his sack and run to get the object until he heard the high-pitched hiss that I had set up as the signal. I fooled him a few times using *th* and *sh* sounds and laterally emitted sibilants before he got so he could recognize the high-pitched hiss of the correct *s* sound; but again he soon mastered the discrimination. Finally, I gave him a good dosing with some isolated and prolonged *s* sounds. I got behind Pete and made a continuous /s/ sound shifting my mouth from side to side. He was to indicate in which ear he heard it loudest. I varied the intensity. Then I told him his left ear was for the /θ/ sound and the right ear for the /s/, and he was to point to the one which represented the sound I was making as I made a series of them in isolation—syllables, words, and sentences. I did all of these activities in a forty-minute session, and at the end of the time I felt Pete had learned pretty well the characteristics of the sound he had to learn to make.

This account of a single therapy session illustrates very clearly how we can help a person define a sound he must learn to make. The speech clinician aided Peter to locate the sound, to isolate it, and to discriminate it from other sounds. She pointed out and demonstrated its distinctive features—how it looked and how it sounded. Instead of hiding it in the swift flow of her speech, she prolonged it and intensified it so that it had some stimulus value. She helped the boy to know the differences between the /s/ and the /θ/ sound he was using habitually to replace it. She could have used many other activities to attain the same goals, but those she used were evidently very appropriate to his needs. If a child fails to perceive the characteristics of his target sound, all the therapy in the world will not help him to acquire it. If a child is to know what his target is, he must learn to cock his ears in such a fashion that he can locate and identify the standard sound he must learn to make. He must learn to analyze the speech he hears in terms of its sounds rather than meanings. He must come to know the characteristic features of this new target sound. The lisper must learn to listen with strange ears, to recognize the high-pitched hiss of his clinician's /s/, to observe how she makes it. He must know when it is distorted and when it is right. He needs a model which he must match. Without such a model, how can he correct himself?

Please note that this is ear training, not mouth training. In this necessary perceptual defining of a standard pattern, the ear training period, we do not ask the child to attempt the new sound. Not yet. First let us be sure that he internalizes the model. In this first phase of therapy for articulation cases, the emphasis is all on listening. It is ear training.

Scanning and Comparing   Now the case must listen to himself. He now needs training in *self-hearing* rather than in listening to the speech of others.

By this time, he should have acquired a clear concept of the target sound. Now he must scan his own speech so that the differences between his own utterance and the standard sound will be made clear. Most of our clients have no idea of how they sound. Many of them do not even hear their errors. This is quite natural. When we speak we have to use our ears to find out what we are saying. Only rarely do we think before we speak. When we were babies, babbling in the crib, we listened to the sounds we were making and found joy therein. But once we learned the magical power of speech in sending messages, in formulating thoughts, in controlling others, we stopped listening to the sounds that emerge from our mouths. We had to keep our ears relatively free for receiving the *thoughts* of others and for scrutinizing our own meanings to see if they were well expressed. Perhaps this is why articulation errors persist. We do not hear them.

Somehow we must open up the invisible channel between the person's ear and his own mouth. We must help him to locate his errors whenever they occur. We must give them new vivid stimulus value. When the laller says a defective /r/ sound, some hidden signal must be triggered off somewhere within the skull. Usually the clinician has to do the signaling first, pointing out when the error has occurred. We have found that it is wise to make these signalings pleasant experiences to prevent the child from hearing echoes of past penalties.

Recalling, Perceiving, and Predicting Errors   In this training in self-hearing, we operate in a time dimension. At first the child recognizes his errors only after they have occurred; next, when they are occurring; finally, he can predict them. The wise clinician understands this natural sequence of recognition and uses it. She signals her perception of the child's error at first only after an interval sufficiently long to let him listen to what his mouth has produced.

In the simultaneous perception of the error as opposed to this delayed perception, one very effective device is to have the clinician read or speak in unison with the case with her mouth to his ear. If at the moment he makes an error, she signals by making the correct sound very loudly, or by stopping her own speaking, or by some other stimulation, he will be brought to notice it instantly. Another device is to have the child record some sounds, syllables, words, or sentences, a few of which contain the target sound, and then to require the child to say them again in unison with his own recorded speech. The clinician turns up the volume of the playback very loudly at the moment of error. There are many other ways.

In predicting errors, the clinician provides sample utterances on each of the various levels and then asks the child to predict whether or not he will make an error on them when he says them. Here is one example:

Clinician: I'm going to say three sounds: first, *mmmmmmmmm;* second, *ssss;* third, *ffff.* In a moment I'm going to ask you to say them but first you tell me on which one you think you might make a mistake: *mmmmm . . . sssss . . . ffff.*
Client: On the latht one.
Clinician: OK, let's see. Try them.
Client: Mmmm . . . th . . . ffff. Oh it wath the thecond.
Clinician: All right. Now let's try these syllables: *eepoo . . . ommee . . . issah.*
Client: Oh, it wath on the latht one.
Clinician: Right! Now try these words: *house . . . ham . . . heavy. . . .*
Client: Houth ith the one.
Clinician: Good. It should have been "house."

Evoking the New Sound   Once we have been able to establish a clear perception of the standard sound and have opened up the circuit of self-hearing so that the child can recognize and identify his errors, we are ready for the next step: learning to produce the new sound. As we have said earlier, this mastery of a new sound must be accomplished on all levels: isolated sound, syllable, word, sentence, and function, but we have found it most efficient to teach it first in isolation by concentrating on its motor and acoustic aspects. There are five different ways of approaching this task. The new sound may be taught by: (1) progressive approximation, (2) by auditory stimulation, (3) by phonetic placement, (4) by the modification of other standard sounds already mastered, or (5) by using key words. Each of these will be described in detail.

Varying and Correcting   Whichever approach is used—and there are times when we must try one then another—the person must go through a process of varying his utterance. Change must occur in the way he shapes his tongue, in the acoustic patterns which emerge from his mouth. One of the basic problems confronting the clinician at this stage of treatment is to provoke such variation. Long-practiced habits are very resistant to change. Often before we can hope to get our client to have a fair chance of hitting his target, we must get him to try new postures, new attacks, new movement patterns. Variation must precede approximation. By this we mean something similar to what happens when a person learns to shoot an arrow at a target. When he shoots and misses, he first must know that his second shot will have some chance of hitting a different part of the target, preferably a spot closer to the bull's-eye. But he must vary and he must try to correct. This same process occurs in articulation therapy. We must get our lisper to try and try again, but to try differently each time so that he comes closer and closer to producing the desired standard sound. Variation must precede approximation.

Progressive Approximation   This method is a trail-blazing procedure. The clinician joins the client and makes the same error the client makes. She then shows the client a series of transitional sounds each of which comes a bit closer to the standard sound until finally the standard sound is produced. Each little modification the client makes that comes a bit closer to the goal is rewarded. Those variations that move away from the target sound are ignored. Through this process, the *degree* of error is constantly determined; and new attempts are aimed at reducing the amount of deviation. The uniqueness of this approach is that it resembles the way that infants seem to acquire normal articulation. They do not suddenly shift from saying *wabbit* to *rabbit*; instead they seem to proceed through a series of gradual and progressive approximations as McCurry and Irwin (1953) have described. This also is the process known to psychologists as *shaping*. Instead of asking the person to exchange a correct sound for his incorrect sound, we help him to shift gradually from where he is to where he has to go. Let us observe some progressive approximation therapy.

Clinician: Now cup your hands like this so they make a channel from your mouth to your right ear. I'm going to talk into your left ear like this. (*Clinician cups her hands and speaks a sound into the person's left ear.*) Now we're going to try to make the new sound. Say *sssssssss*.

Client: Thththththththth. Thath no good.

Clinician: (Still talking into his left ear.): OK, let's do it again. This time I will join you and make the same sound so that we're in tune even if it is wrong. But then I'll change it just a bit and you try to follow me. I'm not going to change it all the way to the correct *sss* but I'll pull back my tongue a little and that will make a different sound. Try to follow me. But we'll start with your sound. Say *sssss*.

Client: Thththththththth.

Clinician: (In unison): **Ththth.** *(And then she makes a slight variation in the direction of the standard sound, and the case varies his sound also.)* Start with your old sound and let's try to shift a bit further like this. . . . *(Clinician illustrates the change the case has already made and a second change that comes even closer to the* sss.*)*

We feel that progressive approximation (shaping) is an excellent method for teaching a new sound. It permits reward for modification instead of reserving it for final attainment of the goal. It helps the identification of clinician and client. It reduces the task. It encourages variation. Even very resistant clients seem to move under this regime. We have found it very efficient.

Nevertheless, there are times when other methods are to be preferred. For example, if a child can make the new sound fairly easily with direct stimulation, we find it easier merely to ask him to imitate us. Again, some clients are unable to perceive tiny variations in auditory experience. They are not at all ear-minded. They have better visual or proprioceptive imagery than auditory imagery. With these we prefer to use the phonetic placement techniques. Finally, there are some children who have been defeated for so long in attempts to correct themselves that it is better to use the modification of sounds they have already mastered.

Auditory Stimulation   This method relies upon simple imitation and demand. An example might run as follows:

Clinician: Now, Johnny, I'm going to let you have your first chance to make the snake sound, *sss.* Remember not to make the windmill sound, *th-th.* This is the sound you are to make: *sss,sss,ssssss.* Now you try it.

If the ear training has been adequate, this simple routine, in which the wrong sound is pronounced, identified, and rejected, then followed by the correct sound given several times, will bring a perfect production of the correct sound on the first attempt. Occasionally it will be necessary to repeat this routine several times before it works, and the child should be encouraged to take his time and to listen carefully both to the stimulation and to his response. He should be told that he has made an error or that he has almost said it correctly. He should then be encouraged to attempt it in a slightly different way the next time. No pressure should be brought to bear upon him; and a review of discrimination, stimulation, and identification techniques should preface the new attempt. He should be asked to make it quietly and without force. The procedure may be slightly varied by asking the child to produce it in a whisper. After the sound has been produced, the cliniican should signal the child to repeat or prolong it and sense the "feel" of it. The attempt should be confined to the isolated sound itself or to a nonsense syllable beginning with it.

Phonetic Placement   The phonetic placement method of enabling a speech defective to produce a new sound is an old traditional method. For centuries, speech pathologists have used diagrams, applicators, and instruments to ensure appropriate tongue, jaw, and lip placement. Children have been asked to watch the clinician's tongue movements and to duplicate them. Observation of the clinician's mouth in a mirror has also been used. Many very ingenious devices have been invented to adapt these techniques for children, and sometimes they produce almost miraculous results. Unfortunately, however, the mechanics of such phonetic replacement demand so much attention that they cannot be performed quickly or unconsciously enough for the needs of casual speech. At best, they are vague and difficult to sense or recall. The positions tend to vary with the sounds that precede or follow them, and to teach all of these positions is an almost impossible task. Dental abnormalities may make an exact reproduction of the standard position inadvisable. Many speech pathologists produce the sounds in nonstandard ways, if, indeed, there is a standard way of producing any given speech sound. Despite all of these disadvantages, the phonetic placement methods are indispensable tools in the speech pathologist's kit; and when the stimulation method fails, they can be used. They are especially useful in working with the individuals with hearing defects, and they certainly help to identify the sound.

Excellent diagrams and descriptions of the various speech sounds may be found in the texts to which references are given at the end of this chapter. The speech clinician should have these texts available and should know the mechanics of articulation thoroughly enough to interpret the diagrams and assume the positions illustrated and described. The clinician should be able to recognize any sound from its description and diagram.

In using methods of phonetic placement, it is necessary that the child be given a clear idea of the desired position prior to speech attempt. If an adult, he should study diagrams, the clinician's articulatory organs in position, when observed both directly and in a mirror, palatograms, models, and the written descriptions of the mechanics whereby the sound is produced. Every available device should be used to make the client understand clearly what positions of tongue, jaw, and lips are to be assumed. It is frequently advisable to have him practice other sounds that he can make easily, using diagrams and printed descriptions to guide his placement. This will familiarize him with the technique of translating diagrams and descriptions into performance.

Various instruments and applicators are used to help the client attain the proper position. Tongue depressors are used to hold the tip and front of the tongue down, as in the attempt to produce a /k/ or /g/, or they may be used to touch certain portions of the tongue and palate to indicate positions of mutual contact. Tooth props of various sizes will help the student to assume a proper dental opening. Thin applicators and wedges are used to groove the tongue. Curious wire contrivances are occasionally used to insure lateral contact of tongue and teeth. Small tubes are used to direct the flow of air. In our experience, they are more dramatic than useful. Enforcing a certain tongue position through some such device produces such a mass of kinesthetic and tactual sensations that the appropriate ones can seldom be attended to. Usually, the moment the instrument is removed the old, incorrect tongue position is assumed.

If these devices and instruments have any real value, it seems to be that of vivifying the movements of the tongue, and of providing a large number of varying tongue positions from which the correct one may finally emerge. Many individuals have difficulty in realizing how great a repertoire of tongue movements they possess, and instruments frequently enable them to attempt new ones. When the correct sound has been produced (and frequently a lot of trial and error must be resorted to before it appears), the client should hold it, increasing its intensity, repeating it, whispering it, exaggerating it, and varying it in as many ways as possible without losing its identity. He should focus his attention on the "feel" of the position in terms of tongue, palate, jaws, lips, and throat. He should listen to the sound produced. Then he should be asked to leave the position intact but to cease speech attempt, resuming it after a long interval. Finally, he should let the tongue assume a neutral position on the floor of the mouth and then attempt to regain the desired position. Sounds produced by phonetic placement are very unstable and must be treated very carefully or they will be lost. Strengthen them as soon as possible and keep out distractions.

Modification of   Another special method for teaching a speech defective a new
Other Sounds   sound involves the modification of other sounds, either those
of speech, those that imitate noises, or those that imitate
other functions such as swallowing. These methods are somewhat
akin to those of phonetic placement, but they have the advantage of
using a known sound or movement as a point of departure for the
trial-and-error variation which produces the correct sound. The modification method may take many forms, but in all of them the sequence is about the same. The client is asked to make a certain
sound and to hold it for a short period. He is then requested to move
his tongue or his lips or jaws in a definite manner *while continuing to
produce his first sound.* This variation in articulators will produce a
change in the sound, a change which often rather closely approxi-
mates the sound that is desired. An illustration of this method may
be given. A lateral lisper is told to make the /θ/ sound and to prolong
it. Then, while continuing to make the sound, he is required to draw
in the tongue tip slowly and to raise the whole tongue, slowly scrape
its tip upward along the back of the upper teeth, and finally bring it
to rest near the alveolar ridge. The /θ/ will change as the tongue
rises, and a rather good approximation to the desired /s/ will be produced. If this is combined with ear training and stimulation, it will be
found to be very effective.

Key Word Method   As we have seen, one of the items in both voice and articulation tests requires the examiner to record all words in which
the usually defective sound is made correctly. Many speech pathologists fail to realize the value of these words in remedial work. They
may be used to enable the client to make the correct sound at will
and in isolation. They are also extremely valuable in getting the client
to make clean-cut transitions between the isolated sound and the rest
of the word. Finally, they serve as standards of correctness of sound
performance. Those with misarticulations need some standard with
which to compare their speech attempts at correct production of the
usually defective sound. Although occasional clients are found who
never make the sound correctly, the majority of them have a few
words in which they do not make the error. The clinician should be
alert enough to catch these when they do occur. Often these words
are those which have the usually defective sound in an inconspic-
uous place—that is to say, the sound occurs in the medial or final po-

sition, or is incorporated within a blend; seldom is it found in an accented syllable. She must train her ear to listen for it in the client's speech or it will escape her. At times it occurs in words in which an unusual spelling provides a different symbol for the sound. To illustrate: A child who was unable to make a good /f/ in any of his words using that printed symbol, said the word *rough* with a perfect /f/ sound. This was probably due to the strong stimulation given by the child's spelling teacher.

These words are worth the trouble needed to discover them. They simplify the clinician's work tremendously, since it is possible to use that sound as a standard and guide and to work from it to other words in which error normally occurs. The experienced clinician greets these nuclei words as veritable nuggets. Similarly, even when the client is highly consistent in his errors, there comes a stage in his treatment when he is saying a few words correctly. These words may be used to serve the same ends as those mentioned in the preceding paragraph.

The procedure used in this method is roughly as follows: The clinician writes the word on one of several cards (or uses a picture representing it). Then she asks the client to go through the series one at a time, saying the word on each card ten times. Finally, the special word to be used is repeated a hundred times, accenting and prolonging if possible the sound which in other words is made incorrectly. Thus the lingual lisper who could say *lips* correctly repeated the word one hundred times, prolonging the /s/. He was then asked to hold it for a count of twenty, then thirty, then forty. Finally, he was required to hold it intermittently, thus: *lipssss.ssss..sss*. The purpose of such a gradual approach is that the sound must be emphasized in both its auditory and its motor characteristics to prevent its loss when the student becomes aware of it as his hard sound. For example, one baby-talker made the initial /r/ in *rabbit* perfectly until told that he did. Immediately the child changed to the *w* substitution and was unable to make the initial /r/ again.

After the child has emphasized the sound a great many times, has listened to it and felt it thoroughly, and can make it intermittently and in a repetitive form, he may be asked to think the word and to speak the sound. It is often wise to underline the sound to be spoken, asking the child to whisper all but the letter underlined. Other sounds and other words may be similarly underlined if a careful approach is necessary. Through these means, the child finally can make the sound in isolation and at will.

Stabilizing the   One of the greatest causes for discouragement in treating an
New Sound   articulatory case may be traced to the parent's or clinician's
ignorance of a very important fact. A new sound is weak and
unstable. Its mechanics are easily forgotten or lost. Its dual phases of
auditory and motor sensation patterns are easily confused. Many
people believe that a complicated skill (such as that involved in a
speech sound) once achieved is never lost, although any musician or
tennis player will tell us that a new stroke or fingering sequence
must be practiced and strengthened a great deal before it can be used
in competition or concert. Many speech clinicians become discouraged and blame the client for his frequent relapse into error or
his sudden loss of the sound he had been taught to make. Many children who can make the correct sound at will never learn to incorporate it within familiar words. All of these unfortunate occurrences are
due to the fact that a new sound must be strengthened before it can
win the competition with the error in the speaking of common
words. A lisper who has said "yeth" for "yes" several thousand
times cannot be expected to say the latter as soon as he has learned
to make the /s/ sound in isolation. Perhaps that sound has been performed only three or four times. Yet parents and teachers constantly
ruin all of their preliminary work by saying some such sentence as
this: "Fine, Johnny. That was fine! You said /s/ just as plainly as anyone. Now say 'sssoup.' " And Johnny, ninety-nine times out of one
hundred, will say triumphantly, "thoup." Most speech clinicians
have to train themselves to resist this urge to hurry. When the child
has been taught to make the new sound, the utmost patience and re-
straint are needed.

When a new sound has just been born, it is a tender thing and
must be carefully treated. It should be repeated or prolonged as soon
as possible, but there should be no great hullabaloo over the achievement or it may be lost again.

During this repetition and prolongation, the client should be
told to keep a poker face and to move as little as possible. A sudden
shift of body position occasionally produces a change in the movements of articulation as well. As soon as the new sound tends to
lose its clear characteristics, the clinician should insist upon some
rest and should then review the procedure used to produce the
sound. Rest should be silent in order to let maturation take place.
Little intensity should be used; and when working with a pair of
sounds such as /s/ and /z/, the unvoiced sound is preferable. Often
sounds such as /l/ and /r/ should be whispered or sung.

After the child is able to produce the sound readily and can repeat and prolong it consistently, the clinician can ask him to increase

its intensity and exaggerate it. He should be asked to focus his attention on the "feel" of the tongue, lips, and palate. Shutting his eyes will help him to get a better awareness of the tactual and kinesthetic sensations thereby produced. Ask him to assume the position without speech attempt and, after a short period of "feeling," to try the sound.

After the client reaches the stage where he has little difficulty in producing the new sound, he should be encouraged to shorten the time needed to produce it. A sound which takes too long to produce will never become habitual. This speeding up of the time needed to initiate it may be accomplished by demanding fast repetitions, by alternating it with other isolated speech sounds, and by using signals. In this last activity, the client should keep his articulatory apparatus in a state of rest or in certain other positions, such as an open mouth; and then, at a certain sharp-sound signal, he should react by producing the new sound immediately.

One of the most effective methods for strengthening a new sound is to include it in babbling and the student should attempt to incorporate the new sound within the vocal flow as effortlessly as possible. It should not stand out and there should be no pausing before it. Doublings of the sound should be frequent. These babbling periods should be continued daily throughout the course of stabilization.

The most important of all strengthening devices is the use of simultaneous talking-and-writing. In this procedure, the client writes the script symbol as he pronounces the sound. The sound should be timed so that it will neither precede nor follow the writing of the symbol, but will coincide exactly with the dominant stroke of the letter. Since this dominant stroke varies somewhat with different persons, some experimentation will be needed. At first the clinician should supervise this talking-and-writing very carefully to ensure clear vocalization of the new sound and proper timing. Later the client can be assigned to hand in several pages of this talking-and-writing every day. The continuant sounds should be pronounced by themselves (*sss, vvv, lll*), and the stops should use a lightly vocalized neutral vowel (*kuh, puh, duh*). Simultaneous talking-and-writing techniques not only provide an excellent vehicle for practice of the new sound, but also give a means of reinforcing it by enriching the motor aspect of the performance. They also improve the identification and, as we shall see, make possible an effective transition to familiar words. For children who cannot write, the sound may be tied up with a movement such as a finger twitch or foot tap. In this case, as in writing, the timing is very important.

Articulation Therapy at the Syllable Level

As soon as the person has learned to produce the new sound in isolation whenever he tries to do so, we move immediately to get him to use it in syllables. You will recall that the second operational level is that of syllabic utterance in the sequence: isolated sound, syllable, word, and sentence.

Beginning with the Syllable   Some speech pathologists prefer to start with this syllabic level—to teach *ree* and *ra* and *roo* rather than *rrr*, because they feel that the syllable is the basic unit of motor speech. They also point out that many sounds such as the plosives /k/ and /g/ can only be produced syllabically and that prolonging an isolated sound distorts its pattern in time and creates unnecessary difficulty in shifting from sounds into syllables and then into words. Why not begin immediately with the syllable and teach *la-lee-lie-lay-lo-loo* instead of the isolated *llll* sound? We will not argue the point with any real vigor, for we have often begun therapy with the syllable in certain cases where the person seemed to produce the sound more easily therein than in isolation. For example, we have known several children who could produce the /l/ sound more easily in a syllable such as *lee* than they could in saying the isolated *llll*.[6] However, since we begin with acoustic ear training rather than with the motor aspect of speech, *the basic unit of auditory perception is not the syllable but the phoneme,* the sound. It provides one target rather than several. It transfers easily to many syllables once it is mastered in isolation so that there is no need to teach each syllable in turn. Moreover, when we have begun with the syllable, we notice that unconsciously our clients kept prolonging and stressing the sound anyway.It is the sound, not the syllable, which is the first target's bull's-eye in traditional therapy.

However, when therapy begins with the syllable, the clinician follows the same basic sequence we have outlined for the isolated sound. The standard acoustic and motor patterns of the various syllables as they occur in the speech of others are defined through ear training. Next, self-hearing of the person's own syllable production is scanned and compared with the features of the correct syllable to define the syllabic errors. Next, the same techniques of progressive approximation, auditory stimulation, and phonetic placement are used

[6] These two sounds, however, are not identical. The /l/ sound at the beginning of a syllable is more fricative and less vocalic than one used in isolation or at the end of a syllable such as *ol*.

196

to teach the isolated syllables. The process is the same; it is the target that differs initially. Moreover, once we have trained the person to make the sound in syllables, we usually return to the isolated sounds, pointing them out within the syllable so that the person comes to recognize the correction he has made.

Strengthening and Stabilizing the New Sound in Nonsense Syllables   Whether we begin with the syllable or the sound, our next major step in therapy is to help our client to use the new sound in all phonetic contexts. This is very important since any sound changes slightly whenever it is preceded or followed by other sounds. The /s/ in the nonsense syllable *seeb,* for example, is acoustically higher in pitch than the /s/ in *soob.* Also the contour of the tongue varies a bit with differing phonetic contexts. Since we must be able to produce the new sound in all possible combinations, we must have some means of teaching these variations. The nonsense syllable provides us with such a vehicle.

Types of Nonsense Syllables   There are three main types of nonsense syllables: *CV* (consonant-vowel syllables such as *la*), VC (vowel-consonant syllables such as *al*), and CVC (consonant-vowel-consonant combinations such as *kal* or *lod*). These syllables can be readily constructed by combining the new sound with the fourteen most common vowels and diphthongs. The first nonsense syllables to be practiced are those in which the transitional movements from consonant to vowel involve the fewest and simplest coordinations. For example, *ko* involves less radical transitional movements than does *kee.* The next nonsense syllables should be those which use the new sound in the final position *(ok)*; and, finally, those in which the new sound is located in the medial position *(oko)* should be practiced. Double nonsense syllables may also be used, but simple doublings are preferred *(kaka).*

These nonsense syllables should be practiced thoroughly before familiar words are attempted. The talking-and-writing technique can be used to facilitate their production if any difficulty is experienced. The client should speak the new sound as he writes the symbol until he gets to the end of the line, then should add the vowel, thus: *s s s s s s saaa.* Signal practice such as that described later in this section can also be used to form the nonsense syllable if it is needed. Generally, however, a simple request by the clinician to repeat the nonsense syllable he pronounces will produce the desired results. This repetition from a model is the usual way in which the syllables are used.

They may also be written by the clinician and read by the client. They may be used to precede each sentence of conversation or used as substitutes for such words as *the* or *and*. Lists of them may be used for practice, and all the various vowel combinations should be employed. The child should practice them finally at high speeds.

Although most young children have no difficulty in using the standard letter symbol for the sound in these nonsense syllables or talking-and-writing, many adults and some young children who have read and written the letter while pronouncing it incorrectly will have difficulty. The letter *s,* for example, means *th* to such a lisper, and he cannot use the usual syllables in talking-and-writing. For these cases, it is wise to use a nonsense symbol in place of the standard letter. In general, the symbols should be parts of the standard symbols, though the child should not realize this fact until later. These symbols should be used for identification techniques and for all strengthening techniques. After he has finally begun to use them in regular words, he may be shown that the nonsense symbol is really a part of the true symbol for the sound.

Nonsense Words The big advantage of using nonsense syllables rather than words is that no unlearning is needed. Were we to use familiar words for this stabilizing, we would immediately find trouble because of the competition of the old error. A child who has said *thoup* for *soup* all his life will find it easier to say the nonsense syllable *soub* than *soup.* Moreover, by giving meanings to nonsense syllables or combining them to form nonsense words we can facilitate transfer to communication and the other functions of speech. The fingers and toes may be given nonsense names. The doorknob may be christened. The clinician can make nonsense objects out of modeling clay, giving them names which include the new sound. Nonsense pictures may be drawn and named. Card games using these nonsense pictures seem to be peculiarly fascinating to almost all cases. Through talking-and-writing techniques, repetition from a model, reading, conversation, questioning, and speech games, these nonsense names can be used repeatedly. The various sound combinations are thereby practiced, and remarkable progress will soon occur. Examples of some of the nonsense pictures are given in Figure 23.

Once we have given meanings to nonsense words, we can immediately begin to use them in the various functions of speech. The child can command us to put the *sooba* in the basket. We can ask him how many red *soobas* are in the box. He can even vent his hostility by calling us a dirty, low-down *poos.* Children enjoy these activities and they are much more effective than drill.

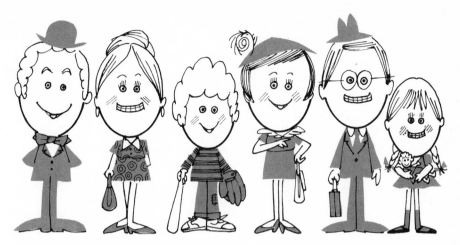

Figure 23 Stabilization of new /s/ sound through use of nonsence names. The *sooba* and *thooba* families.

Articulation Therapy at the Word Level

We are now ready to move onward to our third operational level — the word level. The new sound has now been sufficiently strengthened so that it has a fair chance to hold its own in competition with the error if we can make sure that the odds are in its favor. We must remember that the articulation case has used his old error in meaningful words thousands of times and that it would be unreasonable to expect him suddenly to be able to speak them correctly. We therefore need new techniques to insure the successful incorporation of the newly-acquired sound into his words.

Beginning Therapy at the Word Level   There are times when we even begin our therapy at the word level. We have already discussed how we use key words to provide in-the-mouth samples of the correct sound, and we have emphasized the point that inconsistency of error is much more common than we realize until we do some deep testing. These observations indicate that it might be possible to start therapy immediately by teaching correctly spoken *words* instead of isolated sounds or nonsense syllables. Indeed, most children seem to acquire correct articulation from this type of teaching. This is how parents normally teach a child to speak correctly. The fact that his method has failed with this particular person may not mean that the approach is all wrong, but perhaps merely that it was not correctly administered. Although we have already stated our preference for beginning with the isolated sound for the majority of our cases, we are not prejudiced against using any approach that might be more useful with a particular case. We have taught many children to achieve correct articulation by starting at the word level.

The Key Word as a Nucleus   We suspect that the failure of the traditional parental method of teaching a child words instead of sounds is due primarily to their use of too many words with too many different sounds as stimuli. When the speech clinician begins with the word level approach, she concentrates on teaching only a *few* important words, all of which contain the *same* desired sound. Parents, on the other hand, demand correction of many words containing many different errors. This confuses the child and he gives up trying to conform. The speech clinician tries to create nuclei of standard words and to insert them into the main functions of speech. We try to implant little colonies of these key words within messages, commands, emotional expressions, and even in thinking. Once planted and tended, these nuclei can attract other phonetically similar words. It is vitally important that the child *know* that these key words are ones that he can speak correctly and without error, that when he says these, he is speaking just as well as any other person, big or little. These are his yardsticks. These are his mouth models of correct utterance. He must know that when he says "Yes" he is not lisping. Only those of us who worked long in the vineyard with discouraged children can realize how important it is that such a child can come to be completely certain that he can say at least a few words perfectly. Once he has such a nucleus, he can start a collection.

Creating Key Words   How do we get these key words? Some of them we can find, as we have said, by deep testing, by searching through the child's spoken vocabulary, by checking the lists of assimilation words we can assemble, by varying the conditions of communication. Others we must create out of the sounds and syllables that compose them, using the isolated-sound or nonsense-syllable approaches. Thus, we see that no matter where we begin, we find ourselves sooner or later at the point where we must operate on the word level, creating and collecting key words to serve as nuclei for correct utterance. With most children we find it best to begin with the isolated sound, then move into the syllable and then into key words; with some children, we start with the syllable and move into key words; with a few special children we start with the key words themselves.

Creating Key Words We have two main techniques for creating key words once
from Sounds the child has mastered the sound in isolation and in the non-
and Syllables sense syllable: reconfiguration training and signaling.

Reconfiguration Frequently the reconfiguration techniques must be carried
Techniques out rather gradually. Their purpose is to teach the individual
that words are made up of sound sequences and that these
sound sequences can be modified without losing the unity of the
word. If, for convenience, we use a lingual lisper as our example, the
reconfiguration techniques would follow somewhat the same sequence: (1) the child reads, narrates, and converses with the clinician,
substituting the sound of /b/ for that of /f/ whenever the latter occurs
in the initial position. He reads, for example, that "Sammy caught a
bish with his hook and line." The purpose of using these nonerror
sounds is to make a gradual approach. (2) The child then substitutes
his new sound for other sounds, but not for the error. Thus: "Sammy
sssaught a fish with his hook and line." (3) The child then substitutes another sound for the /s/ in the same material. Thus:
"Bammy caught a fish with his hook and line." (4) The child omits
the s in all words beginning with it. Thus: "—ammy caught a fish
with his hook and line." (5) The child "substitutes" his new sound
for the s. Thus: "Ssssammy caught a fish with his hook and line."
Many similar techniques are easily invented. It may seem to the
young speech clinician that such techniques are far too laborious and
detailed. But, after he has met with persistent error in his articulatory
cases, he will appreciate the fact that careful and thorough training
will produce a thoroughgoing and permanent freedom from error.
Sketchy and slipshod training will enable a person with misarticulations to make the correct sound and perhaps to use it in a few
words when he watches himself carefully, but this is far from the
goal that should be set. Too many speech clinicians have blamed the
child for failure when they should have blamed themselves.

Another group of reconfiguration techniques requires the use of
writing or drawing simultaneously with the utterance. For children
who can read and write, these techniques are often very useful.

Simultaneous The simultaneous talking-and-writing techniques previously
Talking-and-Writing described will be invaluable if used properly. The client
should talk-and-write the first letter, the first syllable, and finally, the whole word. Thus: *s s s s s s·s s s s; s si sick s si sick*, and so
on. Later he can alternate the symbol and the word, and finally he
can write only the symbol as he says the word. Assignments can be

given for home practice. Frequently such a gradual approach is not necessary, and the child need write only the symbol and say any *s* word.

We also ask our clients to draw on paper or trace in the air various figures. The client is trained to associate certain sounds with certain parts of the figures and then to trace continuously through the whole figure, thus producing a word.

Signaling Techniques This group of activities uses preparatory sets to integrate the sound or syllable into the words. Signaling can generate many key words. In this, the child prolongs or repeats the new sound and then, at a given signal, instantly says the prearranged vowel or the rest of the word. The child should be given a preparatory set to pronounce the rest of the word by preliminary signal practice. During this practice he waits with his eyes closed until he hears the sound signal which sets off the response. Thus, during the child's prolongation of *sssssss*, the clinician suddenly raps on the table, and the syllable *oup* is automatically produced. With a preparatory set, the response is largely automatic and involuntary, and thus the new sound is integrated within the word as a whole. Often it is wise to require the child to say the word twice. Thus: *sssssss* (rap) *oupsoup*. Signal practice can also be used with repetition. Thus: *kuh-kuh-*(rap) *atkat*. After some training with this type of signal practice, the child may use other signals, such as those provided by the timing of a rhythm. Thus: *s-s, s-s-soup, s-s-soup*. He may also be required to repeat over and over some nonsense syllable which he can make well, suddenly saying the new word when the signal is given. Thus: *ssi-ssi-ssi-ssi* (tap) *ssip*. The nonsense syllable and the new word may also be used alternatively. The isolated sound may be used in the above exercise in place of the nonsense syllable. Various other combinations may easily be invented.

Difficulties in Forming Key Words from Isolated Sounds or Syllables At times difficulty will be experienced in making the transitions into the words. The child will say *rwabbit* and be confident that he has pronounced the word correctly. The error must be brought to his attention by the clinician's imitation and by the child's voluntary production of the error. Signal practice will help a great deal to eliminate this error.

Another invaluable technique is provided by a signal used in a slightly different way. The client is asked to form his mouth for the vowel which begins the rest of this word; i.e., for the vowel *a* in *rabbit,* then to say the word aloud very swiftly. This preformation of the vowel will often solve the problem. Similarly, the practice of pairs of words, the first ending in the vowel of the second, will be effective. Using pairs of words in which the first word ends with the new sound and the second begins with the same sound is occasionally useful, although the client should be cautioned to keep out all breaks in continuity.

Still another method of eliminating this error is to use some nonsense symbol to represent the part of the word which follows the new sound. Thus, one individual was asked to say *oup* every time he wrote a question mark (?), and after ten minutes of this, he was told to read the following symbols, *t?, kr?,* and *s?.* The last symbol was pronounced *soup* rather than *sthoup,* and no further difficulty was experienced.

Creating Key Words When we decide to forego the isolated-sound or syllable ap-
Directly proaches and to begin immediately by teaching key words, we use the same basic methods described for the other approaches. We must make sure through ear training that the person comes to realize how the *word* sounds when uttered by the clinician. He must also be made to *scan* his own utterance of the word and to *compare* it with that of the clinician. Finally, he must be taught to *vary* his attempts until the correct word is uttered. All the methods used for teaching the isolated sound or syllable can be used also for the word as a whole. Here is an excerpt from an ear-training session in which the clinician is operating at the word level:

The child and clinician are seated at a table. There are a number of little plastic objects on the table and two glass jars, one full of water and one empty.

Child: Put the kitty in the water. *(Clinician does so.)*

Child: Put the baby in the water.

Clinician: OK. Baby have bath.

Child: No, baby drown. All dead.

Clinician: OK. Baby dead now.

Child: Take baby out the water. *(Clinician does so.)*

Child: Baby OK now. You thpank baby bottom. Baby naughty.

Clinician: If you ask me to ssspank her I will, but you didn't. You asked me to thpank her. What's that? *(She holds baby up high.)*

Child (reaching): Thpank her! Thpank her! Thpank her! *(Slaps hand hard on table.)*

Clinician: Thpank her?. . . Oh, you mean . . . sspank her? *(Child nods).* OK. Here goes. *(Clinician spanks baby.)*

Now let us see how we would continue, but using the word level for the therapeutic process of establishing the standard pattern for two key words.

Clinician: No, that's no penthil.

Child: It ith too a penthil.

Clinician: Nope, you said it wrong. You said "penthil" ... th ... penth ... penthil. That's not the same as sss, pensss, pencil. Look, here's a penthil. *(Clinician takes out of the desk a pipe cleaner with two knots and a bolt on it.)* OK, this is your "penthil." Look, it sssinks. The pencil swims.

Child: Oh.

Clinician: Shut your eyes again. I'm going to put the penthil (listen now, I said *penthil,* not *pencil*) I'm going to put the penthil in the water. Can you tell me if it swims?

Child: No. It thinks.

Clinician: You're right. It isn't swimming. But you didn't say *sssssssinks* right. It's *sss, sssih, sssinksss,* not *thinks,* but *sssinks.* You can't peek until you can guess whether I'm saying it right or wrong. OK. Here we go: Which is right, the first or second: The *penthil thinks,* or the *penthil sinks.*

Child: The penthil sssssssinks. . . .

Clinician: And the pencil . . .

Child: Sssssswims.

Not all children make such rapid progress.

We have already indicated in our play-by-play description of this interchange between clinician and child that it is possible to use several operational levels in the same activity. In these stimulation, identification, and discrimination activities, the focus of therapy has been at one time on the sentence, at another on the word, on the syllable, and even on the isolated sound. Sometimes, as our illustration suggests, the child needs little help in producing the correct sound or in incorporating it into words, sentences, and functional speech. A child who gets the words *pencil, swim,* and *sink* in this five-minute period can be taught to use them immediately in commentary, communication, and control, and he should be given opportunity to do so in the interests of stabilization. Here is how it was done in the situation described above.

Clinician: OK. I'll close my eyes, and see if I can guess which one you'll pick up and play with.

Child: I'll pick one up.
Clinician: I bet it's a penthil.
Child: No, it a pensssssil.
Clinician: Is it the yellow one?
Child: Yeth.
Clinician: What are you going to do with it?
Child: I going put it in water.
Clinician: What's it doing now?
Child: It thwims.
Clinician: Thwims? What's that?
Child: It ssssssssswims. You want to look?
Clinician: Good for you. That's right. It's the pencil, not the penthil and it's swimming all right. Now you be the teacher and boss me around with the pencil and the penthil. Tell me what to do.
Child: Put penthil in mouth. (*Clinician does so with pipe cleaner.*)
Child: Put pencil in water. (*Clinician does so.*)
Child: Give penthil a bath. (*Clinician puts pipe cleaner in water.*)
Clinician: Which one do you think will get dry the faster?
Child: The pencil.
Clinician: How many penthils have I in my desk drawer here? (*Child looks.*)
Child: FF . . . no, no. You got none. But four pensssils. I almost forgot. SSS. Pencil!
Clinician: Finish this sentence: I can write with a . . .
Child: Write with a pencil.
Clinician: The only one that sinks is the . . .
Child: It's the penthil.
Clinician: The penthil is heavier than the . . .
Child: Pencil.

Articulation Therapy at the Sentence Level

Once we have taught our client a group of key words which contain the new sound in the initial, medial, and final positions, and he can now correct his misarticulations when he is being careful, we move on to the next operational level: the sentence. Again, we find here some new techniques, but before we describe them, let us tell how sometimes we begin our therapy, not at the sound, syllable, or word levels, but immediately at the sentence level.

Beginning at the   When we *begin* therapy at the sentence level we do so pri-
Sentence Level   marily to provide motivation and hope for those who have
                never felt they could talk normally. Usually, this sentence
level therapy is carried out only after the child has mastered the new
sound in isolation, nonsense syllables, and key words. However,
careful exploration sometimes reveals not only key words but key
sentences, or rather key utterances, in which the usually defective
sound is always spoken correctly. A child with whom we worked
recently and who could not make a /th/ sound in isolation, syllable,
or word, was able immediately to say "shut *the* door!" as a command. He could not say the word "the" or the sound of /th/ or the
nonsense syllable *shuthoo*. We found that by using other commands
of a similar nature, "Shut the window," "Shut that box," in slow motion and echoed speech, we could procure a nucleus of correct utterance from which we could isolate the words, sounds, and syllables
and still have them articulated correctly. Most speech clinicians, if
they *begin* treatment at the sentence level, do so for two reasons: to
convince the child immediately that the correct production of the target sound is not as difficult as he had believed, and secondly, to help
him analyze the correctly spoken sentences to locate the target
sounds, syllables, or words which he must use in the rest of his
speech.

Thus with the lisper who can say "Oh, you're nuts!" perfectly,
we want him to scrutinize this sentence-level expression of emotion
to know that the final *s* sound of the last word was said as well as
any other person on earth could say it; that he has said the syllable
uts and the words *nuts* perfectly, and most important of all, that the
whole insulting utterance was spoken without error. We pair these
key sentences with other sentences in which errors exist and ask the
child to scan them when we say them right or when we say them
wrong, and to scan them again when he speaks them. Thus we locate
the error and target the correct standard pattern.

Creating   As we have said, some of these correctly spoken sentences
Key Sentences   can be discovered by careful exploration and deep testing. It
                is also possible to create them, not only synthetically by in-
corporating sounds into syllables, syllables into words, and words
into key sentences, but as sentence wholes. We have several techniques for doing this: slow-motion speech, echo speech or shadowing, unison speaking, cumulative speaking, and the corrective set.
Each of these attempts to teach sentences as wholes.

Slow Motion Speech   In this technique the clinician and child say the error sentences in unison, but in extreme slow motion. For example: "Iiiiiz-ththththe-pennnnnssssssilll-wwwet?" The clinician should precede this with other slow-motion behavior such as walking, arm-lifting, head-scratching. She sets the tempo and the child follows her slowly shifting model. Often it is important that the clinician sit behind the child with her mouth slightly above his head so as to make the two sound fields similar, and so, by putting her mouth close to the child's ear for the difficult sounds or words, he can be stimulated more vividly.

Echo Speech   There are two forms of this. In the first, *shadowing*, the child tries to repeat instantly and automatically what the clinician is saying, word by word. The child's utterance should follow immediately. This shadowing, or echo speech, seems to be more easily learned by children than adults, and it is curious to find how faithfully they can do it. Once he has learned how to shadow automatically (almost as in echolalia), the child's voice follows not only the words but also the inflections with surprising fidelity.

In the second form of echo-speaking, which they have called "long-echo talk," the child repeats not single words, but a *series* of words or phrases or sentences after the clinician when she pauses and signals for him to catch up and give back the echo. This should be done with a gestural or postural or behavioral accompaniment which the child must also duplicate as closely as possible.

In both types of echo speech it is important that the child try to follow the clinician as automatically as possible. Children who have never produced standard sounds or who cannot do so under direct stimulation in their speech are able to make them easily when doing this automatic kind of echo-speaking. We also teach them to echo themselves.

Unison Speech   In this the child and clinician speak some previously formulated utterances together. It is important that again the child follow the clinician's movements, speech tempo, pitch, and intensity patterns. For this purpose, each utterance is spoken several times. Often the clinician cups her hands and directs her voice into one of the child's ears, while the child listens with the other ear to his mouth with cupped hands, or uses an auditory training unit. This binaural listening permits a simultaneous comparison of correct and incorrect forms. Hand-tapping signals are used to time the moment of attempt and to insure unison speaking. Often, as the same utterance is spoken each time, it is wise to have the child accompany it with a certain head or body movement so that it can be stabilized thereby when the child must speak it alone. We also tape-record some of the child's own speech which is spoken without error and ask him to say it again in unison with himself.

The Corrective Set   We have also found that often a child with an articulation problem can be able to produce his usually defective sound correctly in a whole sentence when he is given a corrective set. The way we usually do this is by saying or doing many things in which our error is obvious and asking the child to correct us and to set us straight. We begin with mistakes which are so apparent that any person would be likely to recognize them. Once the child is thoroughly enjoying our stupidity and mistakes, we slip in some utterance containing his own common errors. Over and over again we have been surprised to find how easily he can show us how to say the sentence without error. Here is an example:

> *The clinician and child are seated at a table. The child lisps and has other defective sounds. The clinician has a bag with various articles in it.*
>
> *Clinician:* I'm going to say and do some things all wrong, and I want you to show me and tell me how to do or say them right. Understand?
>
> *Child:* Uh huh.
>
> *Clinician:* See, here's a comb. I brush my teeth with a comb. (*Pretends to do so.*)
>
> *Child (laughing):* No, No. You comb you heh.
>
> *Clinician:* Show me. (*Child does so.*) Oh, I see, I comb my hair. (*Reaches into bag and pulls out a plastic spoon.*) See, here's a thpoon.
>
> *Child:* Yeth.
>
> *Clinician:* Oh ho! I fooled you that time. I said something wrong and you didn't catch me. I said *thpoon,* not sssspoon. OK. Watch me fool you again.
>
> *Child:* No, you can't.
>
> *Clinician (points to her mouth):* I open my mouf.
>
> *Child (scornfully):* You open your mouth, MOUTH! not mouf.
>
> *Clinician (pretends to cry):* OK, you caught me that time. Oh look, here's a picture of a horth. See the big horth.

Child: No, no. Horsssssssssss! Not horth. Horsssssssey, and it is a little horse, not a big one.

Role-Playing A most curious discovery of many speech clinicians is that some children, when completely immersed in some other person's role, can speak almost perfectly the same sentences that they cannot possibly say without error in any other situation. We use fantasy, children's theater, and creative dramatics to establish these roles and much suggestion and coaching to make them vivid enough so that the child can throw himself completely into them. Identification must be very thorough. Here is a short illustration:

Clinician: All right, let's play bank robbers. Who am I?
Child: You the man at the bank. Thit there at the table with the money.
Clinician: Where's the money?
Child: Here! *(Tears up some paper and gives it to the clinician.)* I'm going out and come in with gun.
Clinician: Don't shoot me when you come in.
Child: Oh hoh. I'll thcare you. You be thcared now when I come in.
Clinician: OK.
Child (goes out, then enters with handkerchief over mouth and pencil in hand. Points it at clinician who pretends to be afraid): Stick 'em up!
Clinician: (lifts two fingers): Like this?
Child (returning to his own role): Naw. Look, when I thay "Stick 'em up" you've got to thtick 'em up like thith. *(Demonstrates.)*
Clinician: Oh I understand. Let's start again.
Child: Stick 'em up now!

Transfer and Carry-Over It is one thing to acquire the ability to use a new sound correctly in isolation, syllable, word, or sentence; it is another to be able to use it habitually and automatically. A person who has thought, commanded, sent messages, expressed himself in lisping speech for years needs special help in making the new unlisped speech habitual. Somehow we must build in this person a control system which will continuously scan the utterance and notice and correct the errors automatically. No one can continually listen to the output of sound from his mouth. We need our ears to hear our thoughts and the thoughts of others. How can we automatize this corrective process? We have three main methods for doing so: (1) enlarging the therapy situation, (2) using the new sound in all types of speaking, (3) emphasizing proprioceptive feedback.

Enlarging the First of all, we must expand the therapy room to include the
Therapy Situation person's whole living space. He must be given experiences in scanning, comparing, and correcting in school, on the playground, on the job, and at home. Here are some of the ways we do this.

Speech Assignments Some typical speech assignments to illustrate methods for getting the child to work on his errors in outside situations are:

(1) Go downstairs and ask the janitor for a dust rag. Be sure to say *rag* with a good long *rrr.* (2) Say the word *rabbit* to three other children without letting them know that you are working on your speech. (3) Ask your father if you said any word wrongly after you tell him what you did in school today.

The clinician should always make these assignments very definite and appropriate to the child's ability and environment. He should always ask for a report the next day. Such assignments frequently are the solution to any lack of motivation the child may have.

Checking Devices Checking devices and penalties are of great value when prop-
and Penalties erly used. Typical checking devices are:

(1) Having child carry card and crayon during geography recitation, making a mark or writing the word whenever he makes an error. (2) Having some other child check errors in a similar fashion. (3) Having child transfer marbles from one pocket to another, one for each error. Many other devices may be invented, and they will bring the error to consciousness very rapidly.

Similarly, penalties are of great service when used properly. It should be realized, however, that painful and highly emotional penalties should not be used, for they merely make the bad habit more pronounced and cause the child to hate his speech work. Penalties used in speech correction should be vivid and good-natured. Typical penalties used with a ten-year-old lisper were: put pencil behind ear; step in wastebasket; pound pan; look between legs; close one eye; say *whoopee*. Let the child set his own penalties before he makes the speech attempt.

Nucleus Situations   Many parents make the mistake of correcting the child whenever he makes speech errors. It is unwise to set the speech standards too high. No one can watch himself all the time, and we all hate to be nagged. As a matter of fact, too much vigilance can produce such speech inhibitions that the speech work becomes thoroughly distasteful. Fluency disappears, and the speech becomes very halting and unpleasant. Then, too, the very anxiety lest error occur, when carried to the extreme, increases the number of slips and mistakes themselves. Other errors sometimes appear.

Therefore, we recommend that parents and teachers concentrate their reminding and correcting upon a few common words and upon certain nuclei speech situations. Use a certain chair as a good-speech chair. Whenever the child sits in it, he must watch himself. Have a certain person picked out who is to serve in the speech situation where the child must use very careful speech. Use a certain speech situation, such as the dinner table, to serve as a nucleus of good speech, and when errors occur in these nuclei situations, penalize them good-naturedly but emphatically. You will find that the freedom from errors will spread rapidly to all other situations.

Finally, we recommend that after a child has mastered a new sound and several words in which it occurs, he be required to say it occasionally in the wrong way. This is called negative practice, and it has no harmful effect. Indeed, it merely emphasizes the distinction between the correct and incorrect sounds.

Negative Practice   By negative practice we mean the deliberate and voluntary use of the incorrect sound or speech error. It may seem somewhat odd to advise clients to practice their errors, for we have always assumed that practice makes perfect, and certainly we do not want the student to become more perfect in the use of his errors. Nevertheless, modern experimental psychology has demonstrated that when one seeks to break a habit that is rather unconscious (such as fingernail-biting or the substitution of *sh* for *s*), much more rapid progress is made if the possessor of the habit will occasionally (and at appropriate times) use the error deliberately. The reasons for this method are: (1) the greatest strength of such a habit lies in the fact

that the possessor is not aware of it every time it occurs. All habit reactions tend to become more or less unconscious, and certainly those
involved in speech are of this type. Consciousness of the reaction must
come before it can be eliminated. (2) Voluntary practice of the reaction makes it very vivid, thus increasing vigilance and contributing
to the awareness of the cues that signal the approach of the reaction.
(3) The voluntary practice of the error acts as a penalty.

The use of negative practice is so varied that it would be impossible to describe all the applications which can be made of it. Variations must be made to fit each type of disorder and each individual
case. There are, however, certain general principles which may be
said to govern all disorders and cases. Make the individual aware of
the reasons for his use of the incorrect sound, for unintelligent use of
the error is worthless. Never ask the client to use the error until he
can produce the correct sound whenever asked to do so.

Set up the exact reproduction of the incorrect sound as a goal.
The use of mirror observation, imitation, and tape recording is invaluable. This is a learning process and does not come all at once.
The clinician should confine all negative practice to the therapy room
until the child is able to duplicate the error consistently and fairly accurately. One should begin the use of this technique by asking him
to duplicate the error immediately after it has occurred—that is to
say, he should stop immediately after lisping on the word *soup* and
attempt voluntarily to duplicate his performance before correcting it.

Using the New
Sound in All the
Various Types of
Speaking
In stabilizing and automatizing the new sound, we find it
wise to provide systematic training which incorporates the
new sound into real live message-sending, social control,
thinking, emotional, and self-expressive types of speaking.

Again we must make deliberate nucleic implants of good
speech in all these various functions. First in the therapy room, and
then in all the person's living space, we must make sure that our
client can use his new standard sounds in all the *kinds* of talking he
must do. When the lisper commands his dog, he must say "Sit
down!" When he responds affirmatively to a question he must say
"Yes!" When he must mentally add four and three, he must think
"seven," not "theven." In expressing his fear, he must say "I'm
scared" not "thcared." He must be able to use good silibants in his
speech of self-display. Until certain correctly spoken sentences are
used automatically in each of these forms of speaking, we cannot feel
our task as a clinician is over.

Emphasizing Proprioceptive feedback is a term which refers to the per-
Proprioceptive ception of contacts and movements and postures. If we place
Feedback a finger on our lower lip, the felt contact is proprioceptive; if
we cock our head to the left or move a foot, the sensations of
posture and movement are proprioceptive. We know what has happened without seeing or hearing. In much the same way, we can
know what is happening in our own speech even when we cannot
hear ourselves speaking. It is quite possible to talk correctly in a
boiler factory. We do not need self-hearing if our proprioceptive
senses are operating well.

We believe that once a person has left babyhood, the most important automatic controls for monitoring articulation are proprioceptive. These controls see to it that we use the right movements, the
right postures, the correct contacts. We feel that when the baby first
learns to talk, self-hearing is most important. That is why he babbles
so much and does so much vocal play. But after he begins to use language and to understand the meanings of others, self-hearing is
given a less important role. Proprioception thus becomes much more
important, so important, indeed, that obvious errors can persist for
years without the person recognizing them auditorially. In articulation therapy, we must first reopen the self-hearing circuits and put
more energy into them so that these errors can be distinguished. But
we must not stop here. We must return to proprioceptive controls if
the child is to use the new sound automatically. No one can listen to
himself constantly. The burden is too great. Too many other functions interfere.

Accordingly, in terminal therapy with a client with misarticulations, we teach him to use the new sound correctly by feel
and touch alone. We put masking noise in his ears so he cannot rely
on self-hearing. We ask him to speak correctly with his ears plugged.
We ask him to speak in a soft whisper and in pantomime. All these
activities decrease the monitoring of speech by self-hearing and emphasize its proprioceptive control. We have found these techniques
invaluable in automatizing the new sound.

In Conclusion As we come to the end of this chapter we fear that you may
be thinking that doing articulation therapy is both laborious
and difficult. It really isn't if the client is a young child whose misarticulations have not become fixed through years of misuse. Most
children respond readily and successfully to a systematic program.
Once they have come to recognize the characteristics of the standard
sound and its error and have been able to produce it in isolation or

syllables, they move swiftly into normal utterance. We have had to describe many more techniques than those normally administered because there are always a few individuals whose problems are more severe. It's fun to work with all these children; it's very rewarding to see a troubled child untangle his tongue and life, to see him grow in self-esteem because he can now talk like other people. Our suggestions are not at all mysterious nor difficult to administer. Many parents and teachers have been able to follow them once they found out from the speech pathologist what they were and why they made sense. Lost children should not have to try to find their way out of the swamp alone. They need a guide who has a map.

References

AUNGST, L. and J. FRICK. "Auditory Discrimination Ability and Consistency of Articulation of /r/," *Journal of Speech and Hearing Disorders*, XXIX (1964), 76–85.

BARRETT, M. D. and J. W. WELSH. "Predictive Articulation Testing." *Language, Speech, Hearing Services in the Schools*, VI (1975), 91–5.

BOWN, J. C. "Technique for Correcting /r/ Misarticulations." *Language, Speech, Hearing Services in the Schools*, VI (1975), 86–91.

CARRELL, J. *Disorders of Articulation*. Englewood Cliffs, N. J.: Prentice-Hall, Inc., 1968.

COSTELLO, J. "Articulation Instruction Based on Distinctive Features Theory." *Language, Speech, Hearing Services in the Schools*, VI (1975), 61–71.

DRAPER, D. J. and J. B. LINGWALL. "Effects of Response-Contingent Consequation on Correct Articulation Responses." *Journal of Psycholinguistic Research*, IV (1975), 123–32.

DRUMWRIGHT, A., A. P. VAN NATTA, B. CAMP, WILLIAM FRANKENBERGER, and H. DREXLER. "The Denver Articulation Screening Examination." *Journal of Speech and Hearing Disorders*, XXXVIII (1973), 3–14.

EDMONSTON, W. *Laradon Articulation Scale*. Beverly Hills, Cal.: Western Psychological Services, 1963.

FISHER, H. and J. LOGEMANN. *The Fisher-Logemann Test of Articulation Competence*. Boston: Houghton-Mifflin Co., 1971.

GERBER, A. *Goal: Carry-Over: An Articulation Manual and Program*. Philadelphia: Temple U. Press, 1973.

GOLDMAN, R. and M. FRISTOE. *Goldman-Fristoe Test of Articulation*. Circle Pines, Minn.: American Guidance Service, 1969.

HARRYMAN, E. and J. KRESHECK. "A Structured Program for Modifying /r/ Misarticulations." *Language, Speech, Hearing Services in Schools*, II (1971), 52–4.

LOCKE, J. J. "Oral Perception and Articulation Learning." *Perceptual and Motor Skills*, XXVI (1968), 1259–64.

LOCKE, J. L. "Short Term Auditory Memory, Oral Perception, and Experimental Sound Learning." *Journal of Speech and Hearing Research*, XII (1969), 185–93.

MANNING, W. H., N. E. KEAPPOCK, and S. L. STICK. "The Use of Auditory Masking to Estimate Automatization of Correct Articulatory Production." *Journal of Speech and Hearing Disorders,* XLI (1976), 143–49.

MARSHALL, R. C. "The Effects of Response Contingent Punishment Upon A Defective Articulation Response." *Journal of Speech and Hearing Disorders,* XXXV (1970), 236–40.

McCURRY, W. H. and O. C. IRWIN. "A Study of Word Approximations in the Spontaneous Speech of Infants." *Journal of Speech and Hearing Disorders,* XVIII (1953), 133–39.

McDONALD, E. T. *A Deep Test of Articulation.* Pittsburgh: Stanwix House, Inc., 1964.

——, *A Screening Test of Articulation.* Pittsburgh: Stanwix House, 1968.

—— and L. F. AUNGST. "Studies in Oral Sensorimotor Function." in J. F. Bosma (ed.) *Symposium on Oral Sensation and Perception.* (Springfield, Ill.: Charles C. Thomas, 1967).

McREYNOLDS, L. V. and D. L. ENGMANN. *Distinctive Feature Analysis of Misarticulation.* Baltimore: University Park Press, 1975.

MILISEN, R. "Articulatory Problems." in R. W. Rieber and R. S. Brubaker (eds.) *Speech Pathology* Philadelphia: J. B. Lippincott Co., 1966, chapter 11.

MORLEY, M. *The Development and Disorders of Speech in Childhood.* Baltimore: Williams and Wilkins, 1972.

MOWRER, D. E. "Transfer of Training in Articulation Therapy." *Journal of Speech and Hearing Disorders,* XXXVI (1971), 427–46.

——, R. L. BAKER, and R. E. SCHULTZ. "Operant Procedures in the Control of Speech Articulation." in H. N. Sloane and B. B. Macauley (eds.) *Operant Procedures in Remedial Speech and Language Training* Boston: Houghton-Mifflin Co., 1968, 296–321.

PAYNTER, E. T. and S. A. WATTS. "Watts Articulation Test for Screening: Evaluation of a Screening Test." *Perceptual Motor Skills,* XXXVI (1973), 721–22.

PENDERGAST, K. *Building Good Speech.* Pittsburgh: Stanwix House, 1971.

——, S. DICKEY, J. SELMAR, and A. SODER. *Photo-Articulation Test.* Danville, Ill.: Interstate Publishers, 1968.

POWERS, M. H. "Functional Disorders of Articulation: Symptometology and Etiology." in L. E. Travis (ed.) *Handbook of Speech Pathology and Audiology.* Englewood Cliffs, N.J.: Prentice-Hall, Inc., 1971.

PSALTIS, C. D. and S. L. SPALLATO. *Programmed Articulation Therapy: Time to Modify.* Springfield, Ill.: Charles C. Thomas, 1973.

RENFREW, C. E. "Persistence of the Open Syllable in Defective Articulation." *Journal of Speech and Hearing Disorders,* XXXI (1966), 370–73.

RINGEL, R. L., K. W. BURK, and C. M. SCOTT. "Tactile Perception: Form Discrimination in the Mouth." *British Journal Disorders Communication,* VIII (1968), 150–55.

RYAN, B. P. "A Study of the Effectiveness of the 'S'-Pack Program in the Elimination of Frontal Lisping Behavior in Third-Grade Children." *Journal of Speech and Hearing Disorders,* XXXVI (1971), 390–96.

SHRIBERG, L. D. "A Response Evocation Program for /ɝ/." *Journal of Speech and Hearing Disorders,* XL (1975), 92–105.

SLIPAKOFF, E. L. "An Approach to the Correction of the Defective [r]." *Journal of Speech and Hearing Disorders,* XXXII, (1967), 71–5.

Swirl Speech Articulation for the /s/, /l/, /r/ and /Θ/. Cincinnati: American Book Co. (1974).

TEMPLIN, M. and F. DARLEY. *The Templin-Darley Tests of Articulation.* Iowa City: Bureau of Educational Research and Service, University of Iowa, 1969.

VAN RIPER, C. and R. ERICKSON. "A Predictive Screening Test of Articulation." *Journal of Speech and Hearing Disorders,* XXXIV (1969), 214–19.

VAN RIPER, C. and J. IRWIN. *Voice and Articulation.* Englewood Cliffs, N.J.: Prentice-Hall, Inc., 1958.

WEBER, J. L. "Patterning of Deviant Articulatory Behavior." *Journal of Speech and Hearing Disorders,* XXXV (1970), 135–41.

WINITZ, H. *Articulatory Acquisition and Behavior.* Englewood Cliffs, N.J.: Prentice-Hall, Inc., 1969.

YOUNG, E. H. "The Motokinesthetic Approach to the Prevention of Speech Defects Including Stuttering." *Journal of Speech and Hearing Disorders,* XXX (1965), 269–73.

7

VOICE
DISORDERS

Although the incidence of voice disorders as compared to those of articulation is low,[1] every speech pathologist is sure to confront them in his practice at one time or another. Some of them will be among the most fascinating of all his clients. Often the most challenging of all the speech disorders, those of voice may reflect not only organic pathology but emotional and even vocational problems. A hoarse voice, for example, may be the first sign of laryngeal cancer in a client who has long disregarded the Surgeon General's warning printed on his packs of cigarettes. Or it may result from habitually speaking at a pitch level too close to the bottom of his pitch range because, as with one of our clients, (a very short, essentially effeminate fellow) who wanted to sound strong and manly. Or perhaps that strained hoarse voice results from communicating in the presence of very loud masking noise. This happened to a foreman in a foundry after he worked in that roaring, banging environment for many months. Voice disorders arise from many different conditions.

While less frequently found than those of articulation, the disorders of voice can be truly handicapping despite the fact that our culture tends to be more tolerant of vocal deviations than those of language or fluency or articulation. Perhaps this is because intelligible communication is still possible even when the voice is harsh or nasal or unduly high-pitched or breathy or of low intensity.[2] Perhaps we may be more tolerant of phonatory deviations because there are so many of them within the normal range. For example, you can recognize most of your acquaintances over the phone by their voices alone. There is no single standard of pitch, intensity, or qual-

[1] Senturia and Wilson (1968) found that about 6 percent of the more than 30,000 school children they surveyed had abnormal voices.

[2] When a client has aphonia, (the complete loss of voice) his messages will be very difficult to understand.

ity. Like noses, voices have to be pretty prominent in their abnormality before they are noticed. Parents and teachers become concerned when a child's language, phonemes, or fluency are different from those of other children, but unless the child's voice is grossly conspicuous and unpleasant they feel no need to seek help. Nor, for that matter, do many persons who themselves should be getting professional voice therapy. The reason for this is that we listen to what we say—to the message we seek to impart—rather than to how we say it. You doubtless were surprised or even shocked when you first heard yourself on a tape recording. Although that recorded voice sounded strange to you, yet it is the voice others hear. Other voices on the same tape probably sounded quite familiar. The discrepancy is due partly to the fact that we sense our own vocal tones through bone and tissue conduction as well as from airborne sound, and also because the sound field is different (our ears being behind our mouths but in front of the mouths of others). The distortions thereby produced, plus our usual inattention to how we sound, probably explains why some people persist in using the unpleasant voices which finally result in real voice disorders.

Chaliapin, the famous basso, once said that going to a party was like going to a symphony played by instruments all of which were out of tune. "All around me are voices blowing discords, squeaks, rasps, whines, grunts, and growls. I can hardly bear it." Fortunately for most of us, our ears are not so sensitive. His observation, however, is more accurate than our calloused ears would be likely to admit. All about us are voices which could be improved, made more pleasant and efficient. And there are some so markedly unpleasant or peculiar that they are referred to the speech pathologist. The singing teacher gets some of these, the speech teacher gets another group, the physician sees the pathological ones, and the speech pathologist is usually called upon last.

Since the human voice varies in pitch, loudness, and quality, the disorders of voice reflect these three features either separately or in combination. With respect to the latter, we remember very well a schoolteacher who lost his first job primarily because his voice was so unpleasant. His pitch level was not only too high; it possessed so little variability that his monotone put the students to sleep. The intensity was so weak that the students in the rear of the room could not hear half of what he said. What was most unpleasant of all, however, was the excessive nasal quality that permeated all of his speech. This weak little whiny high-pitched voice was unbearable, and the man was discharged after only two days of teaching. Like this man, other individuals show disorders of voice that are defective in more than one of the three features of pitch, intensity, and quality; but some of our cases show deviancy in only one of these aspects.

Disorders of Intensity

There are three major disorders in which the basic problem is the inability to produce any voice at all or to be able to phonate loudly enough to be understood. The term *aphonia* is used to refer to the complete loss of voice; the term *dysphonia* to the partial or intermittent inability to phonate. A person whose larynx has been removed because of cancer always becomes completely aphonic,[3] but some persons with a perfectly intact larynx may also show a complete or partial loss of voice. They are those with *hysterical aphonia or dysphonia* and those with *spastic dysphonia*. Besides those two disorders of vocal intensity, there is a third, *phonasthenia*, which refers to a voice which is so soft and weak that intelligibility is impaired.

Hysterical Aphonia   This disorder, the loss of voice due to emotional stress, usually begins suddenly. The person may begin to talk, then suddenly find himself unable to finish a sentence with any phonation. One of our cases went to bed, quite happily he told us later, and arose to find himself unable to speak aloud. A schoolteacher lost her voice in the middle of an explanation of a geometry problem. A preacher who had just conducted the opening exercises and participated in the singing was unable to produce even a squeak of sound when he started his sermon. A housewife about to give her mate a good calling down for coming in late at night found herself unable to say anything except in a whisper. A lieutenant in the jungle of Vietnam started to give the order to his men to enter a particularly dangerous thicket and found that he was not even able to whisper the command, that his mouth moved but no sound came out. Many hysterical aphonias arise from laryngitis or colds, the illness creating the necessary explanation for voice failure, though the real reasons lie deep in basic emotional conflicts. We also meet cases where the aphonia comes and goes intermittently. Here is one:

> Wilma's parents and grandparents had been schoolteachers, and they desired her to follow their profession. Her college educa-

[3] The treatment of this organically-produced aphonia is deferred to the chapter on Organic Disorders.

tion had been financed on that understanding. But Wilma didn't want to be a schoolma'am. As soon as she entered college she became engaged to a young man and thought she might escape the horrible prospect of teaching by becoming a housewife. However, in her senior year, he suddenly decided to enter medical school, a decision which meant that she would have to support him by teaching for several years. She fought the decision but finally acquiesced. It was in her first week of practice teaching that her voice began to go. She would begin her sentences all right, but after saying a few words, she could only whisper. At times longer words would be uttered with the first syllable voiced and the other syllables produced in pantomime. No organic cause was evident. She dropped out of school, and he dropped her; we don't know what happened thereafter.

The medical reports on these clients usually state that no laryngeal pathology is present or that in attempted phonation the vocal folds are bowed. Occasionally the laryngologist will say that though the vocal folds are easily abducted (moved apart), they do not meet in the midline when the patient attempts to produce voice for speech, although they do so in coughing or clearing the throat. Indeed, many of the more naive hysterical aphonics can hum or sing without difficulty. These features indicate that the disorder is not of organic origin, and so also does the use of pantomime speech when it is present. We do not find persons with a true laryngeal paralysis who cannot produce at least a whisper or airflow during attempted phonation.

Treatment of
Hysterical Aphonia   Since this type of aphonia must be viewed symptomatically as a protective device to cope with real or imagined difficulties that have become intolerable, some psychotherapy is often necessary; and the speech clinician may need to refer the patient to a psychiatrist or clinical psychologist and work closely with them. However, there are some cases whose loss of voice persists even after the conflict situation has been resolved; and these provide some of the most sudden and dramatic cures known to speech pathology. At times even in a single session we have been able to help them "find" their voices again and to leave us talking as well as they ever had. When recurrences and relapses occur (and they do not always take place), we can be pretty sure that deeper psychotherapy or environmental change will be required. The largest number of our own clients with hysterical aphonia have been schoolteachers who

just needed a rest from their duties for a time. They often come to us in March when summer vacation seems too far away, and they cannot bear to cope with "the little savages" in their schoolrooms another moment. The speech therapy gains time, and the speech clinician provides understanding and hope; often this is all that is required. Greene recommends the use of breathing and relaxation exercises and some counseling interviews. She says, "Relaxation should be followed by breathing exercises while still lying on the couch, and then an attempt at vocalization made, breathing deeply and sighing, then strengthening the sigh till it becomes an audible sound. The clinician may gently manipulate the lower thorax with the hands or massage the throat to reinforce the suggestion of what is wanted. The confident and convincing manner in which she introduces the exercises is of course far more conducive than the exercises themselves."[4]

Suggestion is frequently used with hysterical aphonias. Physicians often use a faradic current or ammonia inhalation or massage as the culminating procedures in a period of treatment marked by complete cessation of speech attempt and strong cumulative suggestion. In many instances, coughing is used to demonstrate to the patient that voice exists. Persons who have once had such aphonia are likely to have it again unless the cause is removed. In some instances, when the cause cannot be discovered, a relapse is prevented by having the individual perform some simple vocal ritual each day, such as prolonging each of the vowels for ten seconds.

Some quotations from an old article by Sokolowsky and Junkermann will illustrate some of the methods for treating hysterical aphonia:

> First, we administered breathing exercises in connection with a systematic speech and voice retraining . . . (using a humming, or breathy, speech attempt while "pressing together the hands of a nurse standing behind him";) . . . By means of this phonetic reeducation we succeeded in restoring the voice to about 60 percent of our aphonics, a rather meager result considering the relatively tiresome treatment which sometimes lasted several weeks.
>
> Induced by the publications of Muck and his extraordinary results, we then tried his method—the introduction of a pellet or small ball into the larynx between the vocal cords in order to

---

[4] M. C. L. Greene, *The Voice and its Disorders* (Philadelphia: J. B. Lippincott, Co., 1964), p. 154.

bring about a sensation of being suffocated which superinduced a cry of fright. We have to confess that our own results with Muck's ball were not very encouraging.

As soon as the anamnesis pointed to a psychogenic aphonia and the laryngoscopic mirror confirmed this assumption, a short remark such as, "You will be all right quite soon," or, "You will be getting your voice back quite soon," was made. After that the patient was not permitted, so to speak, to "collect his wits." All manipulations such as setting the head in proper position and pulling out the tongue were carried out as quickly as possible, and accompanied by short, crisp and somewhat commanding words. Then followed the deep introduction of the mirror and the attempt to obtain a vocal retching reaction. After this was accomplished, it was brought into the consciousness of the patient with short, crisp remarks, such as "Here we are," "Now your voice is back," or "Do you hear your voice?" After that it required but relatively little effort (the mirror, of course, remaining continually in the throat) to elicit from the patient the unpleasant gag-reminding but nevertheless audible "ah."[5]

In our own practice, we have not needed to resort to such procedures. If the client has had his unconscious profit from the aphonic symptom and is ready to get rid of it because it is a nuisance, we usually can find some way to restore phonation either through sighing, singing, or humming; the prolonged clearing of the throat; or especially through the use of the *vocal fry*. This term refers to the clicking, tickerlike phonation many of us have used while playing lazily with our voices when relaxed. We have found it very useful in modifying many kinds of voice disorders. All students of speech pathology should learn to produce it. For our patients it is wise to set up some home practice in voice-finding, some routines and exercises for voice-strengthening, and to arrange for several appointments in advance so that further opportunity for counseling can be provided and any relapses taken care of. One of the favorable prognostic signs when the voice does come back is the ability to produce it without tension. If the voice is strained or forced, our experience is that relapse is inevitable.

Spastic Dysphonia   In this disorder, we have a mixture of aphonia and a strained, tense, vocalized whisper. The person labors hard to squeeze out some voice. It sounds like the strained speech of some-

[5] R. R. Sokolowsky and E. R. Junkermann, "War Aphonia," *Journal of Speech Disorders,* IX (1944), 192–208.

one performing tremendous strenuous muscular effort and trying to speak at the same time. The mountain labors and produces a mouse of sound. At times there are facial contortions almost as in the severe stutterer. Fear of speaking is present, but usually not fear of words. This is also to be found in the cerebral palsied or some other type of central nervous system disease.

Spastic dysphonia seems to be more prevalent in males than in females and it usually begins suddenly. Here is a description from Boone (1971):

> The patient described what happened when her son was hospi-talized with severe pneumonia: She and her husband went down to the hospital canteen for a cup of coffee. When they re-turned to the boy's room they found that he had died during their absence. In the woman's shock, she was unable to speak for several days. Gradually, over a period of several weeks, her voice returned. Several years later, a second child was hospital-ized, also with pneumonia. While driving the boy to the hospi-tal, the woman experienced severe difficulties in talking, similar to the sort she had suffered after the first boy's death. These voice difficulties persisted with no remission for several years. The patient would speak with a rather placid smiling face, and at the same time would continuously push, or force out her breath. She exhibited no normal phonation except when she laughed, which she would do frequently, using this relatively easy phonation as a "starter" for her verbal responses. Sub-sequent attempts at voice therapy, later combined with psychi-atric therapy, were not successful in changing her spastic dys-phonia. (p. 83)

Not all spastic dysphonias begin in such an emotionally-loaded situation, but once it begins, like stuttering, it grows in severity, spreading from one speaking situation to another.

Unlike hysterical or alaryngeal aphonia, the person with spastic dysphonia often can produce voice at times. Indeed, he may often begin a sentence with easy and normal phonation, then begin squeezing out his speech with progressively greater tension until no sound at all is produced. Thus the term *dysphonia* rather than aph-onia. The disorder has been called "vocal stuttering," and there are several resemblances between it and stuttering. Often the person may be able to sing easily or say non-meaningful asides with good pho-nation, only to strain and struggle greatly on meaningful utterances. Although many authors have felt that spastic dysphonia has an emotional origin, recent studies seem to indicate that it may reflect neurologic lesions probably in the pyramidal tract of the brain and that it may be related to the essential tremor syndrome.[6] Aronson, Brown, Litin, and Pearson found no significant differences between persons with spastic dysphonia and normals on the Minnesota Multiphasic Personality Test.[7] Fortunately, the disorder is rare, for the prognosis is very poor and speech or voice therapy has had little success. We have worked hard with eleven of these persons and completely in vain. Our reason for describing the disorder here is to help other clinicians recognize its distinctive features so they might be spared some of our own heartache at being so ineffective.[8]

Phonasthenia   This term refers to the voice that is too little and too weak to carry the normal burdens of communication. Voices which are not loud enough for efficient communication are fairly common, but they seldom are referred to the speech pathologist. Imitation, overcompensation for hearing loss, and feelings of inadequacy leading to retreat reactions account for most of them. Many pathological reasons for such disorders are common, but they are frequently accompanied by breathiness, huskiness, or hoarseness, or other symptoms sufficiently evident to necessitate the services of the physician, who should rightfully take care of them.

> One individual with a history of prolonged laryngitis, but with a clean bill of health from the physician, claimed that she was afraid to talk loudly because of the pain she had experienced in the past. Something seemed to stop her whenever she decided to talk a little louder. She constantly fingered her throat. She declared that she was losing all her self-respect by worrying about her inability to speak as loudly as she could. Use of a masking noise during one of her conferences demonstrated to her that she could speak loudly without discomfort. Under strong clinical pressure, she did make the attempt, but the inhibition was automatic.

[6] E. Robe, P. Moore, and J. Brumlik, "A Study of Spastic Dysphonia," *Laryngoscope*, LXX (1960), 218–23; R. Luchsinger, and G. E. Arnold, *Voice–Speech–Language* (Belmont, Calif.: Wadsworth, 1965), pp. 328–33.

[7] A. E. Aronson, J. R. Brown, and J. S. Pearson, "Spastic Dysphonia: I. Voice, Neurological and Psychiatric Aspects," *Journal of Speech and Hearing Disorders*, XXXIII (1968), 203–18.

[8] This may be too pessimistic. A *student* of Dr. Robert Erickson (Western Michigan University) was able to help one of these eleven failures of the author to regain completely normal voice several years later. We examined this person very carefully and we are certain of the recovery. All hail to students once again!

When we speak we expose ourselves, and the louder we do it, the greater that exposure is. The insecure, withdrawn person finds even ordinary levels of intensity almost unbearably revealing. His very nature resists the display of self. Usually he has good reasons for his inhibited utterance, although they may remain hidden until counseling makes them bearable and manageable. An emotionally healthy person enjoys a certain amount of display speech. One who is not finds it traumatic. And once again, we find that even when psychotherapy is successful, often there is need for voice therapy to enable the person to use an adequate vocal intensity.

Where there is no organic pathology such as vocal modules, paralysis, or contact ulcers, we can assume that the person does possess an adequate voice. Our task is to help him find it. Often we discover that emotional insecurity lies at the bottom of the problem, and we must provide opportunities for exploration and release of these feelings. These people often are fearful of establishing close relationships, and their barely audible voices reflect this fear. A warm, permissive clinician can make the vocal therapy itself a means of creating at least one nonthreatening relationship. Often the speech therapy is less important than the case's testing of the clinician's acceptance, but we use the vocal exercises as the pathway to reassurance. By extending the therapy to other communicative situations, the person comes to find that the world may not be as threatening as he had supposed.

But there are often habits involved too. Whatever the original cause of the weak voice, these people often show inefficient forms of breathing when speaking. They may habitually exhale much of the inhaled air prior to vocalization (air wastage), or make a series of small inhalations rather than one large one (staircase breathing), or speak on the very end of the exhaled breath, or speak while the chest is expanding (opposition breathing). A certain amount of air pressure is needed for adequate phonation, and these methods of speech breathing make it difficult to speak loudly enough for communication. We seldom need to teach the person how to breath; but there are times when we have to teach him to stop breathing in an abnormal way. Once he knows what he is doing wrongly and recognizes the moments of normal breathing which he always shows occasionally, the normal patterns will return.

Often, the problem may consist of the use of improper pitch levels. The person who speaks at the very bottom, or very top, of his pitch range, for any reason, cannot have normal vocal intensity. We may therefore have to change the habitual pitch. We have had clients referred to us as having weak voices who merely were fearful that if they spoke in their usual way, they would have pitch breaks upward into the falsetto. With these, it was necessary to work on pitch control and to ignore the intensity. Generally, intensity becomes louder as the pitch rises. By prolonging tones and then introducing rhythmic pulses of pitch rises which go higher and higher, the intensity of the pulses becomes louder and louder.

Certain voice quality changes can also increase the intensity. By making the voice less breathy or aspirate through the use of very sudden bursts of sound, the voice becomes louder. Increasing the nasality a bit also helps. We once solved the problem of a foreman in a steel mill who was constantly losing his voice and could barely speak above a whisper due to the constant strain to make himself heard. We trained him to speak with a nasal twang while he was on the job.

Also the duration aspects of voice should be explored. By prolonging the vowels a bit, the carrying quality of the voice can be improved. Most public speakers have learned this technique. Also, a slowing down of the rate and the use of longer pauses seem to aid intelligibility.

Some of these cases are difficult to hear merely because they speak with their mouths almost shut—because they do not articulate with any energy. Putting a stopper in any horn diminishes the loudness of its tones. We teach these people to uncork their mouth openings. Also, by making the plosives distinctly or by stressing the fricative consonants, we can compensate for the lack of vocal intensity. Many of the bad habits of utterance are due to excessive tension in the mouth, tongue, or throat; and by relaxing these focal points of tension, the voice becomes freer and louder. One of the common areas of excessive muscular contraction is the region just above the larynx and below the chin. The larynx is often raised almost into the position for swallowing. When a person habitually assumes this abnormal posture prior to vocalization, it is difficult to produce normal voice no matter what effort is expended. Again, we must identify this abnormal behavior and bring it up to consciousness so that it can be brought under voluntary control and eliminated. Voice should not be squeezed out. It needs an open, relaxed, natural channel. At times we have these persons talk while chewing to discover the normal function. Some of our voice clients have forgotten how to produce voice normally. We must show them.

A few of our voice clients, especially those who have some paralysis of the vocal folds, need more energy rather than less, and they need it in the right places. Certain pushing exercises with the arms or legs, or sudden contractions of the fist may aid if they are accompanied by phonation. Also we have found that certain large body movements facilitate louder and freer voices. One of our clients first found his natural voice while on hands and knees with arms extended forward and his head backward. Once he had found it, he gradually became able to produce it in any position.

Finally, we use masking noise to prevent self-hearing when we feel that the person can really produce normal voice but inhibitions prevent it. We ask such a client to continue reading aloud while we gradually introduce a masking noise from an audiometer or tape recorder into both ears. Usually, the persons's voice grows much louder as the noise level increases. When we feel that sufficient change has occurred we suddenly shut off the noise and he hears himself speaking with a normal voice. One of the author's clients was "cured" when he suddenly emerged from a noisy factory and found himself shouting.

Pitch Disorders

Thusfar we have been describing those voice disorders in which the basic problem is one of loudness or intensity. We must remember, however, that there are two other main aspects of voice which may also be deviant—pitch and quality. Indeed, the professional speech pathologist knows that except for aphonia (in which no voice is present) the majority of his voice clients tend to show abnormality in all three features, though only one is usually most prominent in its deviation. Moreover, he knows too that by changing the pitch level changes in loudness or vocal quality can often be achieved, and often by altering the intensity, or the vocal quality, pitch levels can become more normal. Therefore, when he examines a client with a voice problem he surveys all three aspects of the voice, the intensity, pitch, and quality, and seeks to determine how they may be related.

Suppose, however, that the speech pathologist recognizes immediately that the most noticeable deviation is one of pitch. He then asks himself some diagnostic questions: Is the habitual pitch level too high or too low for the client's age and sex? Is this client speaking in almost a monotone? Do the pitch breaks resemble those of the adolescent male when his voice is changing? Is he speaking with the falsetto? Is the voice tremulous in its pitch? Is the deviation primarily one of stereotyped or peculiar inflections? Is he using two pitches (diplophonia) at the same time? Are there times or conditions when the client's pitch levels are within the normal range?

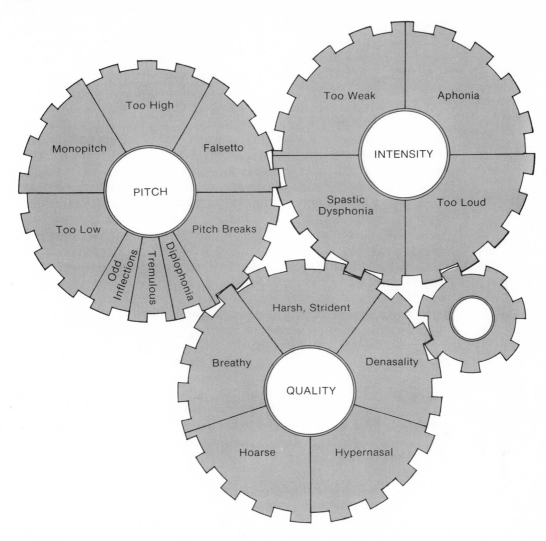

Figure 24 The disorders of voice.

Habitual Pitch Levels   The concept of a habitual pitch level must be clearly under- stood. Except in the case of monotones, it does not refer to a certain fixed pitch upon which all speech is phonated. It rep- resents an average or median pitch about which the other pitches used in speech tend to cluster. For example, in the utterance of the sentence, "Alice was sitting on the back of the white swan," the fun-

damental pitch of each vowel in any of the words may differ somewhat from that of the others. Moreover, certain vowels are inflected—
that is, they are phonated with a continuous pitch change which may
either rise, fall, or do both. Of course, each inflection has an average
pitch by which it may be measured, if the extent of the variation is
also considered. If all the pitches and pitch variatons are measured
and their durations are taken into account in the speaking of the preceding illustration, we shall find that they cluster about a certain average pitch, which may be termed the "key" at which the speaker
phonated that sentence. It should be understood, of course, that different pitch levels will be used under different communicative conditions. Nevertheless, each voice can be said to have a habitual pitch
range in which most of the communication is phonated.

The pitch of the normal human voice presents many mysteries,
and much research needs to be done before we can hope to understand its abnormalities. We know that the voice of a young child is
high-pitched when compared with that of the adult, and that in old
age it tends to creep back again to higher levels. We know that the
major pitch changes occur at puberty, the bottom of the girl's pitch
range descending from one to three tones with an equivalent gain at
the upper limit. Boys' voices usually drop a full octave, and there is a
less marked but noticeable loss at the upper end of the pitch range.
Usually, but depending upon the onset of sexual changes, the voice
changes occur in boys between the ages of thirteen and fifteen with
the girls showing the same basic changes a year earlier. Occasionally,
the change of voice has been known to occur very suddenly (usually
when puberty comes late), but most frequently it takes from three to
six months on the average.

Why do some people fail to make the normal pitch change?
There are several reasons besides delayed sexual development. Some
clients have voices which are high-pitched primarily because of infantile personalities, because they cannot or prefer not to grow up.
This case study may help to make the point:

> Charles J. was first referred to the public-school speech clinician
> for his articulation difficulty at the age of twelve. He substituted
> *w* for *r* and *l, t* for *k,* and *d* for *g.* He had a marked interdental
> lisp. He sucked his thumb and cried easily. He preferred the
> company of very young children and still played with dolls at
> home. He was rejected and despised by boys of his own age
> and bore the nickname of "Sister." He was an only child, pam-
> pered and babied and overprotected by an anxious mother. Al-
> though intelligent, he had failed the third grade twice. He was

absent from school a good share of the time for chronic head-
aches and stomach upsets. The articulation defects were very resistant to therapy, and the child was not cooperative. Consequently, he was dismissed from speech therapy classes and
referred to the school psychologist, who was unable to solve the
home problem because of the mother's attitudes.

At seventeen he was again referred to speech therapy, this time
at a college clinic. No articulation defects were present, but the
voice was very high-pitched, rather nasally whiny, and weak in
intensity. The secondary sex characteristics were present, and he
was quite fat. The personality was still infantile.

In such cases psychotherapy is the indicated treatment, although
vocal training may be used along with it, either to make the psychotherapy more palatable or to help the person to make changes in the
habitual pitch as he comes to accept and solve his psychological
problem.

Another common cause of the high-pitched voice is tension.
The tighter the vocal cords are held, the higher is the pitch of the
tone produced. Tension in any area of the body tends to flow upward
and focus in the larynx. Many individuals who, in their occupations,
are compelled to speak very loudly will raise their voices to make
themselves heard, and this raising also lifts the habitual pitch.
Speech therapy will be of little avail unless the underlying cause of
the tension can be eliminated or reduced. Some case presentations
may help us understand the problem.

Joan P., a high-school senior, referred herself to the speech
clinic after hearing a recording of her voice. "Why, I sound like
a little first grader," she complained. "After hearing that voice
I'll never dare talk to a boy again over the telephone. Please do
something!" Analysis of the average pitch levels used by the girl
showed that she phonated about the pitch of middle C, a level
which is well within the normal range for females of that age.
When the test recording was played back, she said, "That's
funny. That's a little bit higher than I thought I talked but not
so high as the other recording." We then made another recording, in front of a class, and this time the average pitch level did
reach F above middle C. We explained to Joan that most females
hear their recorded voices as seemingly higher in pitch just as
most males hear themselves as possessing a deeper voice than
they expect. We also explained the effect of tension and fear on
the pitch level and the need for learning to adapt to the pres-

sures of confronting a group. A series of experiences in making recorded talks to a group while trying to use the middle-C habitual pitch of her conversational voice proved successful, and no further difficulty was experienced.

Most of us tend to raise the pitch of our voices when communicating under fear or stress, or when trying to speak loudly. In examining a voice case, we must always be alert lest the client's uneasiness give us a false picture.

A boy of seventeen was referred to us as a monotone, and most of his speech was pitched at D above middle C. He tended to use loudness instead of pitch variations to give the meaningful inflections necessary in asking questions, making demands, and so on. For example, he would say this sentence with each syllable pitched at the one note, but saying the last word quite loudly. "Are you planning to GO?" The effect was often one of hostility, which he did not mean to convey at all. The voice quality was rather harsh. Most strange, he was able to sing in a very high tenor voice and sing very well. A series of counseling interviews and examinations resulted in our refusal to accept him for therapy at that time. A year later, he was reexamined and his voice was entirely normal, being pitched at B below middle C, with a range of an octave and a half, and normal inflections and quality. Meanwhile he had started to shave.

As the foregoing case implies, pitch levels are dependent upon many factors. The client mentioned was slow in acquiring the secondary sex characteristics. His larynx, at the time of our first examination, was childlike and underdeveloped. Highly conscious of this, he had endeavored to compensate for the natural high pitch by speaking at the very bottom of his range.

Pitch disorders seem to be more easily recognized than those of intensity or quality, and hence, are more often referred for clinical help as this quotation from Moore (1971) may illustrate:

A consistently high-pitched voice in the late adolescent or adult male is one of the most distressing of voice defects. The resemblance to the female voice suggests a lack of masculinity. It is this implication, with its psychological sequellae, that creates the seriousness of the disorder, since the voice proper does not interfere with communication; nor would it be unpleasant if it were produced by a female. (p. 539)

Similarly, an abnormally low-pitched voice in a girl or woman appears deviant and can cause the person much distress. Though most of our clients with this problem have been adult women who have passed through their menopause and have taken medication containing hormones (testerone compounds) which produced a *virilization* (male sounding) of the voice, we also have had a few young female college students with deep bass voices. They were almost afraid to open their mouths, afraid to talk for fear of the listener reactions which had often traumatized them.

There is much that we still do not know about why we habitually use the pitch ranges that we prefer. The voice of authority in this country is pitched deeply; in Japan, it is very high. Do soprano mothers and tenor fathers beget children with pitch levels higher than their playmates? Are pitch levels determined physiologically or anatomically? Certainly, we find a few clients with very tiny laryngeal cartilages who speak far above the normal range, but most persons with pitch disorders have normal larynges (*plural for larynx*). Why do the deaf tend to have high-pitched voices? Again we do not really know. Speech pathology is full of unknowns.

Monopitch   We have never seen a client whose voice could be viewed as strictly monopitched, although we have known many whose voices were highly monotonous. All of them were capable of some pitch change, and all of them had some inflection. The key characteristic was the narrow range of inflection and pitch change, often no more than one or two semitones. Also, these individuals often substitute a change in intensity for the pitch change, and this creates the impression of deviancy. Many persons whose voices strike us as entirely lacking in inflection are merely those with stereotyped inflections. These are the ones whose voices fall after every pause, comma, or period. There is deadly monotony, to be sure, but not monopitch. Nevertheless, these restricted, lifeless voices are miserable to listen to, and they interfere with communication by sheer lack of variety.

The causes of monopitch are: (1) emotional conflicts, (2) lack of physical vitality, (3) hearing loss, and (4) the use of habitual pitch levels too near the top or bottom of the pitch range. The role of emotional causation in producing the monotonous voice has been described by various authors and researchers. A review of the literature indicates that individuals who are in states of depression and schizophrenics tend to show this type of voice. We have also found it in paranoid or suspicious individuals or those who are barely able to keep their emotions under control, as a defensive mechanism to prevent others from knowing how they feel.

Undernourished, sick, or fatigued persons also tend to show little range of pitch or inflection. They seem to have insufficient energy available for the normal melody of speech. Those who are very hard of hearing also present the picture of monotonous voice, although careful scrutiny often reveals certain stereotyped inflections, most of which are alike and yet unlike those of the normally hearing person. Finally, when the habitual pitch for any reason is either too near the ceiling or floor of the pitch range, we find a tendency toward monopitch. We need voice room to maneuver. If we cannot go downward, we do not go upward. Falsetto voices often show this feature.

Pitch Breaks   Most of us tend to think of the change of voice as occurring abruptly when it does occur, and "pitch breaks" have been the subject for a good deal of humor in our culture. However, recent unpublished research has shown that most children, boys and girls alike, do have these sudden shifts of pitch as characteristic of the period of voice change; and also, some children as young as seven and eight can show similar sudden shifts. We also are prone to think of the pitch changes as always shifting toward the higher notes, but when this does occur consistently, it does so only toward the end of the puberal period. Voice breaks can be downward as well.

The majority of the pitch breaks that do occur are generally an octave in extent in most children. They occur involuntarily, very suddenly, and the child seems to have little control over them, reacting at first with great surprise. The upward pitch breaks of boys start when the word spoken is pitched below the habitual pitch of the moment. It often seems as though, in the attempt to return to the level they feel most natural, they overshoot their mark. In a few children the experience is so traumatic that they resort to a guarded monotone, and develop a very restricted range. According to Damste and Lehrman (1975) we should become concerned about the child's pitch breaks if, after six months to a year, they still persist.

The cause of the puberal pitch changes is not entirely understood, though we do know that profound alterations in the organs of voice occur at the time. The male larynx grows much larger, and the vocal folds grow longer and rather suddenly; the female larynx increases more in height than in width, and the vocal folds seem to thicken. The male vocal folds lengthen about one centimeter, the females only a third as much. At the same time, the child is growing swiftly in skeletal development. The neck becomes longer, and the larynx takes up a lower location relative to the opening into the mouth. The chest expands greatly, and perhaps one of the causes of voice breaks is the greater air pressure that suddenly becomes available. The following case may be illustrative:

> One of our cases was a boy who had been delayed markedly in physical growth until his sixteenth birthday, at which time a great spurt of development occurred. He grew six inches in three months and his voice seemed uncontrollable as far as pitch was concerned, so much so that he developed a marked fear of speaking and a profound emotional disturbance. Speech therapy was ineffective until he was taught by the speech therapist to fixate the chest and to use abdominal breathing as exclusively as possible. Immediately the pitch breaks disappeared, and the technique tided him over the next six months, at which time he returned to his normal thoracic breathing pattern without difficulty.

The above example illustrated another of the characteristics of the truly abnormal voice. Not only did he have many more pitch breaks than does the average boy, but also he showed shifts of pitch which were not of the usual type. Sometimes the break in pitch was of fourteen semitones. The speech clinician can often distinguish a pathological case who will not "outgrow" his adolescent pitch breaks by listening to the type of pitch shift which occurs. Curry cites the following similar case from the German literature:

> Case four is that of a 23-year-old girl with a mutation disorder; since age eight her voice had been continuously hoarse and accompanied by many involuntary breaks. These breaks from a higher to a lower pitch took place so rapidly that the voice was originally diagnosed as diplophonic (two-toned). In this instance, however, the apparent diplophonia is due to a rapid succession of different fundamentals rather than to different rates of vibration of the two individual cords. This case is of especial note because the difference between the two frequencies is not necessarily an octave.[9]

Public-school speech pathologists who have to make surveys of large populations of school children should recognize the fact that the control of pitch during puberal development can vary widely from day to day. Very often there is less control early in the morning than later in the day. We have also found that anger, excitement, fear, and

---

[9]T. Curry, "Voice Breaks and Pathological Larynx Conditions," *Journal of Speech and Hearing Disorders,* XIV (1948), 356–58.

other emotions may give a false picture of the severity of the problem. Laughter, especially if uncontrolled, will also produce an unusual number of breaks.

Too high a pitch in some individuals, either male or female, may be the result of failure to make the necessary transition to the adult voice. The social penalties upon the male with a voice pitched too high are severe in our culture. Indeed, an old name for this voice problem was the "eunuchoid voice." The penalties upon the female are less severe. An occasional male may even find a "baby voice" as attractive as a "baby face." Nevertheless, the high-pitched voice is rarely much of an asset. We have seen some marked tragedies resulting from the disorder. Personalities have been warped by social rejection; vocational progress has been blocked; self-doubts have destroyed the person's ability to cope with the demands of existence. There is nothing humorous about a high-pitched voice.

The Falsetto   All of us have the capacity for speaking in a falsetto voice even if we cannot yodel, but there are some individuals who use it involuntarily. It involves a different way of using the vocal folds. According to Shanks and Duguay (1974) they are shortened and made thinner. Cooker (1972) states that the falsetto register constitutes an entirely different mode of vibration, that in normal phonation "the entire shelf of muscular tissue vibrates whereas in the falsetto only the thin ligaments do. This condition is produced by stretching the vocal ligaments, and at the same time, relaxing the muscles within the folds." (p. 417)

The causes of the habitual falsetto voice appear to consist of (1) emotional factors as a protest against sexual or social maturity, (2) as a defense against pitch breaks, and (3) as a method for preventing the hoarse or husky voice. The first of these presents a problem in counseling and psychotherapy in some cases and professional help may be needed.

R. James S., III, came to us with a very high-pitched falsetto whose only inflection was at the end of his phrases and sentences. He was a fat boy at eighteen, and he was a boy rather than a youth. His divorced mother had spoiled and babied him for years, and he was almost totally unable to cope with his freshman year in the university. She phoned him every evening and wrote to him every day. He refused to eat in the dormitory, he wept easily and frequently and also in a falsetto. We recorded his voice, played it back to him, and then referred him to a psychiatrist. He dropped out of school and we lost track of him for a year. When he returned, he told us that he had continued his psychotherapy, had cut his ties with his mother, and was working as a janitor. His psychiatrist reported that he was now ready for voice therapy. Within a single week he found his deep bass voice. It was one of the easiest bits of therapy we have ever had. Had we attempted to work with Bob, as he had finally come to call himself, earlier, we are sure we would have been unsuccessful.

This case points up another significant bit of information. Abnormal voices can persist of their own momentum and habituation long after the original cause has ceased to exist. They perpetuate themselves by the reinforcement they get from successful consummation of communication.

In some of our clients, the falsetto appears to be the result of a defensive reaction against the traumatic experience of pitch breaks. It is not pleasant to have one's voice flop around, especially when this behavior provokes mockery and social penalty. By using the falsetto, one can prevent these breaks; and some beginning adolescents use it for this purpose, only to find that they have lost the ability to find the normal adult voice. They fear to use the low-pitched voices we can teach them fairly easily, and our problem is to help them realize that the pitch breaks can be controlled and prevented. We use a lot of negative practice in working with these individuals, deliberately practicing the pitch breaks and desensitizing them. Chanting and singing on the lower pitches is useful. These same basic principles are employed when working with a person whose falsetto is a defense against hoarse or husky voice qualities.

Other Pitch Disorders   The tremulous voice may be due to paralysis, muscular dystrophy, or other similar neurological disorders. It may also be due to cerebral palsy on the one hand, or to fearfulness on the other. Referral to medical or psychological services is indicated. Females or children with very low-pitched voices should be referred to a physician before undertaking speech therapy; often glandular and hormonal problems are present. Stereotyped inflections may be due to foreign-language influence, to psychological conflicts, or to hearing loss.

Treatment of When the problem consists of an habitual pitch which is ab-
Pitch Disorders normally high in the male or abnormally low in the woman,
the clinician's basic task is to discover ways of helping his
case produce a more optimal pitch level. First, there must be some
confrontation through tape recording, an experience that often shocks
the case terrifically, for he has not really recognized before how his
voice sounds to others. We have also found the use of the delayed
auditory feedback apparatus very effective in this regard, especially
when longer delay times (at least one second) were used. When appropriate, we have even recorded the voice and then played it back
with strong amplification. This confrontation in other persons must
be done less drastically; but unless the individual really recognizes
his pitch deviation at the time it is occurring, he will rarely have the
motivation to change.

Our next task is to help the person vary his pitch levels, to explore the range of pitches of which he is capable but has not discovered. The pitch of the voice usually varies with the intensity. By increasing the loudness, the tone will usually be made to rise in pitch.
Even high-pitched falsettos will shift downward if a tone is first initiated very loudly, then gradually softened as it is prolonged. Pitch
rises when the laryngeal musculature is tensed, and we can use this
feature in therapy. Tension in almost any part of the body seems to
be reflected and finds some focus in the larynx. By asking the person
to pull upward on the seat of his chair, or to push down on the table,
we can increase the tension of the vocal folds and raise the pitch of a
sustained tone. This works best if the effort is applied in pulses.
Conversely, if we wish to lower a pitch, we can begin by using
strong muscular contractions and let go jerkily in a series of relaxa-
tions.

The self-perception of pitch is still mysterious. We still do not
know why some individuals with excellent hearing seem to be unable to match a given pitch or to locate their own voices on a scale.
They sing off key and do not know it. However, there seems to be
some evidence that pitch perception is tied in somehow with body
postures and kinesthesia. Even little children who have never seen a
musical scale lift their heads and rise on tiptoe when they reach for a
high note. When we try to sing very low, we tuck our chins in, lowering our heads. At any rate, we have found that by having the client
follow our head or arm body movements as we show him how his
pitches are rising or falling or being sustained, we can improve his
faulty pitch placement. Here is a brief transcript of part of a session
with such a person whose pitch breaks were driving him crazy.

Clinician: Now lower your head way down like this, then bring it up
in three steps as we sing together do-me-sol.

Client: doh-fa-la.

Clinician: OK. You went up — but you took too big steps. Raise your
head in smaller steps. Here, I'll hold your head and move it. . . .

Client: doh-fa-sol.

Clinician: That's better. The first and last were all right. You sang do-
fa-sol. It should be do-*me*-sol. Let's make the second movement
smaller. . . .

We stopped the transcript just in time. The case sang, "doh-la-
tee." This is patient work, this voice-retraining — but we have suc-
ceeded often when our first attempts seem to reveal a hopeless prognosis. With real motivation, surprising results may be had. In this
regard, we find that a prime motivation is the opportunity provided
by a permissive clinician for the client's singing. These sour-toned
people love to sing, and they've been penalized and frustrated most
of their lives because their "pear-shaped tones" turn out to be lem-
ons. So we let them sing a lot and do some voice therapy when we
can. Another similar method consists of pitch-writing. We take the
client's hand as he holds the pencil or chalk and tell him to go up
and down or hum or sing his own invented tunes. Then we trace the
variations and provide a graphic record.

Although the above method for teaching a new pitch level is
most effective, there are several others. One frequently employed
uses the vocalized sigh or yawn to produce the desired pitch. These
sighs and yawns must be accompanied by decreasing intensity and
relaxation in order to be most effective. Another method employs ex-
clamations of disgust or contempt in order to provide a lower pitch.
Still another makes use of the grunts and noises symbolic of relief or
feeding. Clearing the throat may also be used to provide a lower
pitch. These methods are often effective with true monotones when
the former stimulation or matching method fails. Many of the techniques included in the stimulation method are combined with the bi-
ological-activity methods in order to provide the necessary stability
of performance.

An example of some actual therapy which produced a change
from a high falsetto into normal male phonation within a single hour
may now be given, though it should be understood that further work
was necessary to stabilize the new voice thereby obtained.

T. J. was a nineteen-year-old boy with a high-pitched mono-

tonal falsetto which was inconsistent in that occasionally nonfal-
setto tones were heard, although they, too, were spoken at the
same high level. After the usual ear-training in identifying the
problem, we had a session in which we demonstrated the following kinds of phonation and asked him to join us and to duplicate what we heard: (1) We asked him to do some vocalized
donkey-breathing, alternately on inhalation and on exhalation,
and very rhythmically. As we produced the model, we occasionally changed the pitch of the exhaled sound, using first the falsetto ourselves and then lower normal tones. Several of his
tones were very good. (2) We asked him to retract his head as
far as he could, then to bring it forward until it dropped down
on his chest, producing a long sigh as he did so. We showed
him and first did what he did so far as sound was concerned,
then gradually let our own pitch fall as the sigh ended. He followed us and ended with a weak, breathy, but very low tone.
(3) We showed him some stretching and yawning and asked
him to join us, saying "Awwwww" in the middle of the yawn.
(4) We placed some tissue paper over a comb and asked him to
buzz it, using a prolonged z sound with his lips against the paper. The tone we used was of low pitch, and so was his. We
then asked him to say zzzeeezzz and zzzooozzz and then
zzzzoooooo as he buzzed the comb. This failed, for he used a falsetto buzz. (5) We asked him to duplicate a vocalized clearing of
the throat as he held his fingers to his ears. It was very low-
pitched and without any falsetto. (6) We then taught him the
clicking vocal fry until he could sustain it for several seconds,
then had him open and shut his jaws and lips during the fry
phonation. In this activity we heard normal phonation along
with the vocal fry. (7) We demonstrated head- and jaw-shaking
from side to side while we produced various vowels of different
pitches. (8) As he duplicated our model by head- and jaw-
shaking in unison with us, we slowly said, "I am using my real
voice," and he echoed it in the new low pitch. (9) We played
back the recording of his voice to him, called it quits for that
session, asked him not to speak very much until we saw him
again, and made an appointment to do so.

Disorders of Voice Quality

There are five major disorders of voice quality: hypernasality; denasality; the breathy, husky voice; the harsh or strident voice; and the

hoarse voice. In addition, there is a peculiar throaty or guttural voice which is probably a low-pitched falsetto.

Hypernasality   This problem is not an uncommon one. It occurs primarily because the back door to the nose fails to close sufficiently. The contraction of the soft palate and pharyngeal muscles which elevate, spread, and squeeze the rear opening to the nasal passages may be said to constitute that door. Research has shown that the closure need not be complete on all sounds to prevent hypernasality, but there are definite limits to the amount of opening permitted. Certain organic conditions reflect themselves in excessive nasality because they make it difficult to close this valve-like mechanism sufficiently. The person with an unrepaired cleft palate shows hypernasality; so does the person whose soft palate has been paralyzed or made sluggish by poliomyelitis or other disease. Investigations have also revealed that hypernasality tends to occur after the adenoids have been removed, a process which leaves a relatively larger channel than had previously existed, due to the adenoid mass.

Hypernasality, when excessive, creates a voice quality which most listeners find unpleasant, although the vocal yokel who loves hillbilly ballads may deny this. It has some virtue in enabling the speaker to get his message across in the presence of masking noise, for it carries piercingly. Auctioneers and barkers at carnival side shows find it useful, if not ornamental.

Assimilation   Hypernasality may be general and exist on most of the vow-
Nasality   els and voiced consonant sounds, or it may be restricted only to the sounds which precede or follow the nasal consonants /m/, /n/ and /ŋ/. This latter type is termed assimilation nasality. Many speakers of general American English show some assimilation nasality in such a sentence as "Any man can make money." This is because of the need for alternate openings and closing of the velo-pharyngeal opening. In the word *man*, the passageway to the nose must be open on the *m*, closed on the *a*, and opened again on the *n*. It's easier just to leave the space open. Also, even on a word such as *and*, we tend to prepare for the *n* opening while we're still saying the *a*, and this may cause a premature lowering of the soft palate, thereby producing the sound nasally. The assimilation may thus be either forward or backward. Hypernasality of either type seems to be more likely to occur on certain sounds than on others. High back vowels such as /u/ and /o/ show less hypernasality than do the lower

front vowels. The consonants /z/ and /v/ tend to show more hyper-nasality on them than do the other consonants. It is possible to have much hypernasality without ever having any airflow coming out of the nose because it is the resonation of the sound, not the airflow, which creates the unpleasant voice quality. The louder the voice, the more prominent the hypernasality appears.

There are other causes for hypernasality besides organic. Through imitation and identification, children can learn the excessively nasal voices of their parents or associates. Low vitality and fatigue also tend to produce more of the problem, for it takes energy to make the swift adjustments needed. Finally, whining children and adults have whining voices; complaint prefers the trombone of the nose. Certain stereotyped rising-falling inflections along with the hypernasality tend to identify this causation. It is different from that shown by the organic cases.

Denasality   This is the voice of the head cold, of the hay fever victim, of the child with enlarged adenoids. The nasal passages are oc-cluded, perhaps by growths within the nostrils, by congestion in the nasal cavities above the roof of the mouth, or by adenoids in the rear passageways. Often some of the nasal consonants are affected, the person saying "Mby syduhzziz are killig mbe." The voice sounds are dulled and congested. Listeners desire to clear their own throats or to flee. Again, as we have found before, denasal voices may be main-tained long after the cause has ceased to exist.

The Breathy,   This disorder often coexists with other problems. It may
Husky Voice   show itself in intermittent aphonia, in cases of weak in-tensity, in conjunction with the hoarse voice. Its major char-acteristic, as the name implies, is an excessive output of airflow along with the phonation. Breathy voices are not whispered, but they are aspirate in quality. Phonation is present, but the rush of air is obvi-ous. At times, the huskiness accompanies the tone; at other times the constricted hissing of the air precedes or follows the tone. There is air wastage. In some cases, a sort of gasping series of short in-halations throughout the person's speech produces the impression of huskiness. When this occurs, the phrases are short and choppy, and the rhythm of utterance is disturbed. From this description it is obvi-ous that there are different types of breathy voices.

Causes   In Figure 25 we present illustrations of some of the organic conditions which can lead to weak, breathy voices. The vocal nodules we have already mentioned, but some persons abuse their voices so much they develop other pathologies. The laryngeal polyp, if it is large enough, not only produces weak and breathy phonation but also a fluttering, tremulous pitch. Usually benign, it can be removed by surgery. Contact ulcers are most often the result of vocal abuse and strain. To aid in their healing, physicians prescribe silence, but unless the person is trained by the speech pathologist in better ways of producing voice, they tend to recur.

The causes of the breathy voice may be either organic or functional. A paralyzed vocal cord may fail to join its twin at the midline for part of its length, thus leaving a gap through which the airflow may leak. A vocal nodule—a tiny corn-like growth on the edge of a vocal cord—may prevent complete closure. Certain diseases may inflame or swell the membranes of the vocal cords so that they vibrate inefficiently. Excessive strain may make them weak—as it does any muscle when overloaded too long. Whenever you meet such a disorder, you should first make sure that the person hasn't just been yelling too long at a football game or has a bad cold, and then, if the condition has persisted or is getting worse, the case should be immediately referred to a physician.

There are also other causes. We have known individuals whose breathy voices were being produced and maintained solely by improper habits of vocal attack. They always began voicing with a preliminary exhalation of air. We had to teach them to start speaking without this preparatory windup. Some persons use a breathy voice because of the fear of being heard or exposed. And a few of them employ it deliberately. The following case illustrates the latter point.

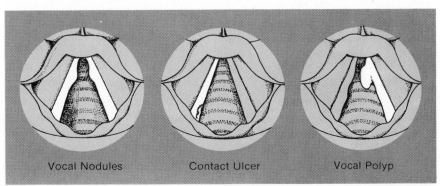

Figure 25   Three organic causes of dysphonia.

Ruth, a rather plain high-school girl, was referred to us by the English teacher, who reported that her voice was so husky she was unable to make herself heard in class. We examined the girl and discovered not only the huskiness but also a low, habitual pitch level with certain inflections which were unmistakable. She could sing well and without any breathiness. A bit of sympathetic interviewing explained the situation. "The boys like this kind of voice," she said grinning. "I'm not too attractive, but a moose is a moose and they come when I call." We found out later that the boys called her "Hot-breath Harriett." We kept her secret.

The male has also been known to mistake asthma for passion.

The Harsh or Strident Voice   There are voices which are so rasping and piercing that they repel listeners. The basic characteristic of these voices is the presence of what is called the "vocal fry," because, perhaps, it sounds like the sizzling of bacon in the frying pan. As we said earlier, it is hard to describe but fairly easy to produce. By opening your mouth and making a ticker-like, crackling sort of sound, you can produce it and even slow it down until the separate clicks can be distinguished. When this vocal fry is fast, however, and accompanied by great tension, we have the basic quality of the strident or harsh voice. It is often accompanied by strain localized about the larynx, and often this structure is pulled up almost to the position used in swallowing. If you will place the tip of a finger against your Adam's or Eve's apple and produce a very harsh voice, you will know what we mean.

Along with these features we also find the presence of what is called the "hard attack." Normally, the vocal folds should be brought together almost simultaneously with the pulse of air pressure. In the aspirate or soft attack, as we have already seen, the vocal folds close *after* the air has begun to flow. In the hard attack, the folds are closed and held tightly prior to the breath pulse. To break them open and start them vibrating from this tight position requires extra effort. If you will squeeze and hold your vocal folds tightly closed and suddenly utter a vowel, you will hear the little strained click that indicates the hard attack. It is not a good way to produce voice; vocal nodules or contact ulcers may result from the strain.

The usual causes of the harsh voice are imitation, personality problems involving hostility and aggression, the need to make one-self heard in the presence of masking noise, and the use of improper pitch levels. We need not belabor the obviousness of the first two of these causes, but some comment on the others is necessary. Strident voices seem to be able to make themselves heard more easily than normal voices, even though the effect is often unpleasant. In this regard they are somewhat like hypernasality. They're harsh but you can hear them. Those of us whose professions demand constant speaking in noisy situations often develop them, and sound more aggressive than we are. One of the nicest persons we have ever known was a lady who was in charge of the woman's swimming classes at our university, and she sounded like a witch until she developed vocal nodules and had to have voice therapy as well as a change of jobs. The only way she had found to pierce the echoing noise of splashing, squealing girls was to scream at them harshly. One of our cases was a foreman in a noisy factory whose harsh straining voice finally gave out due to the formation of contact ulcers near the back ends of his vocal folds. Those of us who become teachers or speech pathologists must remember to take care of our own professional tool, the human voice. It cannot be abused with impunity.

The Hoarse Voice   Acoustically, the hoarse voice may be said to be a combination of the breathy and the harsh voice quality disorders. In it you can hear the air wastage and also the straining vocal fry of the strident voice. When voices suddenly become hoarse, we look for evidence of overuse or abuse. Most of us have become hoarse from too much yelling at one time or another—but not from praying. Usually with rest the hoarseness disappears. You've got to stop calling the pigs from the back forty, Ma. The same situation occurs as the result of a severe cold or laryngitis. Many boys develop a hoarse or husky voice just before puberty in an effort to assume the deep, low tones of the adult male or to demonstrate their toughness. This too shall pass. But we wish to sound a strong note of warning about hoarseness. When it persists long after the abuse or laryngitis has disappeared, and there seems to be no apparent reason for its continuance, referral to a laryngologist should be made. Cancer of the larynx often shows its ugly head first in this form.

A hoarse voice may also be produced through ventricular phonation. By this term we refer to the vibration of the false vocal folds which lie above the true ones. It is uncommon but we have found it in some few bedeviled children who suffer many penalties. The following account by Voelker may illustrate the problem.

One patient complained of dropping his voice at the end of sentences, and it was found that he did not lower his vocal cord pitch, but actually stopped using his vocal cords at the end of the sentence and substituted for them a ventricular vibration. An actor, with an excellent stage voice, complained of hoarseness only in conversation. It was found that in intimate and quiet conversation he used a ventricular voice to "save for his art" his stage voice. A youth was criticized by his parents for having a high and squeaky voice and acquired ventricular phonia in order to lower his voice to a normal pitch. Thus, instead of lowering his voice to a normal pitch of perhaps 150 cycles, he lowered it to one of between 48 to 57 cycles. A similar case was found in which a man thirty-one-years old, who had a deaf wife, became self-conscious about his yelling, and outside his home developed phonation with the ventricular bands to subdue his voice. A college student raised the pitch of his voice to read aloud or to recite but used a ventricular tone in conversation. Sometimes it is found in careless conversation only. A five-year-old boy was kidded by his playmates for having a high voice, and he lowered it by acquiring a ventricular voice. An eighteen-year-old youth, with a eunuchoid quality, substituted ventricular phonation for his weak and strident vocal cord voice and thought his new hoarse voice gave the impression of virility.[10]

Treatment of Voice Quality Disorders

Speech pathologists who have watched professional singers working hour upon hour to perfect their tone, practicing scales, spending long hours with their voice teacher sometimes envy that teacher. To find the same devotion in a person with a voice disorder is unusual. Even when the person has a falsetto or a husky voice due to severe vocal nodules, it is difficult to get him to work hard enough to hope for a favorable result. The reason for this state of affairs seems to lie in the relative lack of attention we pay to our voices. In the expression of emotion, we are more concerned with the cargo of anger rather than the voice vehicle which carries it. In most communicative interchanges, the basic message is carried by the articulation rather than the tones; and unless the voice is so weak it cannot be heard, the fulfillment of communication generally rewards unpleasant voices as well as good ones. It is only in display speech, such as that of the teacher or actor, that a poor voice is a major handicap.

[10] C. H. Voelker, "Phoniatry in Dysphonia Ventricularis," *Annals of Otology, Rhinology, and Laryngology,* XLIV (1935), 471–72.

Identification of   One of the best ways we have found to motivate these clients
the Problem   is to have them hear their own voices on tape recordings, not
once but over and over again. Once we put a schoolteacher
with a very hypernasal voice into a booth, locked the door, and
piped in her own recorded voice a bit amplified for fifteen minutes.
From then on she worked very hard. We also have a delayed-speech
apparatus which echoes what the person says about four seconds
later. But best of all is to have a clinician who can imitate almost exactly the voice he hears. We train our own students in this skill so
that they can be the echo machine. Amplification, by means of one of
the binaural auditory training units, can be very effective, especially
if the clinician joins the person and first uses the abnormal voice,
then shifts to a better one. The same effect can be had by having the
person cup his hands to make a channel from his mouth to one ear,
then the clinician alternately puts his echo and his normal voice into
the other ear as they read in unison. At other times we feed a masking voice into a person's ears from an audiometer as he is speaking,
and then suddenly turn it off so the person hears his voice more vividly. Since much of the inability to hear one's voice comes from the
adaptation to the usual conditions of phonation, almost anything
which alters the usual conditions helps one to hear it as it is. Radio
announcers long ago found that they could hear their own voices better by cupping one ear to alter the sound field. We use this device
and occasionally even employ a hearing aid to help the client identify
his problem. We have often found that having the person plug his
ears with his fingers makes it possible for him to hear his defective
voice more clearly and to modify it.

Analyzing   We often find that the person is unable to recognize the de-
the Deviancy   viancy in voice until he is trained in its analysis. One has to
know what to listen for. One needs training. The clinician
must train the client to do this analyzing, patiently providing examples of what is wrong, checking their occurrence in the person's
voice. Let us give a description of this analyzing process as it would
be done in hypernasality.

Recognition of   In order that the student may learn to recognize the unpleas-
Defective Quality   ant voice quality whenever it occurs in his speech, the vowels
that are least defective should be used. The clinician should
imitate these vowels as the client produces them, and then repeat
them, using excess nasality. The client will readily recognize the difference. He should be required to produce these vowels first normally and then with excess nasality, carefully noting the difference.

Lightly placed thumb and forefinger on each side of the septum, or the use of the cold mirror placed under the nostrils, will provide an accessory check of the presence of the hypernasality. The client should then listen to the clinician's production of his worst vowel, with and without nasality. If difficulty is experienced in recognizing this, the client can correlate his auditory judgments with the visual and tactual sensations received from the use of the mirror and finger-septum contact. Requiring him to close and open his eyes during alternate productions of the vowels as the clinician uses the mirror under his nostrils will soon provide adequate discrimination.[11]

After some of this training has been successfully completed, the clinician should read a passage in which certain vowels are underlined and are purposely nasalized. The client should listen carefully, checking on a copy of the passage all vowels in which he hears the unpleasant quality. Many of the games and exercises used in the ear training of articulatory cases can be modified to teach the client better discrimination and identification of the good and bad voice qualities. Although at first the clinician will need to exaggerate the hypernasality, she should endeavor to decrease it gradually until the client is skilled in detecting even a slight amount of it. After this has been done, the client should read and reread a certain paragraph, making judgments after each word as to whether or not excess nasality occurred. These judgments may be checked by the teacher, and the percentage of correct judgments ascertained. This procedure will serve as a motivating device. The client may also be required to repeat series of words or isolated vowels, using the mirror under his nostrils and making his judgment of normal or nasal voice quality before opening his eyes to observe the clouding or nonclouding of the mirror. Much home practice of this sort can be used.

The same sort of self-scanning should be used with other voice disorders. Unless the person comes to hear what is wrong, he will not correct it. There is one caution we wish to leave with you. Occasionally, a person may feel that he is becoming much worse as the result of this recognition training. All that has happened is that he has become more conscious of what has always been there before; but it is wise, in early treatment, to warn him that this may occur and that it is a good sign of improvement. Similarly, some of our voice cases may become rather emotional and rejecting of themselves as the deviant voice becomes more apparent to them. However, if the

---

[11] There are various devices available to the speech pathologist that display evidence of excessive nasal airflow or hypernasality so they can be monitored by the client. A biofeedback apparatus called the Tonar has been used for this purpose by Fletcher (1972).

clinician is able to share the problem, using the abnormal voice calmly and without anxiety, the person usually soon becomes desensitized to it. We have found it wise from the beginning examination to present the task as a joint endeavor. We explore its causes together, and together we work to modify the voice.

Discovering the New Voice   Each of us is the potential possessor of many voices. We can all vary our pitch, intensity, and quality pretty much at will, although few of us have ever felt that it was possible or necessary to learn a new habitual voice. When this necessity becomes apparent, as a result of the training in awareness, we might think that little further difficulty in procuring cooperation would be necessary. However, a storm of resistance usually arises at this point. This is what one of our clients said to us:

> Yesterday, when we made that tape recording of my new voice and I heard it, I felt all mixed up inside. I told you it sounded much better, and it does. Compared to my old voice, it's a great improvement. But it isn't ME! It just isn't. I sound like a phony or like an actor playing a part. I know it's better, but I don't want to talk so strangely. I just couldn't keep my appointment with you today because I'm so upset about it. I'm even thinking of quitting. I know you said I'd get used to it, but right now I don't think I ever could.

She got used to it, and now it is the old voice which seems unbelievable to her. But this is a problem to be faced. The voice is closely integrated with the personality. Its inflections, volume, and quality have been used since childhood to express emotion. The old voice has a long history of being associated with basic feelings. It does not yield easily to modification, but it does yield. The important thing is that both the clinician and the person with the voice problem must anticipate this resistance and be prepared to cope with it.

Variation   One of the ways to overcome this built-in rigidity and resistance is to begin by exploring all the possible ways of producing phonation. We must share together in free variation, almost in tonal play, trying one vocal variation after another. Van Riper and Irwin describe this process as follows:

> First we can get the case to run through his entire repertoire of possible phonation, locating within it the desired target tones.

Few individuals are entirely consistent in their abnormal voice. Some vowels, for example, may be less nasalized than others; in certain activities, such as sighing, no hard attacks or tension may make the tone strident; in shouting, no breathiness may occur; in humming, a higher pitch level may be used. By varying the postural, breathing, pitch, intensity, or quality factors we may be able to locate within the individual's own phonation the voice we need to use as a standard, or as a goal.[12]

Let us view some of the specific ways by which we might help our voice client vary his phonation in his search for a better voice.

Nowhere will we find resistance to change as tenacious as in voice quality. A habitual voice quality seems as much a part of the person as his nose, and unconsciously the client seems to say, "Keep your therapeutic fingers off my proboscis!" It has been so closely associated with egocentric speech, with emotional expression, with communication, that it is almost a basic feature of the self. Even when the client hates her voice, a better voice sounds so strange and artificial that she tends to sabotage any attempts to change it. We have found it essential to verbalize this, to predict the resistance, and to help the client understand it. It is unwise to ask the person to use new voices in communication, in social gesture, in emotional expression, until this phase of resistance has passed.

Accordingly, our first experimentation with change in voice quality should be confined to play, to fantasy, to imitation of animal noises, or imitation of other people. The clinician must set the appropriate models, and he must be in command of almost as many voices as a professional actor. We have trained our majors in speech therapy in these skills so that they can provide these variations in voice quality. Too many beginning clinicians try too soon to get a better voice quality from their clients. First their clients must discover how many voices they own; first they must vary and play with their own voices.

This variation should first of all involve changes in pitch and intensity, which are easier to accomplish. Then perhaps a falsetto or a hypernasal voice can be attempted. Then a denasal or throaty (low-pitched falsetto) or harsh or hoarse voice can be assumed.

After these gross variations, we have found it useful to go with the client into stores and to study and later to imitate the voices of various clerks. We help the person to learn the technique of silent echo-speaking, pantomiming in subvocal form the speech of the person being heard. Then we use playlets or dialogues, taking various parts

[12] Charles Van Riper and John V. Irwin, *Voice and Articulation* (Englewood Cliffs, N.J.: Prentice-Hall, Inc., 1958), p. 285.

and adopting the voices most appropriate. Again the clinician must share the variation and set the models.

Out of all this variation training comes the firm understanding that voice change is possible. The experiences have been pleasant. The person realizes for the first time that he has not one voice but many—and that he has a choice!

Fixation   Once the person has come to identify his abnormal voice and has learned to vary it, our next task is to get him to locate and fix solidly his new voice. The process is at first a bit like target shooting. He may miss the bull's-eye of the new voice quality more than he hits it. His voice gun tends to wobble. New patterns of muscular contractions and of laryngeal or pharyngeal postures must be learned. It is the clinician's role to help him know how far off the mark his vocal attempts have been. Patiently the clinician makes suggestions, points out the extent of the difference between the voice produced and that desired.

In this process it is helpful if the clinician is able to imitate with some fidelity the client's various voice productions and also to present a model of the voice to be attained. We use a tape recorder more often with voice cases than with any other of the speech disorders. Usually it is possible, even very early in treatment, to get a sample or two of the desired voice. This we isolate from the rest, make a loop of tape bearing the good sample, and use this as our target.

At this phase of treatment every session begins with a playing of this model loop, and we use it often to provide the bull's-eye. We also often make a tape recording which has on it, first a vivid sample of the abnormal voice at its worst, then a series of graduated and numbered voice samples that progressively come closer and closer to the voice desired, which forms the terminal example. After the client becomes familiar with this "measuring tape," he is able, with fair consistency, to evaluate any vocal attempts in terms of its proximity to the desired new voice. Strong motivation is thereby procured.

Progressive   Let us say here again, that speech therapy is not a matter of
Approximation   exchange of one type of speech for another, but a process of progressive approximation. Clinicians who have only *good* and *bad* or *yes* and *no* in their professional vocabularies should exchange them for *closer* and *farther* or *hotter* and *colder* as in the old nursery game. In voice therapy, we work with little shifts, and we reinforce with our approval those vocal attempts that come closer to the

desired goal. This holds for disorders of pitch, intensity, and quality, and for all types of variant human behavior seeking to modify itself.

To aid in getting this concept across (for the client, too, tends to make judgments in terms of black and white) it is well for the clinician to present models of these miniature modifications that change in the direction of the goal. It is the client's task to judge whether they approach or retreat from the goal. By using large changes first, and then smaller ones, the client's perceptions and discriminations are sharpened, and he can then evaluate his own attempts with objectivity.

One of our favorite ways for using progressive approximation in voice therapy is to use a binaural auditory trainer. We then feed in the client's voice into one ear and our own voice into his other ear, thereby permitting simultaneous comparison. We usually begin by joining the client as he reads or phonates a tone, imitating him closely so both voices harmonize in unison, then gradually we change our own voice in small steps in the direction of the desired voice. Perceiving the difference, the client often shifts unconsciously to bring both voices together again, and so a progressive approximation has occurred. Often it is necessary for the clinician to rejoin the client and use the latter's voice again before attempting another shift. But careful training in this way, along with commentary, breaks for relaxation, and suggested corrections, can be very effective. There is also in this procedure a basic psychotherapeutic healing. The client is not alone. Someone is sharing his problem, someone is identifying with him who knows the path out of his troubles.

If no auditory trainer is available, the client may use his cupped hands to bring his voice to one ear while the clinician puts his mouth to the other.

Stabilization   New voices are weak and unstable. They need careful tending at first. We have found it wise to insist that the client use it at first only in therapy sessions where we can concentrate on its motor and acoustic aspects and make it stronger therein.

Once we feel the client has the new voice fairly solidly and can use it consistently in therapy when he's listening to himself, we introduce masking noise into his ears so he can monitor it by proprioception alone, by feeling the vocal postures and muscle tensions. Often at first, this masking tends to create a regression to the old voice, so we introduce the masking noise gradually and intermittently. No one can ever come to use a new voice habitually if he must constantly listen to it. Let's not burden the ears too much. It is also necessary to be sure that the client can use the new voice at his natural tempo or speed of utterance. It must not be labored or too careful. It cannot be confined to a monotone or chant. All these motor and acoustic variations need some attention.

Next we attempt to stabilize the new voice in display speech, and we like to make recordings of the new voice so the person can listen to them and feel good. Role-playing, orating, readings, all can be used for this purpose. Often at this point we ask the person to give us a verbal autobiography, and to use the new voice while doing so. This should run for several sessions. We do this so as to help to identify the new voice with the self. The perpendicular pronoun "I" especially should become colored with the new role. This provides an opportunity for some mild psychotherapy at the same time. However, as we shall see, we prefer at this stage to keep emotional expression fairly innocuous.

Next we like to stabilize the new voice in the thinking aspect of speech. We show slide films, provide problems, and ask the client to keep a running commentary going in the new voice. At times we even have him do a lot of free or controlled association, saying whatever thoughts that come. It is interesting to watch a client whispering and pantomiming, in the new voice. We cannot hear it, but he insists that it is *there;* and when we suddenly signal for him to vocalize, it appears. Pantomimic speech is close to thought.

When we feel definite progress has been made in the foregoing aspects of speech, we stabilize it in communication. We ask the client now to use the new voice outside the therapy sessions—but at first only when he talks to strangers. We do this to avoid the listener's shocked surprise that often greets a voice case when he confronts them with a new voice. The father of a young man who had never known anything but a high falsetto voice stormed into the bathroom one morning to find out what strange man was in the house at seven in the morning. The boy had only said something to the family dog.

Once the new voice has been used easily with strangers, it can be brought out in the circle of acquaintances and friends or family. It is wise to suggest that the person speak of his voice therapy casually or use it as a conversation piece. Most people are very interested. About this time (and perhaps we have protracted the process unduly in describing it, for at times we have changed voices in a single hour), the new voice becomes stabilized and is felt as natural as the old one had been. There will be a few momentary relapses, usually in emotional expression, but the task has been accomplished.

References

ARONSON, A. E. *Psychogenic Voice Disorders*. Philadelphia: W. B. Saunders Co., 1973. (A series of black-and-white sound films presenting different functional voice disorders with commentary.)

——, "Speech Pathology and Symptom Therapy in the Interdisciplinary Treatment of Psychogenic Aphonia." *Journal Speech Hearing Disorders*, XXXIV (1969), 321–41.

BOONE, D. B. "Treatment of Functional Aphonia in a Child and an Adult." *Journal Speech Hearing Disorders*, XXXI (1966), 69–74.

——, *The Voice and Voice Therapy*. Englewood Cliffs, N.J.: Prentice-Hall, 1971.

BRODNITZ, F. S. "Spastic Dysphonia" Annals of Otology, Rhenology, and Laryngology," LXXXV (1976), 210–15.

——, *Vocal Rehabilitation*. Rochester, Minn.: Custom Printing, 1968.

BRYCE, DOUGLAS. *Differential Diagnosis and Treatment of Hoarseness*. Springfield, Ill.: Charles C. Thomas, 1974.

BURKOWSKY, M. R. "Vocal Ulcers in a Seventy-One-Year-Old Male." *Journal Speech Hearing Disorders*, XXXIII (1968), 268–69.

BZOCH, KENNETH B. (ed.) *Communicative Disorders*. Boston, Mass.: Little-Brown, Co. 1972.

COOKER, H. S., "An Introduction to Sound and the Speech and Hearing Mechanism," in A. J. Weston (ed.) *Communication Disorders: An Appraisal*. Springfield, Ill.: C. C. Thomas, 1972.

COOPER, M. *Modern Techniques of Vocal Rehabilitation*. Springfield, Ill.: Charles C. Thomas, 1973.

——, "Modern Techniques of Vocal Rehabilitation for Functional and Organic Dysphonias." in L. E. Travis (ed.) *Handbook of Speech Pathology and Audiology*. Englewood Cliffs, N.J.: Prentice-Hall, Inc., 1971.

DAMSTE, P. H. and J. W. LERMAN, *An Introduction to Voice Pathology*. Springfield, Ill.: C. C. Thomas, 1975.

ENGELBERG, M. "Correction of Falsetto Voice in a Deaf Adult." *Journal Speech Hearing Disorders*, XXVII (1962), 162–64.

FLETCHER, S. "Contingencies for Bioelectric Modification of Nasality." *Journal Speech Hearing Disorders*, XXXVII (1972), 329–46.

FOX, D. R. "Spastic Dysphonia: A Case Presentation." *Journal Speech Hearing Disorders*, XXXIV (1969), 275–79.

FREEDMAN, S. R. and D. C. GARSTECKI. "Child-Directed Therapy for a Non-Organic Voice Disorder." *Language, Speech, Hearing Services in the Schools*, IV (1973), 8–12.

GREENE, M. C. L. *The Voice and Its Disorders*. (2nd ed.) Philadelphia: J. B. Lippincott Co., 1964.

HOLLIEN, H., P. MOORE, R. WENDALL, and J. MICHEL. "On the Nature of the Vocal Fry." *Journal Speech Hearing Research*, IX (1966), 245–47.

Moncur, John and ISAAC BRACKETT. *Modifying Vocal Behavior*. New York: Harper & Row, 1974.

MOORE, G. P. *Organic Voice Disorders*. Englewood Cliffs, N.J.: Prentice-Hall, 1971.

MURPHY, A. T. *Functional Voice Disorders*. Englewood Cliffs, N.J.: Prentice-Hall, Inc., 1964.

OGILVIE, M. and NORMA REES. *Communication Skills: Voice and Pronunciation.* New York: McGraw-Hill Book Co., 1969.

PERKINS, W. H. "Vocal Function: Assessment and Therapy." in L. E. Travis (ed.) *Handbook of Speech Pathology and Audiology.* Englewood Cliffs, N.J.: Prentice-Hall, Inc., 1971.

ROGERS, J. H., J. M. FREDERICKSON, and D. P. BRYCE. "New Techniques for Vocal Rehabilitation." *Canadian Journal Otolaryngology.* IV (1975), 595–604.

SHANKS, J. C. and M. DUGUAY, "Voice Remediation and Alaryngeal Speech," in Stanley Dickson (ed.) *Communication Disorders: Remedial Principles and Practices.* Chicago: Scott, Foresman and Company, 1974.

SHEARER, W. M. "Diagnosis and Treatment of Voice Disorders in School Children." *Journal Speech Hearing Disorders,* XXXVII (1972), 215–21.

STRANTBERG, T. E., J. GRIFFITH, and M. W. HOLLOWELL. "A Case Study of Psychogenic Hoarseness." *Journal Speech Hearing Disorders,* XXXVI (1971), 281–86.

TAUB, S. "The Taub Oral Panendescope: A New Technique." *Cleft Palate Journal.* III (1966), 328–46.

VAN HATTUM, ROLLAND J. *Clinical Speech in the Schools.* Springfield, Ill.: Charles C. Thomas, 1973.

WILLIS, C. R. and M. L. STUTZ. "The Clinical Use of the Taub Oral Panendoscope in the Observation of Velopharyngeal Function." *Journal Speech Hearing Disorders,* XXXVII (1972), 495–502.

WILSON, D. K. *Voice Problems of Children.* Baltimore: Williams and Wilkins Company, 1972.

ZWITMAN, D. H. and T. C. CALCATERRA. "The 'Silent Cough' Method for Vocal Hyperfunction." *Journal Speech Hearing Disorders,* XXXVIII (1973) 119–25.

8

STUTTERING

One of the most interesting of all the disorders of speech is stuttering, a problem which has puzzled clinicians and researchers for centuries. Each new year brings some supposedly new theory of its nature and some new form of treatment (which usually turns out to be one that has failed for centuries to produce permanent fluency). The stutterer is with us still—usually as still as possible. For one of the outstanding features of stuttering is that stutterers don't always stutter. Since they look and sound just like anyone else when they are fluent, they often refrain from speaking if they anticipate difficulty. Because there are more than a million stutterers in this country alone, you are bound to meet or have to work with some of them during your careers. And, if you do not understand the nature of this disorder, you will probably do a lot of things that will make the stutterer more miserable than he already is. So let us be your guide.

The Nature of Stuttering   The essence of stuttering lies in its disruption of fluency. *Stuttering occurs when the forward flow of speech is interrupted abnormally by repetitions or prolongations of a sound, syllable, or articulatory posture, or by avoidance and struggle behaviors.* We stress the word "abnormally" since all of us show some disfluency at times, and yet do not stutter. All of us occasionally repeat and hesitate and filibuster at times of ambivalence or stress or in formulating some difficult thought.

The research shows rather conclusively that stutterers have more syllabic repetitions and sound prolongations than normal speakers. They have more syllabic repetitions per hundred words, and they have more of them per word. We examined one stutterer who repeated one syllable forty-three times on a single word. Normal speakers occasionally hang onto a sound or posture only briefly, but stut-

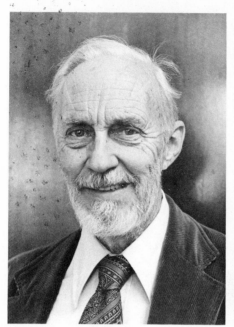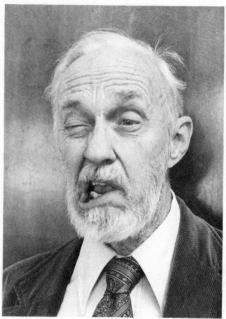

Figure 26   An older stutterer. (The fluent Dr. Jekyll becomes the stuttering Mr. Hyde.)

terers show a long duration on their prolongations. The author once had a silent prolongation on the posture of the first sound of the word "pass" that lasted six minutes by a schoolroom clock, though it was interrupted several times by the need for the intake of air for survival. Normal speakers do not have these experiences. There also seem to be differences in the form of the repetitions and prolongations which distinguish the stutterer from the normal speaker. When a normal speaker repeats a syllable (and he does so only rarely) he uses the correct vowel and repeats it at the regular tempo of his other syllables. He says "Sa-Saturday." The stutterer tends to say "Suh-Suh-Sih-Suh-Suh-Seh-Sa-Saturday," and the variable repetitions occur irregularly and often with tension. Also the syllables in the stutterer seem to be arrested; they are terminated suddenly; the breath is interrupted. These phenomena do not seem to be characteristic of the few syllabic repetitions shown by normal speakers. We say "few" because they are rare. When a normal speaker repeats, he tends to repeat words and phrases, not syllables or sounds. We do not consider the repetition of a word or phrase or the use of pauses, um's and er's, or reformulations as abnormal. We even accept a few repetitions of a syllable. But when a sound or syllable is repeated not once or twice but many times, and when this behavior occurs too frequently, then we prick up our ears and say to ourselves that the speaker stutters. We tend to say the same thing when a sound is prolonged, as in this example: "I think that mmmmmmmmmmy mmmmmmmm-mother wwwwwon't let me go." The tolerance for such prolongations of a sound seems to be much less than for repetitions of a sound or syllable. We have also used the word *posture*. Not all these repetitions and prolongations are vocalized. The stutterer often makes several silent mouth postures before the word is spoken, or he may assume a fixed position and struggle silently with it before blurting out what he wants to say. These fixed postures may be located anywhere in the speech structures. One stutterer may hold his breath with both true and false vocal cords closed tightly. Another may protrude his tongue or twist his lips to one side. Since these silent postures take time, they break up the normal time sequence of speech. Finally, we have included in our definition the terms "avoidance" and "struggle." Although most beginning stutterers show little struggle or avoidance, in the advanced stages of the disorder these reactions may constitute the major part of the problem.

Perhaps some descriptions of these struggle reactions would be useful here. In our speech clinic at the present time, we have a young man who speaks fluently most of the time; but when he does stutter he usually protrudes his lips grossly, makes sucking and clicking noises, then suddenly throws back his head and says the word. This is his characteristic behavior when attempting words beginning with stop consonants; but when he begins a word that starts with a continuant sound such as /s/ or /θ/ or /v/, he protrudes not his lips but his tongue, and this vibrates tremorously. Occasionally he may also simply repeat a syllable several times automatically and without forcing. We also have another man who shows no facial contortions at all but whose stuttering moments are marked by sudden gasps. Sometimes these are so deep that his shoulders jerk upward. A third man shows none of these reactions. He opens his mouth widely agape and neither sound nor air emerge as he exerts a powerful abdominal thrusting in his attempt to break a blockade. These are only a few of the wide variety of struggle reactions to be found in adult stutterers.

We also have some stutterers who show very little of this overt struggle. They duck and dodge their feared words and speaking situations. They have a host of strategies for hiding their difficulty. They may substitute nonfeared words for feared ones. They may just stop talking and pretend to be thinking. They may interject "ah" or "um" or "well" to postpone their expected misery as long as possible. Some of these persons become very skillful in the use of these avoidance tricks but at a great cost of anxiety and tension. Often called interiorized stutterers because most of their stuttering is hidden, they live in a state of constant vigilance lest their disorder be exposed. They scan and plan, trying to anticipate every eventuality. They carry a heavy burden.

Physiological Reactions   Certain important features of stuttering are difficult to see with the naked eye, and yet they can be revealed by instrumentation. Severe stutterers in the advanced stages of the disorder show abnormalities in heart and pulse rate and in breathing. Investigations have revealed changes in blood composition and distribution, states of general or localized tension, tremors, odd brain waves, dilation of the pupils, and many other abnormal reactions. However, these do not seem to form the core of the disorder. All severe stutterers do not show all of them. These reactions occur during the moment of stuttering or during its anticipation. They are especially vivid during the stutterer's efforts to escape from the fixations or oscillations. They are probably no more than the reflection of the stress he feels. They are the physiological correlates of his struggle or fear. They do not occur on the shorter unforced stuttering. They do not appear in the young stutterer whose automatic repetitions and unforced prolongations do not seem to bother him. But for the older, more severe stutterer they form a major part of his internal distress. They contribute much to his feeling that something terrible is happening to him. The brain that controls the mouth is flooded with static from the viscera. The normal automaticity and monitoring of utterance is thus doubly beset. It is more difficult to talk.

The Origins of Stuttering   Although the disorder has been studied intensively for years, we still have not found any adequate answer to the question: "What causes stuttering?" Some authorities, usually psychiatrists, feel that stuttering is a neurosis and originates in deep-seated emotional conflicts. Others, mainly psychologists, insist that stuttering is learned behavior and the result of classical or operant conditioning or both. Some workers, presently in the minority, are certain that stuttering has an organic or constitutional basis sometimes called *dysphemia*. Most speech pathologists, including this author, maintain an eclectic point of view. We feel that stuttering may have different origins in different individuals, and that the original causes are not nearly as important as those that maintain the disorder once it has begun. The river of stuttering does not flow out from only one lake.[1]

The Development of Stuttering

Stuttering usually begins to show itself between the years two to four. In some children the onset comes later, about the time they enter school, and we have known a few persons whose stuttering began after they became adults. The picture of stuttering at its onset is usually quite different from that shown by the person who has stuttered for years. Although we have often been able to arrest the disorder in its early phases when we had the opportunity, in other cases we have seen it grow in complexity and abnormality as the years went by. We have seen little children stumbling occasionally in their speech, repeating syllables and prolonging sounds quite effortlessly and without apparent awareness; and then we have seen them again some years later with facial contortions, complete blockages of utterance, and deeply troubled by the feeling of stigma. One of the essential evils of stuttering is this tendency toward increasing abnormality. In seeking to cope with the breaks in his speech, the stutterer habituates many coping behaviors which complicate his problem. Under stress, he uses certain tricks of avoidance and postponement to hide or escape his difficulties. When caught in verbal oscillations and fixations, he employs various devices to interrupt them and to release himself from their hold. These coping behaviors soon become automized components of the stuttering, and the stutterer feels that they are involuntary, that he cannot keep them out.

Different stutterers show different courses of development. The majority seem to run a course in which the initial, effortless syllabic repetitions and sound prolongations become full of tension and struggle and then in turn the interrupter or avoidance reactions begin to develop. Paralleling this overt development, we find a change from unawareness to surprise, to frustration, and finally to fear and shame. This seems to be the most common developmental track, but there are also others. Some stuttering, as we have mentioned earlier, begins suddenly with complete blockages and immediate struggle; and

[1] For a detailed discussion of the differing views concerning the nature and causes of stuttering, see C. Van Riper, *The Nature of Stuttering* (Englewood Cliffs, N.J.: Prentice-Hall, 1971).

the fears and shame develop swiftly. In other stutterers, the growth is very gradual, and no struggle symptoms appear.

It should be understood that not all beginning stutterers show this morbid growth. Indeed, we have fairly good evidence that about four out of every five children who begin to stutter seem to regain or attain normal speech with or without therapy. Moreover, the progressive development even in those who continue to stutter is oscillatory: It is not linear. When we see a child struggling or avoiding, we are concerned; but often a few weeks or months later he may return to the effortless repetitions that characterized his initial difficulty. These swings in developmental severity are usually viewed as indicating a good prognosis. Some stutterers may swing all the way back to normal speech long enough to escape from the clutches of the disorder. Unfortunately, too many do not. They get caught in the whirlpool of self-reinforcement; the disorder becomes self-perpetuating.

Our most important job, therefore, is to prevent this morbid growth of the disorder, to keep it in its early stages, to prevent the struggle and avoidance that are the result of communicative frustration and social rejection. The speech pathologist, if he can get the child early enough and can get the parents to cooperate, is usually very successful with young stutterers. The older, confirmed ones present a much more difficult problem because fears, frustration, and shame have come to be ever-present. It is important that all who work with stutterers understand the role played by these negative emotions.

The Role of Fear   We always hate to see a young child stutterer begin to fear the act of speaking, for we know that he is in grave danger of getting worse. By fear we mean the expectation or anticipation of unpleasantness, and most of that unpleasantness comes from two sources: from the experience of being punished, rejected, mocked, or pitied by his listeners, or from the experience of momentarily being unable to communicate, of feeling his utterance blocked, or finding himself unable to inhibit the compulsive repetition or prolongation of a sound or syllable. Here are some of the things different stutterers have told us about the first of these sources of fear.

What hit me worst of all and something I've never forgot or forgiven was how the parents of other kids would yank them away from me when they would hear me stutter. They wouldn't let me come in their yard to play. They told me to go home and stutter somewhere else. They didn't want their kid to get infected.

Elsie was the worst. She was always teasing me, calling me "stutter-cat" or "stumble-tongue" or mocking me. She was so slick at it that hardly anyone but me noticed it. She'd say it as she went by my desk, under her breath, so only I got it. I could have killed her if I hadn't been so hurt and helpless. And I couldn't hit her, because boys can't hit girls, not even out on the playground.

Whenever I'd stutter, Dad would slump down behind his paper, or if he didn't have any, he'd just look away and pretend to think. Sometimes, he'd just drum on the table with his fingers or hum an absent-minded little tune, as though to say, "I'm not listening so it doesn't count." He never teased me or said anything about my stuttering. No one did. It was as unmentionable as Sex. My father, as a small town minister, believed in letting sleeping dogs lie. I grew up feeling that stuttering was somehow pretty sinful.

My nickname was "Spit-it-out-Joe," or "Spitty" for short. I got it from my third-grade teacher, an impatient, aggressive old dame who couldn't bear to hear me block. Every time I did, she'd yelp, "Spit it out, Joe!" and the kids picked it up and I've carried the tag for years. I still have dreams of killing the old hag.

My mother only did one thing when I stuttered. She held her breath. She never teased me, punished me, or seemed embarrassed. Her lovely face was always serene. But she held her breath. She was entirely patient, sweet, and understanding. She gave me the feeling that she was proud of me and was completely confident that everything would turn out all right. But she held her breath every time I stuttered. That breath-holding sometimes sounded louder than thunder to me.

It is from experiences such as these that most young stutterers begin to expect unpleasantness in the act of speaking. This expectation may at first be specifically focused on a single word, the one on which the unpleasantness occurred. Or it may start with a more general fear of a certain situation, such as talking over the telephone, or speaking to a hard-of-hearing grandmother. Stuttering fears are of two main types: situation fears and word fears.

Word Fears The first word fears arise from two main sources: (1) from words which are remembered because of the severe frustration or vivid penalties experienced when uttering them, and (2) from words which, because of their frequent use under stress, accumulate more stuttering memories upon them.

> The question words have always been hard for me to say, ever since I can remember. What? Where? When? Why? How? My folks were always so busy. I always had to interrupt something important they were doing. They either answered without paying any real attention so I had to say it again, or else they told me not to bother them, or they told me to stop asking so many questions.

> My own name is my hardest word. Too many big people have asked me, "What is your name, sonny?" I've had to say it too many times when I got into trouble. I've said it so often and stuttered on it so often that I almost think it should be spelled with more than one *t*, like T-T-T-Tommy.

> I believe I remember the very first time I stuttered or at least it was the first time I ever noticed it. I was in the second grade, in the third row, last seat. The teacher asked me several simple *times* problems in multiplication, and I stuttered and she got irritated and asked me something simpler until finally she said, "Okay, dummy, how much is two and two?" and I couldn't say "Four." I've been afraid of that number and of all *f* words ever since.

These fears, starting from such simple instances, grow swiftly. Often their growth almost seems malignant, constantly invading new areas of one's mental life. A child begins by first fearing the word *paper*. He has had an unpleasant experience in uttering it. He sees it approaching and expects some more unpleasantness, either frustration or penalty. He finds more difficulty. Soon he is fearing many *p* words besides *paper*. He recognizes *pay* and *penny* as hard words to say. Then the fear generalizes or becomes fastened to other features of the stuttering experience. It spreads to other words having similar visual, acoustic, kinesthetic, tactual, or semantic features.

The visual transer, for example, may be in terms of spelling cues. Because of his fear of *p* words, he may see the word *pneumonia* as dreaded, even though the actual utterance begins with a nasal sound. Or, to illustrate the acoustic transfer, he may come to fear the *k, ch,* and *t* sounds because they, like the *p,* are ejected with a puff of air. Or tactually and kinesthetically, he may soon be fearing all the other lip sounds, starting with the *b,* then spreading to the *w, m,* and even the *f* and *v* sounds. The spread of fear can take several directions. The following example illustrates how the cues precipitating fear of stuttering can spread semantically.

> I had never, so far as I remember, had any real trouble on words beginning with a *w.* Oh, I might have had some, I suppose, but generally I considered them easy sounds to say. And I had very frequently used the word, "well," as a sort of handle, saying it as a kind of way to get started. Sometimes, of course, I might have to say it three or four times before the next word came out, but anyway, I could always say "well." It was a handy trick to cover up and postpone. Then one day I had an experience which ruined that word for me forever. To this day, "well" is a hard word for me to speak without stuttering, and it all happened because of that one experience. It happened like this. I was in a grocery store, asking for five pork chops, and I got blocked in saying the name of the meat. It was a long one with hard sticking in my throat, and I kept trying to break it by saying "well." I must have used too many of them because a man behind me impatiently shouted, "Well, well? You aren't well, young lady. Get out of here and go home to bed. You're sick. Not well, sick! Do you hear, sick!" I fled without the pork chops, but I can never use the word in the sense of healthy without blocking completely. I sometimes can use it as a starter, but if I happen to think of it as the antonym of "sick," I block on it immediately.

Situation Fears We have been describing the stutterer's conflicting urges to utter and to avoid the utterances of a given word. Shall he or shan't he attempt it? He scrutinizes the word for cues which might indicate danger, for resemblances to other words formerly provocative of great unpleasantness. The same sort of process occurs on the situation level. Sheehan puts the matter as follows:

> At the *situation* level there is a parallel conflict between entering and not entering a feared situation. The stutterer's behavior toward using the telephone, reciting in class, or introducing himself to strangers illustrates this conflict. Many situations which

demand speech hold enough threat to produce a competing desire to hold back.[2]

Often in word fears there occurs an actual rehearsal of some of the expected abnormality. Breathing records show that even prior to speech attempt the stutterer's silent breathing often goes through the same peculiar pattern that he shows when actually stuttering. In situation fears this is not the case. Situation fears are more vague, more generalized, more focused on the *attitudes* of the listener and the stutterer than upon the *behavior*. Situation fears can range in intensity all the way from uncertainty to complete panic. We have known stutterers to faint and fall to the floor in their anticipation of a speaking situation. The fear fluctuates in intensity from moment to moment. It is often set off by the stutterer's recognition of certain features of an approaching speech situation as similar to those of earlier situations in which he met great penalty or frustration. Stutterers learn to scan an approaching speaking situation with all the concentration of a burglar looking over a prospective bank. Like word fears, situation fears generalize. They may begin from a simple recognition on the part of the child that he was having much difficulty in talking to a certain storekeeper. Remembering this, he may begin to fear speaking in any store; or to take another tack, he might begin to fear talking to all strange men, or to mention still another, he might fear having to relay any message given him by his mother. Situation fears are like word fears in another way, too. Avoidance increases them greatly. The more the stutterer runs away from a given speaking situation, the more terrifying it becomes.

Both situation and word fears can serve as *maintaining* causes of the disorder. By constantly reinforcing them by avoidance, the stutterer keeps his stuttering "hot." Any therapy worthy of the name must have as one of its basic aims the elimination of this avoidance. Stuttering begins to break down and disappear as soon as the stutterer ceases his constant reinforcing.

Avoidance Behavior   The stuttering picture shown by those who have progressed to this latter stage in the development of stuttering can best be understood in terms of avoidance and escape. Let us be very clear about what is being avoided and escaped. It is the experience of finding a part of the body mysteriously oscillating or fixating; it is the experience of having communication blocked and retarded; it is the experience of behaving in a way which other people penalize.

[2] J. G. Sheehan, "Conflict Theory of Stuttering," in J. Eisenson, ed., *Stuttering: A Symposium* (New York: Harper & Row, Publishers, 1958).

No one likes to have feelings of frustration, anxiety, guilt, or hostility. When these feelings appear in conjunction with repetitive or prolonged interruptions in the flow of speech, those interruptions will be viewed as highly unpleasant. The stutterer will seek to prevent, avoid, or escape from repetitions which keep repeating, from prolongations of a sound or posture which persist. It is very important that we understand that, to the secondary stutterer, this repeating and prolonging appears to be involuntary, uncontrollable, mysterious. When this behavior is anticipated, the stutterer tries to avoid it; when it has occurred, the stutterer tries to escape from it.

How the Stutterer Avoids Stuttering   Since, in this stage, the secondary stutterer has learned to scan approaching speech situations for clues that indicate he will probably have difficulty, and since he has also learned to scrutinize the formulation of his sentences for "hard" words and sounds, he naturally tends to avoid these words and situations. One of our child cases just stopped talking altogether; one of our adults became a hermit in the Ozarks. But most stutterers cannot use this drastic solution to their problem. They continue to talk, but they talk as little as possible in these feared situations, and avoid or alter them if possible. It is often difficult for the nonstutterer to realize that much of the abnormality he witnesses in examining a stutterer is due to the latter's efforts to avoid unpleasantness. The desire to avoid stuttering may lead to such jargon as "To what price has the price of tomatoes increased today?" when the stutterer merely wished to say "How much are your tomatoes?" Dodging difficult words and speech situations becomes almost a matter of second nature to the stutterer. He prefers to seem ignorant rather than to expose his disability when called upon in school. He develops such a facility at using synonyms that he often sounds like an excerpt from a thesaurus. He will walk a mile to avoid using a telephone. And the tragedy of this avoidance is that it increases the fear and insecurity, makes the stutterer more hesitant, and doubles his burden.

Postponement   Procrastination as a reaction to approaching unpleasantness is an ordinary human trait, and the stutterer has more than his share of the weakness. We have worked with stutterers whose entire overt abnormality consisted of the filibustering repetition of words and phrases preceding the dreaded word. They never had any difficulty on the word itself, but their efforts to postpone the speech attempt until they felt they could say the word produced an incredible amount of abnormality. One of them said, "My name is . . . my name is . . . my . . . my . . . my name is . . . my name . . . name . . . name . . . what I mean is, uh . . . uh . . . my name is Jack Olson." Others will merely pause in tense silence for what seems to them like hours before blurting out the word. Others disguise the postponement by pretending to think, by licking their lips, by saying "um" or "er." Postponement as a habitual approach to feared words creates an anxiety and a fundamental hesitancy which in themselves precipitate more stuttering.

Starters   Stutterers also use many tricks to start the speech attempt after postponement has grown painfully long. They time this moment of speech attempt with a sudden gesture, or eye-blink, or jaw-jerk, or other movement. They return to the beginning of the sentence and race through the words preceding the feared word in hope that their momentum will "ride them over their stoppages." They insert words, phrases, or sounds that they can say, so that the likelihood of blocking will be lessened. One of the stutterers hissed before every feared word, "because I get started with the *s* sound which I can nearly always make." Another used the phrase "Let me see" as a magic incantation. He would utter things like this: "My name is Lemesee Peter Slack." Another, whose last name was Ranney, always passed as O'Ranney, since she used the "oh" as a habitual device to get started. Starters are responsible for many of the bizarre symptoms of stuttering, since they become habituated and involuntary. Thus, the taking of a deep breath prior to speech attempt may finally become a sequence of horrible gasping.

Antiexpectancy   The antiexpectancy devices are used to prevent or minimize word fears from dominating the attention of the stutterer. Thus, one of our clients laughed constantly, even when saying the alphabet or asking central for a phone number or buying a package of cigarettes. He had found that, by assuming an attitude incompatible with fear, he was able to be more fluent. Yet he was one of the most morose individuals we have ever met. Other stutterers adopt a singsong style, or a monotone, or a very soft, whispered speech so that all words are made so much alike that no one will be dreaded. Needless to say, all these tricks fail to provide more than temporary relief, and all of them are vicious because they augment the fear in the long run.

The Role of   It is intensely frustrating to try to say someting and not be
Frustration   able to say it. Or to find oneself helplessly repeating a syl-
        lable prolonging a sound. If you have ever had to use a type-
writer or piano in which the keys stuck, you may have some slight
awareness of the frustration a stutterer experiences over and over
again every day. Or perhaps you have tried to talk on the delayed
feedback apparatus, a machine which returns an amplified echo of
what you have said a fraction of a second after you have said it. If so,
you probably found yourself "stuttering" or experiencing some uncontrollable repetitions or prolongations. In either event, you will
know in a faint way the intense frustration with which the stutterer
lives out his life.

As we have said earlier, the experience of finding one's mouth
repeating a syllable uncontrollably or discovering one's tongue or lips
frozen in a fixed posture is not only unpleasant but almost terrifying.
There is an overwhelming desire to escape from this experience, to
"break the block," to "get free from it," to find release. These are the
stutterer's own words. Williams has clearly expressed this common
experience of the mysterious something which holds the stutterer in
its mysterious grip.[3] Undesired perseveration in any activity is
traumatic. It makes one doubt one's will. It violates the integrity of
the self.

Interrupter Devices   The fast little vibrations called tremors which first appear
        during the third stage are very prevalent in secondary stutter-
ing. They are produced by highly tensing the muscles that form a
fixed posture, often an abnormal one. When triggered by a sudden
ballistic movement or surge of tension, the tremors come into being.
The stutterer doesn't know what they are, or how he sets them off.
All he knows is that some part of him is vibrating, and it scares him
as it would you. In some stutterers several structures will be vibrating at the same time—the lips, the jaw, and the diaphragm, and often at different rates. The client attempts to free himself from the
tremor by increasing the tension or by using some interrupter device
similar to the starter tricks he has used to initiate speech attempt after prolonged postponement. He tries to wrench himself out of the
frozen vibration of the tremor by sheer force. Even as he closes the
articulatory door of the tongue or lips and holds it tightly shut, he

[3] D. Williams, "A Point of View About Stuttering," *Journal of Speech and Hearing Disorders*, XXII (1957), 390–97.

strives to blow it open with a blast of air from below. When the opposing forces are equal, nothing happens except the quivering of the muscles. Oddly enough no stutterer tries to open the speech doors voluntarily; he must break them down with a surge of power. As in transitional stuttering, the random struggling often results in out-of-phase movements of the vibrating structures which cause a release from tremor and make possible the utterance of the word. One stutterer may squeeze his eyes shut; another will jerk his whole trunk; another may suck air in through his nostrils. These peculiar reactions have become habituated through their chance presence at the moment of tremor release. The anxiety reduction, the freedom from punishment, give them their compulsive strength. The stutterer comes to feel that only through using them can he ever escape from the dreadful feeling of inability which the tremor creates in him. Even when they do not give release, he will try them over again, sniffing, not once, but twenty and thirty times in his desperate effort to free himself from the mysterious closure that his opposing efforts have produced. There are easier ways to terminate tremors than these, but few stutterers ever find them without the aid of a therapist.

Other Reactions of *Escape*   It is obvious that the same devices used to interrupt tremors can also be used to interrupt repetitions or prolongations of sounds, syllables, or postures. A few stutterers split their words, giving up the attempt to produce an integrated word and finishing it after a gap. They would say "MMMMMM . . . other." More frequently the stutterer responds to the experience by ceasing the speech attempt and making a retrial, often only to find himself again in the same predicament. He may stop upon feeling an interruption in speech flow and try the entire word again: he may stop and use some starting device on the retrial, stop and use a distraction, stop and assume a confident behavior, stop and postpone the new attempt for a time, stop and avoid the word, or stop and wait until almost all breath is gone, subsequently saying the word on residual air.

Stuttering as a *Self-Reinforcing* *Disorder*   We have said that usually when stuttering develops into its final stage, little hope can be held that it will be "outgrown" or disappear. Even when the environment is changed so that it is permissive and free from fluency disruptors, the person continues to stutter. A few individuals are able to escape even after they enter this stage only because their morale is powerfully strengthened through other achievements. But usually, once fear and frustration, avoidance and escape have shown themselves, the disorder becomes self-perpetuating. As a response, it becomes the stimulus to other stuttering responses. It is necessary to understand how this comes about.

The Role of Guilt   In addition to his fears and frustrations, the confirmed stutterer is also beset by feelings of guilt, shame, or embarrassment, their intensity depending upon how other people have responded to his communicative difficulties. Some parents still try to "shame" their child out of his stuttering and certainly his playmates will occasionally make fun of his impediment. Moreover, many listeners look away when a person stutters, a reaction which he usually interprets as meaning that he has done something that he shouldn't have done. These feelings of guilt and shame are commonly felt by most confirmed (advanced) stutterers and in some of them they are very intense. Here's what one of our clients wrote:

> The fact that I am Chinese is very important in my stuttering. We are trained from infancy never to do anything which would cause our families to lose face. I cannot tell you how strong this need is, but maybe you can understand by my telling you how I cut off part of my tongue when I stuttered in front of my father, when I was only five. I almost bled to death. I don't think at all about my own trouble, only about what a disgrace I am to my family. I fear stuttering more than anyone I have ever known. I am even afraid to talk to myself sometimes. I sleep on my face so I will not speak in my sleep. And the more I think about it, the more I stutter. The more I try to hide it or avoid it, the worse it gets. . . .

We hope that when you encounter a stutterer you will not add to his burden of fear, frustration, and guilt.

Stuttering as a   There are several vicious circles, or rather spirals, which char-
Self-Reinforcing   acterize the confirmed stutterer. The more he fears, the more
Disorder   he avoids certain words or situations, and with each avoidance his fears increase. Also, the more he struggles as he tries to escape from his communicative frustration, the more abnormal a picture he presents, and again, the more he stutters the more guilt he feels. Once caught in this trap—or whirlpool—stuttering seems to be able to maintain and to perpetuate itself with a tenacity that normal

speakers find difficult to understand. Nevertheless, competent speech pathologists can do much to alleviate the difficulties of even the most severe stutterer and enable him to become reasonably fluent. They prefer, however, to work with the young child and his parents as soon as possible, knowing that if they can prevent the disorder from becoming self-reinforcing, the prognosis will be much more favorable and the stutterer can be spared much distress.

Summary   Perhaps the best way we can summarize this material is to use the picture or map in Figure 27. Stuttering has three sources; the major one represented by the largest, Lake Learning, into which the stream from Constitutional Reservoir flows. Neurosis Pond is also one of the sources of stuttering, but it is smaller. Its contribution to the flow also occurs further down the river's course. Stuttering can come from any of these three sources.

As the stream leaves Lake Learning, it flows slowly and many a child caught in its current may make it to shore by himself or with a bit of parental or therapeutic help. Some of them are cast up on Precarious Island and become fluent for a time, only to be swept away

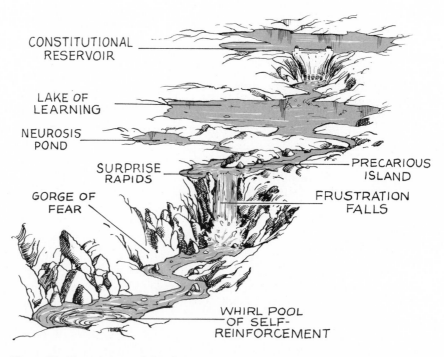

Figure 27   The origins and development of stuttering.

again by the swift-moving emotional currents from Neurosis Pond. The second stage in the development of stuttering is represented by Surprise Rapids, and the stutterer begins to know that he is in trouble. It isn't hard to rescue him, however, if you know how to do it.

Once he is swept over Frustration Falls, however, he takes a beating from the many rocks that churn the stream. Despite their random struggling, a few make it to shore even at this stage, the third, but they usually need an understanding therapist and cooperative parents to help them. The river flows even faster here, and soon it enters the Gorge of Fear. This is the worst stretch of the whole stream of stuttering, for below it lies the Whirlpool of Self-reinforcement. Once the child is caught in its constant circling, there is little hope that he will ever make it to shore by himself. Only an able and stout swimmer who knows not only this part, but all of the river of stuttering, can hope to save him. Where does the river end? King Charles the First knows.[4]

The Treatment of Confirmed Stuttering

One of the fascinating things about this disorder is that literally hundreds of methods for successfully helping stutterers have been reported. Many of these are mutually contradictory; some of them, on first glance, make no sense whatsoever. Yet we do not doubt the honesty of these reports. Some stutterers have been helped and even cured by each of these many diverse procedures; the same procedures applied to other stutterers have failed.

> We know an elocutionist who cures stutterers by drill in mental multiplication. We have seen a few of them before treatment and afterward. There is no doubt that they were helped. We have also seen some of her cases who showed no improvement and who actually got worse. We would explain her successes as the result of the increased motivation. The children who improved were deprived, young, rather dull children. They had few personality assets, and their initial morale was low. They were not severe stutterers. Their situation and word fears were mild and infrequent. Most of the penalty they had received was for their poverty and poor grades in school. They had not reacted very much to their stuttering by frustration, anxiety, guilt, or hostility. No one had expected much of them, nor had they

[4] He had his head cut off and was completely cured.

expected much of themselves. Fortunately for them, the elocutionist is an older woman, child-hungry, unmarried, and she gave these children her love and time and faith without measure. She was very patient with them. She believed that they would be cured if they could only learn how to multiply in their heads; and they also came to believe it. She did not penalize their stuttering. She ignored it. As a result of her drilling, they became able to astound and astonish their schoolmates, their parents, and their teachers with their often-paraded ability to solve these problems. Their stuttering decreased and finally disappeared. The elocutionist believed it was the mental multiplication that was the healing agent. Our own belief is that it was the morale, motivation, and self-confidence they had attained.

Two stutterers with about the same amount of stuttering may have completely different problems so far as therapy is concerned. Because of his habitual avoidance of speaking, one stutterer's situation and word fears can be very intense; another stutterer may show the reverse. It is the clinician's task to study each individual stutterer until she knows which *factors* are especially important in the picture he presents and then to work especially hard to weaken or strengthen these, while not forgetting the others.

We especially wish to emphasize the plural of the word *factors.* The weakness of most therapy with stutterers is that it has concentrated on only one or two of these. The psychiatrist who works to relieve anxiety, guilt, and hostility may do his job well; but the person will still stutter if his stuttering still brings penalty or frustration, or if his situation and phonetic fears have not been decreased by speech therapy. And morale alone, like love, is not enough for many stutterers. It may be for a few special ones, such as the occasional television or movie star who says he formerly stuttered—but not for most stutterers. We need a many-pronged therapy if we are to help most of our stutterers. A one-pronged therapy will help the special few who present equations in which the factor hit by the prong is of major importance. It will fail with the others. There are too many factors operating in stuttering.

In the light of what we have just said, let us look at some of the ways stuttering has been treated. One of the earliest accounts goes back to ancient Greek literature, and it tells of one Battos who went to the Oracle of Delphi to find out how he could be freed of his stuttering. The Oracle gave him this prescription: "Exile yourself forever to a foreign land and never come back." We have had a few ornery clients to whom we were tempted to offer the same advice. But there is a fighting chance that Battos was helped by the Oracle's prescription. A change of environment often decreases situation fears and also permits an escape from some of the sources of conflicts in the original life situation. Or perhaps he found a Parthian maiden who loved him completely even unto the elbows, and so his self-esteem soared. Let us hope that Battos was cured, but if he was, let us understand why.

During the Middle Ages, the tongues of stutterers were burned; and even as recently as sixty years ago they were sliced surgically. Cures were reported. Once, long ago, the French government paid several hundred thousand francs for the secret stuttering cure of a Madame Leigh, who was said to have phenomenal success in treating stammerers. Her secret, when finally exposed, consisted of a small pad of cotton rolled up and held under the tongue during speech. Bizarre? Of course, but even apart from the faith healing and confidences which might have been engendered, we can see why a few stutterers might have been helped at least for a time. If your mouth and tongue were hurting or if you had to hold a pad under it, you'd have a hard time pressing that tongue hard enough to precipitate a tremor. You'd find yourself not struggling so hard. You'd find yourself expecting to have some long hard blocks and then having little ones or not having any. And so the frustration would go down, and so would the fears of words and sounds. And so would the stuttering.

About 150 years ago, a man called Columbat treated stutterers by having them say each syllable of their speech as they waved their arm or tapped on a table. This method is still in use today, even though it has had a long history of failure. But doubtless, like every other method, it has had a few successes, because, for the moment, it can reduce or eliminate most of the stuttering in most stutterers. What it does is to make all words very much alike. It reduces phonetic fears by distraction. It reduces the communicative meaningfulness of speech. It is an antiexpectancy device. Like most distractions, however, as soon as it becomes habituated, it loses its power to distract and often becomes a part of the compulsive symptomatology. There are better ways to reduce the fears of sounds and words.

Relaxation has also been used as a basic treatment for stuttering. In the late 1800s, Sandow trained his stutterers to achieve states of calm relaxation and serenity and found that much of the stuttering disappeared. (He reported some difficulty in transferring the relaxed states and the consequent fluency into situations outside his clinical facilities.) Since deep relaxation is incompatible with fear or struggle, dramatic decreases in stuttering occur in the safe situations of the therapy room; but outside, in the world of knives, it is difficult to stay relaxed enough to maintain the fluency. Nevertheless, relaxation therapy for stutterers has been used for many years all over the world.

During the last years of the nineteenth century and the first years of the twentieth, most of the treatment offered stutterers was carried out in residential centers or homes called "stammerers' institutes," usually under the direction of some former stutterer who had managed to achieve some fluency. Exorbitant fees were charged, and guaranteed promises of cure were offered in the advertisements of these institutions. The author of this text attended three of them in his youth, and he remembers wryly that the guaranteed cure at one of them was qualified by the condition that the stutterer must follow all instructions. Instruction number nine was that the stutterers must not stutter! At these institutes, group therapy was offered, the stutterers doing breathing exercises for hours, reciting isolated sounds and word drills, chanting and singing, relaxing, and speaking each syllable or each word in unison with a wide arm-swing or a finger-tap. Strong suggestion, almost hypnotic in nature, was made that if the stutterer followed the secret method, he would be completely cured. Each moment of stuttering was immediately punished and fluency was rewarded. Under this ironclad discipline and the safe protection of isolation from the real world that was provided by the institute, most of the stutterers became remarkably fluent; but the precarious fluency so attained disappeared as soon as they returned to their homes. With the advent of the new profession of speech pathology, most of these commercial institutes disappeared from the scene; but many of their methods, alas, are still in use today.

Current Methods for Treating Stuttering[5]

At the present time there is no one form of treatment for confirmed stuttering that has gained general acceptance by all speech pathologists. Some of them, relatively few, use only psychotherapy, hoping that psychological counseling will lead to the lessening of the negative emotions that created or continue to play a part in maintaining the disorder. Another group of workers concentrate their efforts on conditioning the stutterer not to stutter. A third group, using what has been termed traditional therapy, trains the stutterer to respond without struggling or avoidance to his fear or experience of being

[5] The text by C. Van Riper, *The Treatment of Stuttering* (Englewood Cliffs, N.J.: Prentice-Hall, 1973) gives a detailed account of the various methods used for treating confirmed stuttering and examines the claims of success for each.

blocked, that is, to learn to stutter easily and fluently. Since all of these approaches have some successes and some failures, students should be wary of the many claims of cure or improvement for some ostensibly "new" treatment for stuttering. Confirmed stuttering is a tough nut to crack. It is very easy to get even a very severe stutterer to be fluent for a short time, but keeping him that way is an entirely different matter.

Psychotherapy   There is some psychotherapy inherent in all forms of stuttering therapy because the close relationship between the clinician and his client provides an opportunity for the ventilation of emotion and an opportunity in a permissive setting to explore new ways of coping with stress. Most speech pathologists confine themselves to providing this supportive relationship, and refer their stutterers elsewhere when they discover deep-seated emotional conflicts that are not speech-related. Some stutterers, mainly the affluent, are referred to psychiatrists; others to psychologists or to counseling centers. At present the field of psychotherapy is in flux with literally hundreds of different kinds of treatment being offered, and so speech pathologists need enough background in psychotherapy to be able to make the proper referrals.[6]

We wish to emphasize, however, that most stutterers, despite the constant emotional stress under which they live, are pretty normal individuals. Most of the research has shown that they are no more neurotic or psychotic than normal speakers. Their anxieties, guilt, and frustrations seem to be the result of their stuttering, not the cause of it, and once they become fluent, their emotional upheavals usually disappear. Deep psychotherapy is for the relatively rare stutterer whose stuttering stems from and is maintained by basic emotional conflicts.

The "Don't Stutter"   The second major form of treatment currently being used for
Approach   the confirmed stutterer in this country is based upon the belief (or supposition) that the stutterer's fluent speech can be strengthened sufficiently to enable him to withstand any threat of stuttering. Zero stuttering is the goal, certainly one to be desired if it is possible to attain. There are many variants of this kind of stuttering therapy but all of them use some technique to produce some non-stuttered speech, and then some program is administered to re-

---

[6] A discussion of the role of neurosis in stuttering is given in C. Van Riper, *The Nature of Stuttering*, Englewood Cliffs, N.J.: Prentice-Hall, 1971, Chapter 11.

inforce and maintain the precarious fluency evoked in the therapy room. All of the ancient techniques, such as rate control by metronome or delayed feedback, relaxation, unison speaking or shadowing (echoing), speaking while sighing or using passive breath control, various forms of suggestion (including hypnosis), rewarding fluent speech and punishing stuttering, prolongation of the vowels or syllables, and many others are still being used despite their long history of failure.

Why does this situation exist? The first reason is that most stutterers can be made temporarily fluent by any of these procedures; the second is that they are relatively easy for the clinician to administer. We repeat: All stutterers can speak fluently under special conditions and not one of them stutters on every word of every sentence every time he speaks. He can speak normally when he is unafraid or calm or relaxed or when he feels confident and assured or has faith in the clinician's presumed competence. His stuttering also tends to disappear if he is asked to speak in a way that is markedly different from his usual manner, such as using a falsetto, drawling his words at a very slow rate, using a sing-song kind of utterance, adopting a dialect, or making the voice very nasal and so on. By concentrating on any of these strange ways of talking, the stutterer temporarily can distract himself from the fears of words and sounds that usually precipitate his stuttering, and, for a short time, become fluent. Unfortunately, these strange ways of speaking prevent stuttering only as long as they are novel. When they become habitual they lose their distractive value and back come the fears and the stuttering. Most speech pathologists are aware of this situation but many of them (especially the advocates of operant conditioning) feel that no matter how the first fluency is obtained it can be reinforced sufficiently and any stuttering punished contingently, so that the person will be able eventually to speak normally. When relapses occur, as they tend to do no matter how the stutterer is treated, booster sessions are provided for those who return for further help. Many, alas, do not return.

Modification of
Stuttering Approach
The third way of treating a confirmed stutterer seeks to make him fluent by training him to stutter without struggle or avoidance. Believing that most of the stutterer's abnormality and communicative deviance consist of learned responses to the threat or experience of breaks in the speech flow, many speech pathologists seek to reverse the vicious developmental spiral, and to teach the stutterer to stutter as easily and as effortlessly as he did when the disorder first began. Even the most severe stutterer will oc-

casionally exhibit some of these easy early stutterings, and if his characteristic stuttering behaviors can be modified and shaped to resemble them, most of his abnormality will disappear. Certainly, he will not get many penalties or feel much frustration if all that he shows are a few easy syllabic repetitions or a slight lagging prolongation of a sound. In short, the speech pathologist does not penalize stuttering or try to get the stutterer to avoid it. Instead, he encourages the stutterer to stutter if he must but in a new and different way, one that will not interfere with his communication.

What usually happens is that the amount as well as the severity of stuttering dramatically decreases once the stutterer finds he can cope with his fears or his feeling of being blocked, once he discovers that he is no longer helpless, that he can be fluent even though he does stutter. Advocates of this approach believe that only a few advanced or confirmed stutterers can ever be made permanently fluent by strengthening their normal speech or by punishing their stutterings or by merely undergoing psychotherapy. They believe that the stutterer needs to know what to do when he fears he may stutter or finds himself doing so.[7]

All three of these therapeutic approaches involve learning and unlearning. The person undergoing psychotherapy learns to recognize the presumed sources and nature of his disturbing emotions and inappropriate or self-defeating behaviors and to substitute new adjustive responses in their place. In the second approach the clinician seeks to extinguish the stuttering behaviors and to reinforce fluency. In the third major form of treatment, new responses to the threat or experience of stuttering are taught and learned. We should remember that there are different strategies that can be used to facilitate this learning and unlearning, and that most clinicians use all of them at one time or another in the course of their therapy. Insightful or cognitive learning emphasizes the devising and revising of behavioral planning on the basis of new perceptions. In classical conditioning, the emotional responses to certain stimuli or cues associated with stuttering are weakened or extinguished. In operant conditioning, maladaptive behaviors are systematically punished or extinguished and fluency is reinforced. All of these kinds of learning and unlearn-

[7] The student should be aware that the author is probably biased in favor of this third approach. Psychoanalysis helped him solve many personal conflicts but left him stuttering as severely as ever. A number of different experiences in being made temporarily fluent through the use of rate control, new breathing patterning, relaxation, etc., all resulted in failure to maintain the fluency obtained thereby. It was only after he stopped trying to avoid stuttering, but instead learned to stutter openly but easily, that he was able to solve his problem.

ing probably take place in any stuttering therapy, no matter which one of the three approaches is being administered.

A Psychotherapy Session   To help you understand what really goes on in the therapy room during these various ways of treating confirmed stuttering we provide some word pictures. The first of these is an excerpt from a tape recording of a psychotherapy session.

Clinician: "When you phoned me last night you said that you had discovered something pretty important? What was it?"

Stutterer: "Well, I, I don't know now if it was or not . . ."

Clinician: "Tell me about it."

Stutterer: "Well, OK. I had a pretty miserable experience yesterday afternoon. I was in a drugstore downtown. Wanted to get me some Gillette razor blades. I'd prowled all around trying to locate them but couldn't, so had to ask the clerk. And I stuttered terribly on 'Gillette'. Couldn't get it out. Jumped around and made faces. Awful! . . ."

Clinician: "A really bad blocking, eh?"

Stutterer: "Yeah, but that wasn't the worst of it. There was this little old lady, see. Right beside me. And she . . . she put her arm around me, damn her, and said, 'Poor boy, do you always have to stutter like that?'"

Clinician: "And you didn't want anyone pitying you . . ."

Stutterer: "No, God damn it. I could have killed the old bitch. I wanted to slap her old face right there. . . ."

Clinician: "You were furious. She had no right to smear you with her pity . . ."

Stutterer: "That's right. That's right. I can't help it if I stutter but they got no right to . . . But you know, a strange thing happened. I flung her arm off me and said, 'No, you nosy old biddy. I only stutter when I talk!' That's what I said and you know what? I said it fine. Without a bit of stuttering and right to her face, I did . . ."

Clinician: "And you're wondering why you were so fluent when you let her have it. . . ."

Stutterer: "Yeah, yeah. And that's what I've been thinking about ever since. How come I was so fluent when I was sarcastic like that? And why, why did I get so mad at that little old lady? She probably meant well, but I still get really angry even thinking about it. Wish I'd really hit the old buzzard. And you know, that's not

like me. I don't hit back or talk back. Just take it and get the hell
out quick as I can.''

Clinician: "You don't usually express your anger. You just store it up
. . .''

Stutterer: "That's right. . . . Humm. . . . You know I'm just full of
anger really. A volcano, kind of! No one who knows me would
ever believe that, but it's true. I hold it in, but it's there. Always
there under the surface. *(Laughs)* And everybody thinks I'm
such a quiet sweet kind of guy. Hell, I want to hit everybody I
know. . . . Everybody I talk to, anyway. Hey! Maybe . . . Maybe I
hit people with my stuttering. Punish them with it, and they
got to take it and can't hit back? Hey, suppose that's true?
Doesn't make any sense but why didn't I stutter when I let that
old gal have it? And why am I so angry, so full of hate all the
time?''

This small glimpse of a small part of only one of many sessions
illustrates the basic methodology of the pyschotherapy approach.
With a highly permissive clinician, the stutterer verbalizes his feelings and perceptions at deeper and deeper levels and, on the basis of
the insights so achieved, becomes able to accept and change himself.
For example, the stutterer who provided the interview we have just
used showed a marked change in personality by the end of a year of
weekly psychotherapy sessions. He became much more aggressive
and outgoing. He no longer avoided opportunities to speak, and
while his stuttering remained, its severity had decreased markedly
both in terms of duration and visible struggle or contortions. And he
felt that he had been greatly helped.

A Classical   Now let us describe how classical conditioning was used by a
Conditioning   speech pathologist to help another stutterer overcome his in-
Session[8]   tense fears of speaking before a group. This stutterer—Bill—
      had always been excused from any recitation or oral book re-
ports throughout his elementary and secondary school years because
his parents so insisted. Bill was not a very severe stutterer, but his
panic in a public-speaking situation was devastating, and he knew
that he could never enter the professions of law or teaching unless he

[8] For further information concerning this approach see L. M. Webster and G.
Brutten, "The Modification of Stuttering and Associated Behaviors," in S. Dickson (ed.)
Communication Disorders (Glenville, Ill.: Scott, Foresman, 1974), Chapter 4.

could handle such speaking situations. Again, we provide a picture of only one of many sessions.

> After some preliminary interviews to explore the nature, history, and intensity of his fears of public speaking, the clinician then trained Bill in relaxation. He had the stutterer first clench his fists, then relax them during a prolonged exhalation of the breath until the hands hung limply at his side. Then the same process was used to procure relaxation of the toes, then the legs and arms, then the shoulders, and finally all of them at the same time. During this training the clinician repeatedly suggested calmness and quietness and the lack of any tension. Moreover, Bill had to learn how to relax not only in the therapy-room chair, but while standing, walking down the hall, opening the door to a classroom, entering it, and standing before the lecturn.
>
> Once the clinician was satisfied that Bill had learned the basic technique of relaxation, he then devised the following hierarchy of situations in which Bill had to *imagine* himself while being thoroughly relaxed: (1) Sitting quietly in his chair in the therapy room; (2) Hearing the clinician say, "It's time to make that speech. Let's go."; (3) Walking down the hall to the classroom; (4) Opening the door and walking to the lectern; (5) Hearing the clinician say, "This is Bill Jones. He's going to talk to you today about his stuttering."; (6) Looking at the prettiest girl in the class and saying, "Most people don't know much about stuttering, so let me tell you something of my history."
>
> As Bill was imagining himself in each of these situations, he was asked to signal by raising a forefinger whenever he felt some tension arising. When this occurred, as it first did when imagining himself hearing the clinician say "Let's go . . .", Bill was to go back to an earlier step on the hierarchy, relax more thoroughly, then try the new step again, always in his imagination. It took about four sessions before Bill was able to remain relaxed while imagining all six situations. Then the clinician had Bill act out, rather than imagine, the first five steps while maintaining the relaxed state he had learned to create. Then two new sub-steps were inserted: (5-a) Bill was to imagine himself saying his first sentence when there was no one except the clinician in the classroom. Then (5-b), in which Bill had to imagine that two of his friends were in the audience as well as the clinician. The whole six step hierarchy was again imagined in sequence and then acted out, but this time Bill found himself in the classroom full of students. Much to his surprise, he did very

well. Indeed, he spoke to the class for over half-an-hour and with very little stuttering. What was more important, he experienced none of the terrible panic or fear that had so long beset him. As he said to his clinician afterward, "Hey, that was sure fun. I really enjoyed it. I bet I'll never be afraid of talking to a group again." (The clinician crossed his fingers. And also his toes!)

An Operant Conditioning Session   Now let us provide a picture of a speech pathologist using operant conditioning strategies with a stutterer. You will remember that the essence of this approach lies in the use of contingent reinforcement to strengthen desired behaviors and contingent punishment to weaken them. This clinician was attempting to get his client not to stutter.

The session was divided into two parts, the first half-hour being spent in an interview during which the clinician positively reinforced all the stutterer's statements that seemed favorable to therapeutic progress and either mildly punished or ignored those verbalizations which indicated helplessness or self-defeating attitudes. Here is an illustrative portion of that interview:

Clinician: "How did things go over the weekend?"
Stutterer: "Oh, good and bad, I guess. You see there's a girl I've been wanting to date for a long time, *(Clinician nods approvingly)* but until yesterday I never really had the nerve to call her. But I did . . . I really tried to . . . *(Clinician says, 'Good!')* . . . I mean I tried but, oh God, I made a mess of it. The person at the phone desk in the dorm couldn't understand who I wanted, I stuttered so hard, and kept saying, 'Who are you calling? Who are you calling?' And then she hung up on me. Jeez, I felt low as dirt. Couldn't eat any supper. *(Clinician looks away.)* Then I thought, maybe I should try again using that slow kind of speech . . . *(Clinician says, 'Good!')* that we were practicing on the Delayed Feedback machine Friday but I couldn't bring myself to do it. *(Clinician looks at his watch.)* No, I couldn't! It would be worse than my stuttering. They'd think I was nuts talk—ing—like—this." *(Clinician shakes his head almost imperceptibly but negatively.)* Oh, I know I've just begun to learn how to talk without stuttering, *(Clinician nods.)* After all I've only been here four times. Yeah, I've got a lot to learn yet. *(Clinician says, 'That's right.')* Got to learn to control myself. *(Clinician nods approval.)* Probably tried to dance before I'd learned to walk. . . ."
During the second half of therapy hour, the first ten minutes

were spent in having the stutterer read aloud into the microphone of the Delayed Feedback apparatus, saying each new word simultaneously with the amplified echo of the one he had just spoken. The machine was set so that the echo arrived in the stutterer's earphones two seconds after he had uttered the word, thereby achieving a base rate of about thirty words per minute. The reading passage was divided into 100 word segments and the clinician underlined on his copy all stuttered words and at the same time signalled their occurrence by setting off a loud buzzer which continued for the duration of that moment of stuttering. Also, whenever an entire sentence was spoken without any stuttering the clinician gave some expression of approval such as "Fine!" or "Good!" At the end of the ten-minute period, the stutterer was having less than two stutterings per one hundred words, and so the clinician turned off the machine and instructed his client to continue reading at the same slow rate. An increase in stuttering frequency occurred at this point, but very soon,

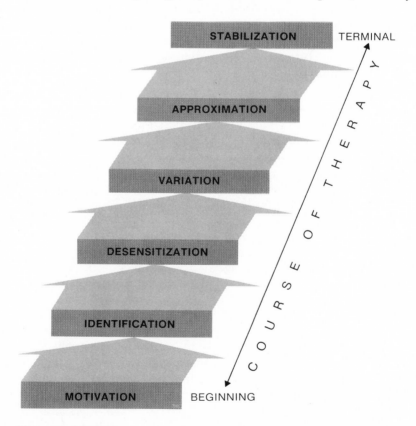

Figure 28　MIDVAS

under the clinician's contingent reinforcement and punishment, the stutterer achieved the same level of fluency he had experienced when on the apparatus.

Then the same procedure was repeated, but instead of oral reading, the stutterer had to tell of some of the most enjoyable experiences he had ever had. This proved to be more difficult. Several times he had to return to talking on the delayed feedback apparatus before he was able to regain the slow speech rate free from stuttering. The clinician then engaged the stutterer in conversation but this proved to be too big a step. The very slow rate control seemed intolerable in conversing. The clinician, therefore, returned the stutterer to the delayed feedback machine, but this time he gradually decreased the delay between utterance and echo so that the mandatory rate was speeded up to about one word a second or sixty words per minute. Again oral reading and narration were used, both with and without the delay, always with the buzzer and the clinician's approval. Then again some conversation was attempted and this time more success was achieved. That ended the long session.[9]

Modifying the Form of Stuttering

We now describe the third approach to the treatment of the confirmed stutterer. This we shall do in some detail since it is the kind of therapy this author has found most successful. In many ways it is eclectic, combining psychotherapy, classical and operant conditioning, and insightful therapies. Its major focus is on the stutterer's fears and frustrations and the avoidance and struggle behaviors they generate. In this approach the stutterer is encouraged to seek out stuttering rather than avoid it or try to talk without stuttering. And he is trained to modify that stuttering so that, if it does occur, little abnormality will be exhibited. In other words, we try to shape the stuttering into a more fluent form.

The stutterer already knows how to speak normally but he does not know what to do when he fears or finds himself stuttering. We simply teach him better ways of coping. The stutterer's fluency increases because once he stops being terrified of stuttering or ashamed of it and once he finds that he can stutter easily and ef-

---

[9] This account, though it accurately reflects what happened in an actual therapy hour—one of many—must not be seen as representative of all applications of operant conditioning to stuttering. For a more detailed account see G. Shames and D. Egolf, *Operant Conditioning and the Management of Stuttering*, Englewood Cliffs, N.J.: Prentice-Hall, 1976.

fortlessly the number of his stutterings decrease in both frequency and severity. Advocates of this approach feel that psychotherapy alone ignores the abnormal speech behaviors which constitute the essence of the disorder. They also feel that trying to extinguish the stutterer's fears by classical conditioning or merely strengthening the fluent speech or punishing the stuttering usually results in relapse and eventual failure. They believe that merely experiencing the *absence* of fear or having a period of fluency does not solve the stutterer's problem. He has had many such experiences before. What he needs are new and better ways of coping with fear and stuttering when they beset him.

The Sequence of Therapy   To understand how the speech pathologist of this persuasion goes about the task of making the confirmed stutterer fluent you should know something of the program's sequence. We have coined an acronym, MIDVAS, to help you remember. Each separate letter of this word refers to the goal of a particular phase of therapy, and they follow the order of the letters of the word. *M* is for motivation; *I* is for identification; *D* for desensitization; *V* for variation; *A* for approximation; and *S* for stabilization. This is the sequence of our therapy. We structure our therapy plan so that each new phase has a special emphasis, but all preceding goals are continued. New experiences are added but the old are reviewed. It is cumulative therapy. For convenience of exposition, we shall describe the treatment as though it were being administered to severe adult stutterers. Modifications must of course be made for young children or for the very mild stutterer, as well as for the special needs of any given individual. All stutterers present special problems. All need special treatment, but there still are general principles and practices which help all of them.

Motivation

One who has not worked much with confirmed stutterers would expect to have little trouble motivating them to do the things necessary to find relief. Certainly, the interruption to communication, the social implications and deprivations, and the struggling and the fear are unpleasant. Why then do we find so much resistance? For we certainly do. We think there are two answers. First, it is always difficult to confront one's abnormality, to expose it enough to modify it, and this resistance is found in healing all emotional ills. Indeed, unless resistance occurs in psychotherapy, we can be pretty sure that any apparent insight and improvement in adjustment is superficial and temporary. Secondly, the fact of the stutterer's fluency when alone or in nonstressful situations makes him feel that no major overhaul is needed. But deep in his bones he knows he has a tough job to do, that the seizure-like behavior and the panic of his fears are not going to yield to any waving of a savior's hands; yet it is only human to hope for easy miracles. We keep in our desk a little bottle full of pink aspirin with a label reading: "One of these will cure stuttering forever." In an early session, we always hand a new stutterer the bottle. He always grins and hands it back. We have never had one so much as open it in thirty years. They know.

The Role of the Clinician in Motivation   When the confirmed stutterer first comes for therapy, he usually speaks with great difficulty; and we have found it wise to begin by revealing our own role and competence. We don't tell him how good we are; we let him find that out. But we do define our role, not as a teacher or preacher or medicine man, but as a guide and companion on a joint quest. We do this in the initial interview, explaining why we ask the questions we do, and sharing with him the implications of his answers. When he stutters, we provide a running commentary of our own objective evaluations of his behavior. When he avoids, or postpones a speech attempt on a feared word, or uses some trick to start his utterance or disguise the stuttering which occurs, we recognize and identify what he has done with complete acceptance. This always seems to surprise the stutterer. He always seems to feel that his little devices for avoiding or escaping from his difficulty are his own personal secret. And he is always surprised at the acceptance. The only listener responses he has remembered are those of rejection or embarrassment or pity. Suddenly he finds not only a permissive listener but one who understands. This is one of the crucial experiences in all successful therapy. Often, at this point, he will begin to stutter very severely as if to test the genuineness of the clinician's acceptance, and again he is surprised to find that the behavior is welcomed, rewarded.

Another crucial experience which the stutterer should have as soon as possible is that of observing his clinician actually *sharing* his abnormality. Here is the transcript of one such experience:

Clinician: You had a pretty long and complicated block on that word "people." Let's see if I can duplicate it. First of all you squeezed, then protruded your lips like this. Then I think you gave a quick little gasp like this . . . and then. . . . No, I don't have it right. Let me have another bad one so I can learn what you do.

Stutterer: Pppeople. That time it came out easy.

Clinician: Yes it did, but I wish you could show me a more severe one, the kind that make you panic, as you said a moment ago. I've got to feel it in my mouth to know what you do so I can understand what the problem is. You've got to teach me.

Stutterer: Yyyyou mmmmean you want me, you want me, you want me to teach you to sttttt . . . stttttttttutter like I do?

Clinician: To know how you feel, to know what you do, I've got to do it too. And not just here but in real speaking situations. As soon as I've learned how you do it, I'll make a phone call and try it out, and you can tell me how close I am, and if my feelings are similar to yours.

Stutterer: Holy C-C-Cow!

We do not only repeat the stutterer's behavior; we also share it as it is happening. By pantomiming what he is doing as he is doing it, we become a human mirror for him. When he first experiences this, old memories of the mockery of playmates long ago flood back and suspiciousness is aroused, then allayed as he finds that the clinician is actually trying to understand and share his burden of abnormality. This interaction not only helps to produce a close relationship between the stutterer and the clinician but it also partially extinguishes some of the persisting evil effects of old traumatic wounds.

Another important experience occurs when the clinician reveals that he is interested and desires to share not only the outward behavior of the stutterer but also to understand his inner feelings. We find it wise to begin with the feelings created by the immediate moment of stuttering. A few stutterers are able, with skillful counseling, to express these feelings, but most are not. The stuttering itself interferes with expression. As Fenichel put the matter in a nutshell, when speech, the healing tool of psychotherapy, is itself infected the task of the clinician is hard. We have therefore found it wise to verbalize the stutterer's feelings for him. We do this tentatively and ask for corrections and additions. Here is a portion of the transcript of a session in which this took place:

Clinician: When you were stuck that time, what were your feelings?

Stutterer: I don't know. All, all mmmmmmmmmmmmixed up, I gggggguess.

Clinician: You probably felt helpless . . . sort of as though your mouth had frozen shut. . . .

Stutterer: And, and and I cccccouldn't open it. Yeah.

Clinician: You couldn't open it. It was almost as though you had lost the ability to move a part of yourself when you wanted to. . . . Sure must be frustrating. . . .

Stutterer: Sssure is. BBBBBurns me up. I, I, I, jjjust hate mmmmm . . . Oh, skip it . . . I don't know.

Clinician: (acceptingly): It almost makes you hate yourself when you get stuck like that.

Stutterer: Yeah, dih-dih-disgusted with mmmmmyself and everything else. . . .

Clinician: Some stutterers even find themselves hating the person they are talking to.

Stutterer: Yyyyea. I, I, I, I, I, wwwwwas huh-huh-huh-hating yyyyyyyyyyyou just then.

Clinician: Uh huh. I know.

Stutterer (blurting it out): How, howcome you know all these th-things?

If these three crucial experiences, which will be repeated many times in many different forms, are scrutinized, it is apparent that we are already at work on the stuttering equation. The client finds for the first time that stuttering is not being penalized, but encouraged. Frustration declines a bit as he discovers that his clinician is in no hurry, that this ear is always open no matter how long the blockings last. He learns that here he can pour out a bit of anxiety, guilt, and hostility with impunity. In the therapy situation, communicative stress is reduced. It is easier to talk here. Moreover, since stuttering is actually sought and encouraged, the fears are reduced. We do not fear that which is rewarded. Finally, and perhaps most important of all, there comes an increase in morale as the stutterer finds that he is not alone, that someone who seems to understand his problem has faith that he can solve it. Moreover, burdens which are shared are thereby divided. The load lightens. All of these changes reflect themselves in increased motivation.[10]

Goal Orientation   But the clinician is not only an understanding companion sharing part of the load; the stutterer soon comes to feel that this person is also a competent guide. At least he seems to know one way out of the swamp. Let us outline how we help him to come to this conclusion.

[10] A series of eight videotapes showing the entire course of therapy with Jeff, a severe stutterer, is available from the Speech Foundation of America, 152 Lombardy Road, Memphis, Tennessee 38111.

First of all, we try to provide some person whom he can see or hear who has been able to conquer his stuttering problem. Usually we have several around who are determined, despite our usual discouragement, to become speech pathologists. We also have the tales of many others on tape, tales that often exaggerate a bit the difficulties encountered, and we must use them with care so that the new sprout of hope will not be withered by the frigid windiness of their exaggerated accounts of what they had to do. We use films for the same purpose.

Next we try to help the stutterer realize that he possesses in his own present speech both a certain amount of fluency and also, what is more important, a certain amount of stuttering that does not interrupt communication unduly or show much abnormality. This latter item is of utmost importance. All stutterers have some moments of stuttering which are unforced and unaccompanied by struggle or avoidance. We point these out when they occur and often make a tape in which many samples of these fluent, normal stutterings are combined. We ask the stutterer to listen to this tape frequently. Also in our pantomimic sharing of his stuttering, we often repeat again and again these fluent stutterings so that he can see them, and we ask him to repeat them also. We point up this easy, fluent sort of stuttering as a goal object. Even a rat runs a difficult maze better when he has a taste or smell of the cheese to be found at the end of that maze.

At this point the stutterer often objects.

Stutterer: Yyyyou mean, you mmmmmmmean that it's possible to stutter easy like that even when you're scared green?
Clinician: You feel it isn't possible. (*nods acceptance of the feeling.*)
Stutterer: Oh nnnnnnot when you're really petrified, nnnot wheh, when you can see th ... em c-c-c-coming and the ffffffffffear builds up.
Clinician: Real hard fears are bound to throw you into long hard blocks. . . .
Stutterer: Yeah, but mmmmmaybe, maybe not. Maybe it is ppppppossible to let them kind of leak out, hey? MMMMaybe I c-c-could lllllearn. . . . (*He shakes his head.*)
Clinician: But you have your doubts. . . .
Stutterer: SSSSStill those other gggguh-guys say they can stutt ... stutter. . . . Hey, I'm doing it right now. I just had an easy bbb-block on sssss, on sssssssstut. . . . Why can't I say it now? On ssssss-stutter. I, I, I, dddddid have one, dddddidn't I?
Clinician: Sounded like it.

Stutterer: And, and, and mmmaybe the ffffears wwwwwwwon't al, al, al, al, always be so strong. Even already I dddddon't seem to bbbbe quite ssssssssssso sceh, scared. YYYou know it's true. I, I, I, I dddddo have dddddifffferent kkkinds of bbbbblocks.

At some such moment it is possible to help the stutterer to have another very important experience: the realization that it is possible to stutter in many different ways and that some ways may be better than others. We make it possible for him to observe and duplicate the kinds of stuttering shown by other stutterers. We also ask him to experiment a bit in modifying his own.

Clinician: I notice that usually on a word beginning with *b* or *p* you squeeze your lips tightly and then open them and suck in a little air just before the release comes—like this. . . . *(Therapist demonstrates.)*

Stutterer: YYYYeah, and it, it, it, it mmmmakes a ssssssssssssssssssuck-ing sound I don't like.

Clinician: You hate that sucking noise.

Stutterer: Yeah. *(It is evident that he is not going to pursue the subject further.)*

Clinician: Then let's see if you stutter on words like that without sucking.

Stutterer: Huh?

Clinician: Let's see if you can say these names in the phone directory beginning with *P* and try to keep the sucking noises out.

Stutterer (doubtfully): OK. PPPP *(suck)* Partridge; PPPPPP *(suck)* Parsons . . . I can't.

Clinician: OK *(acceptingly)*.

Stutterer: LLLLLLet me rrrrreally try th . . . is tttttime . . . PPP-Puh-puhparparpartridge. Hey! I did it! What do you know! Yyyyou mean I, I, I, I don't have to ssssssuck?

Clinician: Looks like it.

This is another of the crucial experiences which are the mile markers on the road to freedom. There are many of them.

Mapping the Route to the Goal   It is also necessary that a clear picture of the course of ther-apy be given to the stutterer. He needs some kind of a map before he becomes willing to undertake a journey, even though he now knows he has a guide. We have found it useful to give him some understanding. This first phase of therapy requires the imparting of information. The stutterer is usually as ignorant of the nature of his disorder as he is of the behavior he uses so compulsively. He needs to know something of the causes of stuttering and the way it develops, and we also help him to find information about the way stuttering has been treated in the past as well as how it is being treated by other clinicians. We do not believe in blind therapy. We want him to know where he's going, where he is, and what he has to do. We find that we get a better motivated client this way.

The Second Phase of Therapy: Identification

As soon as possible we move directly into the second phase of our therapy, in which the basic goal is the identification and evaluation of the various factors in the client's *personal* stuttering equation. There is no emphasis on trying to speak more fluently. Just the converse. The stutterer is to seek out stuttering experiences and to analyze the behavior and identify the forces which created it. This is the period of self-study, of self-exploration. (Note that this goal-structuring increases the approach and decreases the avoidance vectors in the approach-avoidance conflicts.) The objective observation of the stuttering behavior gets down to what the semanticists might call "first-order facts." The more the stutterer stutters, the more opportunity he has to make his observations. The clinician shares and rewards these discoveries. He also provides structured experiences which will make them possible.

Speech Assignments   One of the unique features of this type of therapy is the use of the speech assignment. In addition to the stutterer's own attempts in self-therapy, certain required activities and experiences are devised by the clinician to provide guidelines and models for what the case should be doing himself. Some stutterers need few of these; others need many; but the emphasis is always on self-therapy. The devising of self-assignments is constantly and vividly rewarded. Usually, the clinician-formulated speech assignments are given more frequently in the early phases of therapy, and especially during the phase of identification. Reporting the experiences *and feelings* evoked by these experiences is a very necessary part of the clinical routine. This may be done orally either in private sessions with the clinician or in group sessions with other stutterers, or the reports may be written in certain instances. Often we use both oral and written reports. The mere act of preparing and handing in reports of self- and clinician-assigned experiences gives a sense of achievement which has profound and cumulative effects. Moreover, these assignments often provoke the resistance and testings of the relationship between stutterer and clinician; that when worked through, create new insights and energies for healing. They make it possible for the clinician to share significant moments in the stutterer's life; they reveal the basic feelings which can then be accepted and reflected upon. They help the stutterer to know where he is and how much he is doing and how much he still must do. They provide an objective account of the course of therapy. We have found them very useful.

Typical Assignments in Identification   Since this is a general and introductory text in speech correction and not a manual for stuttering therapy, we can do no more than provide one or two typical assignments for each of the subgoals involved. There are hundreds of other possible assignments which might be more appropriate for a particular case. The stutterers themselves often invent better ones than we can design. Since the basic goal of this phase of the therapy is the identification of the various factors in the stutterer's personal equation, the illustrative assignments will be organized about these factors. Often, in a single day's work, the stutterer will perform one of the clinician's assignments for each of the factors, and also a self-invented one of his own for each of them. There are also times when he may do nothing. He gets the clinician's warm approval for the first of these responses, and the other is accepted as part of the difficulty. However, if the client proves entirely unwilling to work, therapy is terminated. Even a psychoanalyst has to get them on the couch now and then.

Penalties   Many secondary stutterers have become a bit paranoid about the reactions of listeners to their stuttering. Even when no overt rejection is evidenced, they think the listener is merely covering up a punitive or embarrassed reaction. It is vitally necessary that they do some reality testing. Some assignments which could begin this testing might run like this:

> Keep track of the number of listeners who frown or show objective signs of impatience when you stutter. What proportion do not? Get a sample of ten strangers with whom you stuttered obviously to determine the proportion.

How many store clerks did you talk to before you found one who showed signs of mirth or mocking when you stuttered? Try a minimum of five.

If possible, ask one of your friends how he really feels when you stutter to him. Ask him to tell you the truth. Report what he said and whether you think he was honest.

Here is one stutterer's own self-assignment report:

> I've been wondering maybe I've been blowing this fear business all up. Maybe most people don't really give a damn whether I stutter or not. Maybe they figure it's my problem, not theirs, and they let it go like that. Then I got to thinking how many people I can remember who really did laugh in my face when I stuttered and you know I couldn't remember a single one except Wilbur Ketchum when I was a kid and he was goofy anyway and laughed all the time. So I got to thinking and thought I'd try something out. I called on the phone a whole mess of people and asked them things like "Is Wilbur home?" or "May I speak to Jane, please?" and I stuttered plenty but I cocked my ear to see if I could hear any laughing or giggling. I just got one who did. It was a little girl who answered the phone. All the rest just waited till I got it out. I was sure surprised. Maybe I have been exaggerating.

And here is another:

> Had a lulu of a penalty today. It threw me. Was talking to a stranger, a man about sixty, and asked him how to get to the bank. He got mad when I stuttered. He said, "If you can't talk any better than that don't ask questions." And turned away. Felt like quitting right there. Made me feel dirty mouth. But I said to myself why does he act like this? What kind of a guy is this? So I follow him around and listen. He gets some tobacco in a store and he raises hell with the clerk for not having his kind. Then he goes to another place and gets his tobacco but growls at that clerk. I tailed him into Gilmore's, and there he was giving some other clerk hell for something. So I guess I got a bad one and it wasn't just my stuttering. Felt pretty good after.

These assignments happen to revolve about the speech disorder itself, but we wish to make clear that we explore all penalties, not just those evoked by stuttering. Punishment of any kind seems to add an increment of stuttering. During this phase of treatment the client tries to locate and assess the importance of all penalties, present and past. He becomes aware of sources of rejection other than his stuttering. One girl changed her hairdo and bought new clothes and a red hat instead of the mousy-looking apparel she had been wearing. A boy learned how to dance when he found he could get dates easier for such affairs than for the movies. As a result of some vivid experiences, one man began to see that he was getting more rejection for his aggressive sarcastic reactions to other speakers than for the fairly mild stuttering which he exhibited. And he also found that his stuttering began to decrease. One of our college students wrote an essay on "My History of Penalty" and won a prize for the composition. Often, in group sessions, the memories of past penalties are ventilated, and again not just those concerning stuttering. In this phase of therapy, we make no attempts to eliminate the behavior that provokes the penalty but merely to explore and to define it, and often the stutterer starts making some changes anyway. The emphasis at this phase of therapy is merely to *identify* those penalties which contribute to stuttering.

Frustration In exploring this factor the stutterer compiles an account of the frustrations characteristic of his present situation and also a history of those of the past. He also thereby becomes aware of basic drives and needs other than to speak fluently. Many stutterers become so focused on stuttering that other major problems are completely disregarded, even though they contribute to the disorder and may be more easily rectified. In the identification phase of therapy, the whole target, not just the bull's-eye of stuttering, comes into view. Here is the report of a self-initiated assignment in exploring the frustration factor.

> My roommate in our girl's dormitory has a nasty little habit that's been driving me to distraction. She sniffs. She sniffs when she's studying. When it's quiet all I can hear is that sniff, sniff, and I almost go wild. It's a tic or something. I used the radio for a while to cover it up, but she says she can't study with it going. I asked her if she couldn't stop it and she said no, that if it didn't bother her why did it have to bother me? I told her it still did and she said that's too bad. Lately I've been doing all my studying at the library, but that's pretty inconvenient. Well, I've been thinking about frustration and how it may affect my

stuttering, and I know her sniffing makes me jittery so I said to myself, "All right, let's see if you can learn to bear it." Ruth's a very nice girl in other ways and we have lots of fun together. So I said to myself, "Let's measure how many sniffs you can count before you get nervous, and then you can give her one stutter for every five sniffs." That made me grin to myself. Well, I stuttered eleven times to her before we went to bed, ten for her sniffs and one for myself. It actually took fifty sniffs and three hours of studying before I couldn't stand it any longer. I guess I can get used to it if I can only use a little psychology on myself.

Anxiety, Guilt, For some stutterers only professional counseling can help to *and Hostility* ease the pressures of these emotions. There are clinicians who are qualified to do such counseling. Other clinicians cannot and should not do it, and the patient must seek help elsewhere. Professional psychotherapy for the stutterer whose disorder is primarily neurotic in nature is a must. But most stutterers, in our opinion, do not fall in this category. Yet they all have some anxieties and guilts and hostilities which need ventilation and release. Fortunately, the speech assignments and experiences usually bring about the expression of many of these feelings.

Communicative Here we confront the stuttering directly. In this phase of *Stress* treatment, the stutterer explores and identifies the types of communicative stress to which he is most vulnerable. Again he is *seeking* speaking experiences instead of avoiding them, which is healthy in itself and a reversal of old practices. Here are some typical assignments.

Which of these two audience reactions seems to produce more stutterings: (1) interruption by having the listener finish what you are trying to say, or (2) having him look away when you're stuttering? Collect two experiences of each kind and report.

Read a passage aloud to some other stutterer very swiftly; then another of equal length at a normal rate; then another at a normal rate; and finally a fourth at a fast rate. Using hand counter, have him count how many blocks you have under fast and ordinary speaking rates, averaging the two trials for each. How much of a factor is speed in producing more stuttering? Report your findings.

Tell a joke to some friend. Do you have more stuttering on the words that carry the key meaning, or on the punch lines? Why?

Analyze four speaking situations which produced different amounts of stuttering and attempt to identify the kinds of communicative stress present in each.

Read aloud the names on one page of the telephone directory to some other person and have him indicate which ones you stuttered on most severely. Were some of these strange unfamiliar combinations of sounds such as occur in foreign names?

What kinds of attitudes shown by your parents when you were trying to talk to them seemed to produce the most stuttering when you were a child?

Situation Fears   In exploring these, the stutterer should not only identify those of the present and the past but also attempt to assess their intensity. He should also try to discover what he specifically dreads. Many very important insights come from this sort of investigation. He may even find that he doesn't know what he is afraid of. The stutterer should also study the relationship between situation fears and the amount of actual stuttering that does occur. He may find that the correlation is not as high as he thinks it is. We find that experiences of this sort are very salutary because they weaken the *fear of fear*. Often these people seem to be more afraid of the fear than of the stuttering itself. By seeking out what is dreaded, by exposing and analyzing it, the evil subsides a bit.

Some typical assignments are as follows:

Before you enter five different speaking situations, predict on this five-step scale how severely you will stutter. Then, after you have left the situation, record how badly you actually did stutter.

What three speaking situations in your whole life do you remember as being the worst? Why were they the worst?

Apply for a job at some restaurant. On your way downtown, try to identify and remember the kind of thinking you were doing and what you were especially dreading. Report this in writing.

Word Fears   This factor, as we have said, includes not only fears of specific words but also the phonetic fears of sounds. It might be objected that by focusing the stutterer's attention on them, we only make them that much worse. All we can say in this regard is that any increment of this sort is negligible. They already have their full strength based upon a thousand memories. Stutterers also fear these phonetic fears; they attempt to distract themselves from them, to re-press them, to escape from them. We have found it healing to look them plumb in the face.

The Morale Factor   We also feel it very important for the stutterer to study his own variable feelings of self-worth. As we have said, stutterers are focused so much on their stuttering that they fail to see their other difficulties. In much the same fashion they are also unable to evaluate with any objectivity the other assets they possess. In this phase of the treatment they learn objectivity, and it is important that they apply it to the favorable factors as well as to the unfavorable ones. While much of the increase in ego strength comes from the sense of achievement gained by working on their stuttering and from the identification with a strong clinician, nevertheless we find that certain assignments can have a real effect. Here are some samples:

> Prepare a list of all your personality assets and liabilities. Shyly we suggest that you include stuttering among the latter.

> Write up an account of all the things for which you have received approval from others.

> Keep a mood chart in which you assess your feelings of morale four times a day: after breakfast, lunch, and dinner and before you go to bed. Make a graph of your mood swings for an entire week of a five-step scale with these values arranged on lines from top to bottom: (1) Whoops! (2) Feeling good. (3) Uncertain. Don't know. (4) Depressed. (5) Mighty, mighty lowdown.

> Who are the people who have evidenced some faith in you? Why do you suppose they evidenced this faith?

Exploring Fluency   Only his stuttering seems to have stimulus value for the stutterer, the quite evident amount of fluency he also possesses does not. Again we must help him assess the real state of affairs. At this stage he has become morbidly conscious only of his abnormality, not of his normality. Also, most confirmed stutterers have an exaggerated concept of what constitutes normal fluency. They do not realize that normal speakers are also nonfluent, at times of stress very nonfluent. This area must also be investigated.

> On what percentage of words do you really stutter? Make tape recordings of yourself (1) reading to another person, (2) explaining something to a friend, and (3) making phone calls. Count

the words spoken and the stutterings, and find out how fluent you are in each.

Listen to the conversations of other people, and be able to show us all the different kinds of nonfluencies they demonstrated.

In this section describing the *identification* phase of therapy we have tried to show how we help the stutterer recognize the scope of his problem as expressed in terms of the various factors that make his stuttering better or worse. We would like to reemphasize here that this exploratory phase by itself often produces immediate decreases both in the amount of stuttering and in the intensity of the fear and avoidance. As in motivation, identification experiences will continue throughout therapy. We find, however, that we have more success when we stress it early in the treatment.

Desensitization Phase of Treatment

The third major phase in the treatment of confirmed stuttering we have termed "desensitization" because our major goal in this part of the therapy is to toughen our client to those factors which normally increase the frequency and the severity of his stuttering. Human beings are wondrously adaptable. They can exist in the Arctic Zone and on the equator. They can even live in big cities. They can endure anything once they put their minds to it. Rats can be trained to bear electric shocks of great intensity with proper schedules of reinforcement. Surely, we can hope that our stutterers can improve in their ability to resist and endure the stresses they must encounter. In this phase, we are raising the thresholds of breakdown. It is very necessary that the stutterer understand why this is being done. But there are immediate rewards from desensitization. He will soon learn that as he becomes more hardened, he stutters less and suffers less. As he becomes tougher, he finds that penalties do not throw him so quickly; that frustration has a less evil effect; that he can tolerate more anxiety, guilt, and hostility than he could before; that communicative disruption and fear do not precipitate stuttering as frequently as once they did. And the morale factor rises, as any soldier knows, once he has learned what he can endure.

It is obvious that the administration of this phase of therapy takes some skill and empathy on the clinician's part. By now he should have gained a clear picture of his client's sensitivities and the energies the latter might marshal to modify them. He must not overload. Indeed, often the clinician must keep the client from overloading himself. But there must always be present the faith that comes from realizing the enormous potentials that all humans seem to possess, and the support which only a loved and respected clinician can give. Evidence must be provided that the clinician can also share these experiences, can also bear the stress, can also suffer but endure. Often he must become the receptacle for the hostile attacks that result from the hurt the stutterer experiences when he tries and fails. But the clinician knows that if he can accept these, the stutterer can try again. And he knows, as does Britain, that you can lose a hundred battles and still win a war.

Again, assignments are given which provide opportunities for desensitization to occur. Again, the stutterer is prevailed upon to construct his own assignments and to bring to the clinician for sharing and analysis all the trophies and the failures which result. Group therapy provides an excellent situation for sharing these accounts, and the stutterers vie with each other and support each other. For example, we have found, in such a group, that if one girl shows she can make progress, all the males have to do more. Also, as they often do assignments together, a sense of comradeship is established which relieves the feeling of isolation so many stutterers know so well.

Usually, we begin fairly gradually to introduce the stress challenges, and the clinician sets models for the client to follow. We have found it wise to enter a store or similar speaking situation and to fake a very long stuttering block in the presence of the stutterer or stutterers. And we show we are not upset, that we remember exactly what the clerk did and how he reacted. We also verbalize our own feelings honestly. And then we do it again. We have found this often to be another crucial experience in the stutterer's life. The fact that another human being, a normal speaker perhaps, would be able to undergo such an experience and remain well-integrated and relatively unperturbed, seems to impress the stutterer greatly. After a few of these demonstrations, he is willing to try himself. We now list just a few illustrative assignments and experiences.

Penalty

Keep making phone calls and fake one long repetitive block until one listener hangs up on you. Time the faked stuttering with a stopwatch, and report how many people you called before one did hang up.

Ask one of the other stutterers to yell at you "Stop that damned stuttering!" every time you do so as you read a paper aloud.

Ask one of your friends to laugh at you every time you stutter in a conversation. Explain that you are trying to be able to resist going to pieces when such reactions occur.

Keep your collar buttoned, but do not wear a tie all morning. Report all actual and suspected penalties.

Frustration

Prewrite everything you say before you say it for an entire morning. Report your feelings of frustration but try to hold to the assignment despite the desire to talk without the annoyance of putting it down.

Do not smoke at all today.

During the noon hour, before you say the first sentence of any conversation, tap your toe once for each word within it.

Anxiety, Guilt, and Hostility

Deliberately stutter to one person in a mildly hostile fashion, and then to another in a very hostile fashion. Smear him with a little of it, then with a lot of it. Report his reactions and your feelings.

Verbalize some of your worries about the future to five different listeners, one at a time. Say the same things each time. Report your feelings.

Using a hand counter, click it every time you feel ashamed during your conversations at meal times. Do this for three days in a row and see if the number doesn't decrease.

Communicative Stress

Find someone who habitually interrupts your attempts to speak or finishes the words for you on which you are stuttering. Every time he does either, go back to the beginning of your sentence and repeat the whole thing. Report what happened.

Ask your roommate to heckle you as you explain something. Try to keep from hurrying or getting upset. And do not stop moving forward even though you stutter. Do not stop or repeat. Have him heckle only a little at first, then turn on the heat.

Situation Fears

Make twenty-five phone calls before you go to bed tonight.

Stop at every residence in one block; go to the door and ask if someone with your own name lives there. Stutter at least once, real or faked stuttering, at each house.

Remembering one of the worst speaking situations you've ever had in the past, try to invent another which has some resemblance to it, and enter it.

Word Fears

Prepare a reading passage containing your most feared words, and make a tape recording of four readings of this material to the same listener.

In speaking to a friend, repeat each stuttered word either until you no longer stutter on it, or until you have tried it ten times.

Make a list of five of your most feared words and deliberately introduce them into conversations. Write each word on a small slip of paper and hold each of these in your hand until it has been used.

Purposely fake repetitions of the first feared sounds of words until you find yourself calm, then say the word. Collect ten of these.

Let us repeat that these are merely illustrative speech assignments, any one of which might be entirely inappropriate for certain stutterers. Moreover, we have not indicated — and cannot indicate — the wide variety of assignments possible under each heading. Each clinician and each stutterer must invent his own. We have found it wise to keep the busywork at a minimum, to ask for as little performance as possible and yet enough to produce some impact. Assignments must be so structured that an objective report can be pro-

303   *Stuttering*

duced. They must provide enough stress to permit desensitization to occur. For any given case, their difficulty must be so tailored that more success than failure ensues, but failure is not to be avoided entirely. Indeed, in the sharing period with the clinician or other stutterers, often the failures when expressed and accepted do more good than even the successes. But there must be clinician approval and reward for meeting these challenges. And constantly we must emphasize the basic purpose these desensitization experiences are designed to fulfill: the building of a thicker hide on the stutterer's sensitive soul.

The Variation Phase of Treatment

It is not enough to motivate, to identify, and desensitize, although these bring reductions in the frequency and severity of stuttering. In this new phase of therapy we begin to change, to modify the reactions to the factors that determine stuttering. Our purpose is to break up the stereotypy of the stutterer's responses, to attach new responses to the old cues. Much of the strength of habitual compulsive reactions lies in their stereotypy, in the consistency of their patterning. Varying them weakens them. Until new responses are made available, the stutterer has no choice except to yield to the old ones. We must help him to know that he has this choice. We cannot persuade him through intellectual argument. Only by behaving differently can he know that it is possible to behave differently.

This variation phase of treatment is usually short in duration because it passes directly into the next one of approximation, in which we seek to help the stutterer learn not just *new* responses to old pressures, but *good* responses. By "good" we mean only that new responses can be learned which will facilitate fluency rather than reduce it. There are always better ways of responding to penalty, frustration, word fear, and all the other evil factors than those the stutterer has habituated to compulsive automaticity. We must help him learn new responses which do not continually reinforce his stuttering as his old responses do. But before these new ways of behaving can be learned, the old ways must be weakened. Variation must precede approximation. The stutterer must realize that he has a choice of responses before he can pick out and master a better one.

Again we seek to provide for the stutterer experiences in which this learning may occur and to motivate him to seek such experiences himself. Let us reverse our usual sequence of presentation and begin with the factor of word fear.

Varying the
Reactions to Word
Fear

Read a passage omitting all words on which you anticipate any stuttering.

On every other word on which you stutter, be sure to stutter repetitively but slowly on the first syllable. Do this to three listeners.

Underline the feared words in a reading passage and substitute (or add) a tremor in your right leg for each one that you find in your lips or tongue.

In a phone call, when you find yourself using such stallers as *a . . . a . . . a . . .*, vary them so that you also use *um, uh, ub, oops,* and *Ozymandias.* Your job is to vary the way you usually postpone.

During three moments of stuttering attempt to shift the focus of the tension from where it usually resides to some other parts of your body. Report what you did.

Instead of gasping as an interrupter of your tremors, try blowing out a puff of air on four of your stuttering blocks.

Since you usually lower your head whenever you stutter, watch yourself in a mirror with an observer, and raise it instead.

Instead of shutting both eyes as you usually do when stuttering, try shutting only one. Work before a mirror until you get ten successes.

Varying the
Reactions to
Situation Fears

You have said that when you enter a phone booth to make a call, you hurry too much and go all to pieces. Today, enter five phone booths, stay in each for two minutes before you call me. When I answer, just make noises and hang up. Report your feelings.

You report that when you must do an errand, you rehearse over and over again what you plan to say, picking out easy words and revising sentences. Today, do three such errands with a friend but you are to say only what he tells you and to say it exactly as he does. He is not to tell you what to say until the last minute. Report your experiences.

Ordinarily you walk around the block several times before entering a store to ask for something. Today, ask questions in three stores, but stand absolutely still looking in the display window for as long as it would take you to walk around that block. Then go in and ask for it. Report your introspections.

Varying the Reactions to Communicative Stress

Get a companion and hunt for the noisiest places you can find. Try not to speak more loudly to your friend but speak more slowly and distinctly.

Ask some acquaintance to do you a favor you know he will not grant. Do not apologize or appear uncertain. Just ask him.

Criticize your roommate for some of the behavior you do not like. Speak very slowly as you do so.

When one of your listeners looks away while you stutter, speak more loudly or do something different so he will look at you.

Varying the Reactions to Anxiety, Guilt, and Hostility

You say you find yourself worrying vaguely about everything and find it hard to get to sleep. Tonight, assign yourself to worry on purpose and do so aloud in self-talk just before you hop into bed. Worry aloud about everything you can possibly think of.

You've reported that when you've felt ashamed about something you did or didn't do, you found yourself biting your fingernails to the quick. Keep a pocketful of peanuts and remember to bite one of them (only one) instead whenever you start to nibble a fingernail or find yourself feeling guilty or ashamed.

You've reported how frequently you keep reviewing your wrongs and hates. This evening before you go to bed, write out as many of them as you can on toilet tissue, read them again, then flush them down the drain.

At the beginning of each hour, by your watch, verbalize to yourself a statement of one anxiety, one guilt, and one hostility. Try not to repeat yourself. Do this for each hour of the afternoon.

Varying the Reactions to Frustration and Penalty

Every time you feel frustrated this evening, smile and continue to smile until the frustration has subsided.

Whenever a listener interrupts you or finishes a word on which you are stuttering, say to him, "Don't interrupt me. I've got a hard enough time talking anyway."

As we write this chapter we are constantly aware of the inadequacy of our presentation of such assignments in reflecting what actually occurs in therapy. These assignments by themselves have no value. Only when shared with the clinician and when feelings are expressed and when rewards are appropriately timed, do the experiences they evoke have potency in modifying the attitudes and outward behavior of the stutterer. It would be easier and perhaps safer to resort to statements of vague general principles, but students seem to profit more from specific examples. So be it!

The Approximation Phase of Therapy

Once the stutterer has learned that his habitual reactions to the factors which make stuttering worse can be varied, we try to help him learn *new responses which will diminish that stuttering.* We now seek not just different responses but the best responses, those which tend to extinguish stuttering rather than reinforce it. Why do we call this phase the approximation phase? Because we feel that new responses are acquired, not by sudden exchange, but by gradual modification. You just don't stop stuttering severely and suddenly begin to stutter easily. Again, it's like learning to target-shoot. You shoot and miss; then you change a bit of your behavior and shoot again. Your attempts result in a coming closer, in an approximation to the behavior needed to hit the bull's-eye consistently. By approximation we mean the progressive modification of behavior toward a goal response.

The basic goal then of this phase of therapy is to learn how to stutter and to respond to stress in such a fashion that the disorder will not be reinforced. The clinician's responsibility is to see that rewards are felt whenever the stutterer moves closer to this goal. Approval is contingent upon *progress,* not merely upon performance. Happily, the relief from communicative abnormality seems to follow the same course, and provides even more powerful reinforcement. The goal is getting nearer now.

In our discussion of this phase of therapy, we will confine ourselves to the exposition of what we do with the fears and experiences of stuttering itself. It must be remembered, however, that the characteristic responses to penalty, frustration, and all the other disturbing factors must also be modified in the direction of nonreinforcement of the stuttering. There are better responses to penalty, to communicative stress, than those the stutterer first brings to us; and these he can also learn by progressive approximation. However, here we will concentrate on the stuttering behavior.

Stuttering in Unison   One of the best ways we have discovered to help the stutterer learn an easier, nonreinforcing kind of stuttering is to do it with him. He watches us and hears us as we join him in his stuttering, duplicating the first of his behavior, but then we ease out of the tremors, cease the struggling, and smoothly finish the word. Often at first, the contrast between his continued struggles and our smooth utterance tends to shock him, but gradually he begins to follow our lead and to stutter as we do. He finds us sharing his initial behavior but then diverging. We make the changes gradually, at first setting models of minor changes which he may be able to follow, and rewarding them when they appear. Once he can make these minor changes (e.g., stuttering with his eyes open rather than closed), he gets no more approval until a further change occurs (e.g., lips are loosened from their tensed closure), and so on. We move only as far as the client is ready and able to go in any given session. It is vitally necessary that this training be done under some stress, stress that can be felt but not stress that overwhelms. To sum it up, we share and show him how to shift, how to change his responses. Verbalization of feelings is always encouraged, and this phase of therapy often produces some new storms. But the mere fact of the sharing, the fact of the clinician's faith, the fact of his patient acceptance of failure as a necessary part of learning—all these create a favorable climate for change and growth.

Cancellation[11]   As soon as any change in the stuttering behavior has been learned, the stutterer is encouraged to use it in cancellation. By this term we mean that the stutterer stops as soon as a stuttered word has finally been uttered; pauses; and then says it again, this time using the modification he has learned in unison stuttering with his clinician. He still stutters this second time, faking, if he must, a duplication of the same stuttering he has just experienced; but now he modifies it in accordance with the new behavior he has learned. Then he finishes his sentence. Communication stops once he stutters, and it continues only after he has used a better stuttering response. This is also powerfully reinforcing.

Pull-Outs   This awkward term, stemming from the stutterers' own language usage, refers to the moment of stuttering itself and what the stutterer does to escape from his oscillations or fixations. Evil pull-outs are the jerks, the sudden exhaling of all available air. These only increase the penalty and all other factors that make for more stuttering in the future. There are better ways of terminating these fixations and oscillations, and once these new ways have been learned in unison speaking with the clinician, and practiced frequently in cancellations in all types of speaking situations, the stutterer should begin to incorporate them within the original moment of stuttering itself. Any change for the better should be incorporated as often as the stutterer can manage it. Thus the new behavior moves forward in time, from the period just following the stuttering into the moment of stuttering itself.

Preparatory Sets   Our next step is to move it even further forward, into the period of anticipation, into what has been called the "prespasm period." Usually, in response to word or phonetic fears, the stutterer actually makes little covert rehearsals of the stuttering abnormality he

[11] An illustration of a complete operant conditioning program for getting the stutterer to use cancellation, pull-outs, and preparatory sets will be found in Speech Foundation of America, *Conditioning in Stuttering Therapy* (Memphis, Tenn.: Fraser, 1970).

expects. These preparatory sets to stutter often determine the kind and length of abnormality which result. Therefore, once the stutterer has shown that he can incorporate the new change not only in cancellation but also during the actual stuttering behavior, he is now challenged to incorporate it within his anticipatory rehearsals, to plan to stutter this new way. Often we can help him by rehearsing for him and by getting him to duplicate our model before he attempts the word he has indicated he will stutter upon. Again, we reward the successes and disregard the failures. Again, we reward progressive change.

As each new modification of stuttering is learned and starts up the series of experiences in cancellation, pull-outs, and preparatory sets, new modifications are being born, either with the help of the clinician through unison stuttering or through self-discoveries. With each new change comes a decrease in the severity and often in the frequency of stuttering as well. Fears of words, then of situations, lose their intensity. The stutterer's self-confidence begins to grow with each new achievement. The fluency factor grows larger. He becomes able to tolerate more communicative stress. It is also interesting to watch how he applies the same therapeutic principles to his other inadequate behaviors. He begins to modify his old inadequate reactions to penalty and frustration; and the ways he handles his anxieties, guilts, and hostilities improve. Progress comes swiftly on all fronts. Instead of avoiding stuttering experiences, he hunts for them so he can try out his new skills. Avoidance declines.

Perhaps some glimpses of the actual interaction between clinician and stutterer would be helpful here, although it is impossible to indicate the changes in behavior which occur. The student will have to use some imagination.

> This stutterer, when he attempted a feared *p* or *b* or *m* word, characteristically assumed a wide-open-mouthed posture, invested it with a strong tremor, then attempted to release himself from it by a sudden movement in which the head went up but the jaw went down. The final utterance of the word always emerged from one of these jerks. Often he would have to use two or three of the latter before release occurred; and if one failed, he then returned instantly to the tremorous highly tensed, open-mouth posturing.

Clinician: Today, let's see if we can't learn to stutter a bit more easily than you've been doing it on that feared *p* sound of yours.
Stutterer: GGGGGGGood. I'm rrrrready.

Clinician: On these cards I have written some *p* words that you have often stuttered on, and I'm hoping that you'll stutter on a few of them at least.

Stutterer (opens mouth and has his characteristic abnormality): . . . *(jerk)* Probably!

Clinician: Well, I won't need the card, I guess. I'll ask you a question now, and if you stutter on the answer, I'll join you, do just what you do at first, but then do something differently too. Try to follow my lead. Here's the question: Do you think you'll have some stuttering on these words?

Stutterer: (Open mouth in same tremorous posture, which the clinician duplicates almost exactly; but clinician slowly closes mouth while continuing the tremor so that finally the tremor is occurring on the lips alone. The stutterer also closes his lips as he watches and follows the model; but just before he says the word "Probably" his mouth again opens suddenly, and the head-and-jaw jerk of release precede its utterance. The clinician's utterance finally emerges from the closed-lip position, so the two performances, at first fairly identical, later diverge.)

Clinician: Good. You made some change. Not enough, but at least you managed to produce the only posture that the first sound of "probably" can use. Here's what you did . . . *(demonstrates),* and here's what you always have done in the past . . . *(demonstrates),* so you can see that you made some change for the better. Nobody can say "probably" with his mouth as far open as your Grand Canyon of the Colorado. Now show me both ways. Show me, by faking if you must, how you usually stutter on the word, and then how you just changed it a bit.

Stutterer (demonstrates old way): . . . *(jerk)* Probably. . . . Hey, that . . . *(jerk)* bbecame real! *(Clinician grins, and the stutterer then demonstrates the changed stuttering pattern.)*

Clinician: Pretty good! Now let's try some of these *p* words, and be sure to get your mouth closed and hold it closed a bit before you jerk it out. Remember I'll be joining you every so often . . . not always.

They work on eight different *p* words this way. The clinician gives approval intermittently but only for lip closure during the stuttering. Then he says:

Clinician: Now let's hear about that job you have with the *Gazette.* Forget about doing anything about any other stutterings, but if you have one of your old unchanged blocks on a *p* word, stop immediately, pause until I give you the signal, and then cancel it by stuttering again on the word but in the changed way.

Stutterer: OK. Well, I, I, I dddddelivered ffffffffforty . . . *(jerk)* papers. . . . *(Clinician signals and client stops. Clinician pantomimes changed stuttering pattern, then nods, and client cancels in the new way)* . . . ppppppp . . . *(jerk)* papers. How's that?

Clinician: Attaboy. Good. Let's do some more cancelling. Tell me some more about your deliveries. *(The stutterer begins but forgets to cancel on the first p word.)*

Stutterer: Oooops, I fffforgot.

Clinician: It's hard to remember when you're interested in what you're saying. *(The stutterer gets some more cancellations, and then he uses his new change in the first attempt on another p word.)*

Stutterer (surprised): Hey, I used it in the mmmmmmmmmiddle.

Clinician: Good. Good! How about trying to get some more of those in the middle of your stutterings? Look, here's how you do it. . . . *(Clinician demonstrates.)* You don't *have* to keep your mouth open when you try to say a *p* word.

They collect several more experiences, some successful, which the clinician rewards, and some failures, which he ignores. Several times the client failed but then cancelled. This was reflected and rewarded. Once, he successfully rehearsed it before succeeding.

Clinician: How do you feel about this experimenting?

Stutterer: MMMMMan! It's ffffffffffascinating. I, I, I, I think I'm gggggetting the idea. MMMMaybe I can do it easier, hey?

Clinician: Want to try changing it a bit further?

Stutterer: Sure.

Clinician: OK. Now, let's see if you can stop jerking just before the word comes out. Look, here's what you do *(demonstrates)*. . . . Can you also do this? . . . *(demonstrates the elimination of the jerk release and shows how the utterance could come directly from the tremorous lip posture.)*

They then work on this new change in the same way. Now the clinician only rewards the new changes. The session ends in some fairly potent expression and reflection of feelings revolving about the stutterer's fear of hoping too much and his many doubts about the future.

We cannot end this section on approximation without reminding the student that most of the progress made must be due to the stutterer's solo efforts. Many speech assignments are devised to provide the necessary opportunities for progressively modifying the stuttering behavior under stress.[12] But this is how we begin.

Stabilization

The final phase of stuttering therapy we have called stabilization. For lack of a clear-cut program of this sort, many stutterers have experienced frequent relapses and despair. It is not enough to bring the stutterer to the point where he is fluent, where he can speak with little struggle or fear. We must stabilize his new behavior, his new resistance to stress, his new integration. Anxiety-conditioned responses are very difficult to extinguish entirely. New adjustments must be made, new responsibilities undertaken now that the stuttering excuse is no longer valid. Terminal therapy must be done carefully. It must be done well. We always keep in fairly close touch with our confirmed stutterers for two years after formal therapy is terminated. Many of them occasionally avail themselves of our counsel for many years, often on matters other than stuttering.

Often stuttering seems to go out the same door it entered. More of the easy and unconscious repetitions and prolongations appear; periods of fairly frequent small stutterings alternate with periods of very good fluency. Sudden bursts of fear and even avoidance occur. Under moments of extreme stress an occasional severe blocking may be evident. It is important that the stutterer understand this and accept it as part of his problem. Often the clinician must be available for the verbalization of these traumatic episodes and receive the confession of avoidance and compulsive behaviors with accepting reassurance and remedial measures. However, it is possible to prevent much of this stress by an organized program of terminal therapy.

Fluency   Even when the stuttering disappears, there remain gaps in the flow of speech where the stuttering formerly occurred. These people have had so little experience in smooth-flowing speech that some training is needed to provide it. One of the best ways we have found to do this is through echo speech or shadowing, in which the stutterer, while watching TV or observing some fluent speaker,

[12] A booklet, *Therapy for Stutterers,* published by the Speech Foundation of America, 152 Lombardy Rd., Memphis, Tenn. 38111, provides many illustrations of these assignments.

follows in pantomime the speech that is being produced, saying it silently as it is being spoken aloud. Often we train the stutterer to repeat whole sentences exactly as the speaker spoke them. We also ask him to cancel whole sentences of his own in which gaps or hesitancies appeared so that they can be made to flow more smoothly. We persuade him to do much self-talk when alone. We emphasize display speech of all types so that he can get the feel of fluency. At the same time we also show him that even excellent speakers have some nonfluencies and that these are different from the residual breaks which come from a long history of broken speech.

Faking   We also train our stutterers to fake easy repetitive or prolonged stutterings, to put these into their fluent speech casually in certain situations every day. We ask them, too, to demonstrate an occasional faking of a short block of the old variety and then to follow it with a cancellation. Occasionally it is wise to fake a pullout or some of the modifications of postures and tremors so that these basic skills may remain fresh for use in emergencies. Most stutterers dislike doing these things, and they will not do them unless the activities form a basic part of the stabilization phase of treatment.

Assessment   The practice of taking an honest daily inventory must be encouraged. In this phase of treatment, we help the stutterer to learn to survey his own personal stuttering equation, to assess the variations in strength of the various factors, and to be honest in his evaluations. Here the accepting attitudes of an understanding clinician are most essential. He hears the confession and turns it into an inventory, for these are not sins but the natural residues of a severe disorder of communication.

Resistance Therapy   In this final phase of active therapy, we work especially hard to help the stutterer learn to maintain his new methods of fluent stuttering and fluent speaking in the face of pressures of all kinds. When he first comes to us, the stutterer has but two choices: to stutter on the feared words or to avoid them. We now have given him a third choice, the ability to stutter in a relatively fluent and unabnormal fashion. It is necessary not only to stabilize his new behavior of this third choice under conditions of stress but also to give him a fourth choice — to resist stuttering.

In helping the stutterer to resist communicative stresses of all kinds and yet maintain his new ways of short, easy stuttering, we deliberately create conditions in which the pressures to stutter in the old way are strong, and then the stutterer does his utmost to resist them. We seek out and enter the feared situations of the past; we look for more and more difficult situations. By programming this stress so that the stutterer is largely (not always) able to beat it and yet can stutter easily when he does stutter, we enable him to strengthen the new behavioral responses to the old cues, to the old stresses which once set off the old abnormal responses of avoidance and struggle. This stress strengthening is even good for concrete beams; it is good for stutterers in the terminal stages of therapy.

But there is another form of resistance therapy which goes further and which holds the promise of curing stutterers and not merely making them fluent. It provides the fourth choice we mentioned earlier. Stutterers have long known a curious experience, namely, that occasionally they are able to summon up their powers and just refuse to stutter. It sounds unbelievable, but most stutterers will so testify; and often this occurs under conditions of great stress. They do not know what happens, nor do we. However, we have found in the terminal stages of therapy, when avoidance has been pretty well eliminated, and when, if difficulty does come, it can be handled without great distress, we can train the client to resist his urge to stutter. Let us illustrate.

A simple procedure is to have the stutterer read in unison with the clinician. Under these conditions he will be very fluent. He is also very fluent in automatic echoing or shadowing. But then the clinician deliberately introduces some stuttering into his own speech and challenges the stutterer to resist him, in other words, to continue to speak the words as fluently as when the clinician was using fluent speech.

This is a strange and a new challenge. It is possible to resist the clinician's behavioral suggestion that he must stutter! There is no avoidance of feared situations, words, or sounds here. There *is* the resistance to suggestion, a resistance which stutterers need badly. Why should they always yield? By judiciously using the principles of desensitization therapy and introducing just enough stuttering in the model so that the stutterer wins more often than he loses, it is possible to teach him to battle rather than succumb. There's no virtue in stuttering if you can resist the influences which tell you that you must. In this technique there is no avoidance, no running away. The challenge is proffered and accepted. No postponement, starting tricks, or other devices are permitted. The stutterer is simply to say the

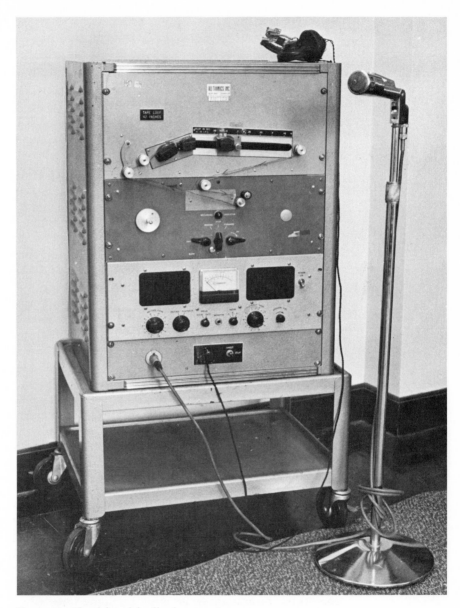

Figure 29   The delayed feedback apparatus.

word if he can without stuttering, at a moment when the clinician is trying to make him have some stuttering. Once the principles of this resistance therapy have been mastered, the stutterer, through speech assignments and self-therapy, continues to battle the suggestion that if he has fear, he must stutter. Other ways of resisting stuttering involve the monitoring of speech by proprioceptive feedback and the use of masking noise or the echo device called the delayed auditory feedback apparatus.

Treatment of Early Stuttering [13]

You have observed that there is considerable disagreement about how speech pathologists try to help the confirmed stutterer overcome his disorder. Fortunately, this situation does not hold for the beginning stutterer, one who has not developed fears and other negative emotions, one who has not learned to respond to the interruptions in his speech by struggling. As we have said, most of these young children simply repeat some syllable or prolong some sounds and have little awareness of what they are doing. Indeed, they have a lot of fluency. Moreover, since many of them seem to overcome their stuttering with or without help, most speech pathologists prefer to concentrate their efforts on prevention. If the young stutterer can be kept from developing situation and word fears, if he can be helped to withstand the communicative frustration, if he does not become ashamed or troubled by his simple repetitions and prolongations, then he has an excellent chance of becoming as fluent as any other child. Therefore, most of the speech pathologist's efforts are devoted to reducing the environmental penalties upon stuttering, to building frustration tolerance, and to strengthening the normal speech the child already possesses.

Penalty Reduction The stutterer's negative emotional states, as we have seen earlier, result from the rejecting and punishing reactions of his early listeners. Accordingly, much of the speech pathologist's time may be spent in counseling parents to help them understand that these vulnerable children need permissiveness rather than punishment, and that it is unwise to make the child feel he has done something wrong when he stutters. Sometimes when he quits getting punished for stuttering, he quits stuttering.

[13] Two films, *Identifying the Danger Signs* and *Family Counseling,* dealing with the problems of beginning stuttering and its prevention may be rented or purchased from the Speech Foundation of America, 152 Lombardy Road, Memphis, Tenn., 38111.

Penalty Reduction   Our task, then, is to reduce the penalties they are ex-
                       periencing, not only those which parents are placing on the
speech interruptions, but all penalties. They need more permissiveness
and less punishment.

> One of our young stutterers who showed the behavior of the
> first stage was having a very bad time with his speech. The first
> word of almost every utterance was spoken with repetitions or
> prolongations. Often the repetitions would continue for several
> seconds. He would say, "Ca-ca-ca-ca-ca-ca-ca-ca- can I go
> now?" His frantic parents, who had been asking him to "Stop
> that!" or to "Stop and begin over again!" followed our advice
> and ceased these admonitions. The reduction of this penalty re-
> duced the stuttering, but too much still remained. We then dis-
> covered that they were also breaking him of the habit of suck-
> ing his thumb. As soon as we persuaded them to stop their
> efforts in this regard, the child stopped stuttering completely.

Reducing   Children in the early stage of the disorder usually experience
Frustration   little frustration so far as their stuttering is concerned. It
                comes in a bit later when the major reaction is the occasional
expression of surprise and bewilderment, and the repetitions become
faster, more irregular, and end in prolongations of a sound or posture. The child, without knowing why, is beginning to sense that
speaking is hard work at times, that it isn't easy. But the major frustrations come from other sources, from the daily business of living in
a world geared to the needs of others as well as to one's own needs.
One of the sad things about our culture is that the age of speech-
learning is made to coincide with the application of so many taboos.
During the preschool years, there are so many things that a little
child must learn he mustn't do. The frequency of usage of the word
"No!" by mothers of children of this age is probably exceeded only
by that of the expression, "Oh dear!" All children of this age hear a
hundred "No's" each day of their lives, and some children hear
more, or feel the sharp slap of a heavy hand on their bottoms. We do
not wonder that the age of three is a negativistic age; the demands
for conformity are especially heavy then. All this means frustration.
The child must indeed learn to behave the way our culture says he
must. But he can't help feeling plenty of frustration.

In counseling our parents we must help them to understand the
role of frustration in precipitating stuttering. We cannot ask them to
stop being culture carriers. Their own needs for a peaceful, reason-

ably quiet, and orderly home life would then be frustrated. They know that each of us much learn to inhibit some of our infantile urges if we are to live in a civilized society. A child must learn to re- spect the needs of others. A totally ungovernable and spoiled child is an excrescence in any household. Are we then caught in a dilemma? On the one hand, to reduce the stuttering, we must reduce the frus- tration; on the other, if we do so, we create a continuing annoyance in the home which will provoke penalty outside the home if not within it.

The solution to the dilemma is simply to help the parents do two things: (1) *reduce* the number of the child's frustrating experi- ences, and (2) build up his frustration tolerance. There is no need to eliminate all frustration; we merely need to decrease it. Indeed, since life is always bound to hold many frustrations in store, it is wise to help our children learn to tolerate them.

> In counseling the mother of another of our very young stutter- ers, we first got her to express most of her own frustrations not only in child rearing but also in other areas. Then when the river ran dry we explained a bit about the role of frustration in stuttering, gave her a little hand counter and asked her to click it every time she used a forbidding "No!" to the boy. The first day's total was 186; the second day's 132; the third day's 71; and on the fourth day she brought back the counter, saying that Ju- nior had stopped stuttering.

We need not and we cannot eliminate frustration; but we always can reduce it.

Increasing Many an adult should learn the lesson that it is possible to *Frustration* increase one's tolerance for frustration. The inappropriate in- *Tolerance* fantile behavior shown by our frustrated friends (never our- selves!) is evidence that somewhere along the growth line, many of us fail to learn this lesson. Perhaps it is because we have never had the teacher we needed. There are two major ways in which we can build up frustration tolerance. One is through the empathic understanding of the needs of others; the second is through desensi- tization or adaptation. We shall not go into the first of these save to say that children should learn that parents have rights too, and to give one illustration.

> Willy was an *enfant terrible*. He had conquered his parents. He controlled them. The mother, a frantic, neurotic wisp of a woman, was very infantile herself and totally unable to cope

with his nagging, his defiance, his temper tantrums. She even feared the little stuttering monster, for once he had chased her up the backstairs with a butcher knife. The father was a weak, colorless individual whose response to his miserable home life was to stay away from it as much as possible. We managed to get them to send the boy away for the summer to a camp, and for the rest of the year to an uncle's family where the laws of the Medes and the Persians and of the parents were clear and enforced. He had a bad time of it at first, but his stuttering disappeared as he learned to curb his pampered infantile urges and become a member of society. He had learned to recognize the needs of others.

The second way to build frustration tolerance involves conditioning. It follows one method for breaking a horse. First you put a cloth on the horse's back, then later a sand bag, then a saddle, then a brave little boy, and then you can jump aboard. It takes time and patience and plenty of gentling and loving along the way, but some horses are taught to accept their riders this way. Through parental counseling and observation of the child, the major frustrating factors are defined. Then they are introduced into the child's life very gradually, but persistently, and only to the degree that he can tolerate them. The consequence is that the child will adapt and gradually be able to tolerate more and more frustration.

Grant was almost four years old when volleys of stuttering appeared and went away in their usual fashion. For a week he would be very fluent; the next, he could hardly say a sentence without many repetitions. After several months of this, the repetitions began to come out irregularly and faster. Often they would end in a prolongation that rose in pitch. He did not seem to be aware of these interruptions, perhaps because he was so anxious to talk. He talked incessantly to anyone who would listen and to those like his elder brother and sister who often would not. The slightest loss of the listener's attention or any sign of the listener's impatience or any interruption seemed to precipitate a burst of stuttering. The periods of remission were shorter and further apart. He was in real danger. Occasionally he would stop and look bewildered. Talking was getting hard.

The parents fortunately were both understanding and cooperative. They loved the boy and there were no penalties to be decreased. There was little communicative stress in the picture. If anything, they had created conditions which made his communication too easy. If he began to talk, they stopped their own conversation. They asked few questions, talked slowly and simply, and gave him the floor whenever he wanted it. We could discern little evidence of emotional conflicts, anxiety, guilt, or hostility. It was a wonderful home. Even the brother and sister seemed to understand, and they made things easier for Grant than most children would. The boy had simply developed an abnormal appetite for attention and for communication. He had been a bit delayed in speech and still had some errors in articulation. Perhaps, once he learned the magical power of speech, it was too good to lose. He had logorrhea. The more that appetite for speech was fed, the bigger it grew, and the less he could bear to have it frustrated.

We asked them to institute a progressive change in policy. First they were to give him their complete attention but gradually to introduce a few mild interruptions, a consciously averted glance, a slight delay in answering his questions, or in doing what he wanted. They were to do this judiciously so that the amount of his frustration would not be sufficient to precipitate stuttering. But they would put a bit of pressure on him. They were to return to the former policy of giving him complete attention, putting an arm around him and listening intently. Then they were to give him another dose of communicative frustration, a little larger one if possible, but again returning to the complete attention. We asked them to do this eight or nine times a day, gradually increasing the dosage of their inattention. Within a week they reported that Grant was now able to wait his turn, to accept delay in responding, to tolerate an occasional interruption. Within a month the stuttering was gone. We had increased his ability to tolerate frustration. Frustrations other than those in speech can be handled in the same way. It is possible to build up frustration tolerance.

There is also another way of breaking a horse. You can jump on his back, drive in the spurs, and break his spirit to your will. We do not advocate this method for children, but we have known a few instances in which parents used this policy to teach their children to bear frustration. And again we have seen the stuttering disappear. But we do not advise this method. We want our children free, not broken.

Reducing Anxiety, We can reduce these reactions by reducing the penalties and *Guilt, and Hostility* frustrations which beget them. Secondly, outlets other than stuttering should be made available. Thirdly, the beginning stutterer needs extra reassurance that he is loved and accepted. We have already considered the first of these three sources; now let us discuss the second.

We find many homes where the need to express one's feelings of anxiety, guilt, and hostility is neither understood nor accepted. If a child reveals that he is afraid of big dogs, thunderstorms, going to bed, or anything else, he is subjected to ridicule and "shamed out of his silly fears." His confessions of guilt and shame evoke a slap or a smile or parental embarrassment. His expressions of hostility are punished. He soon learns to keep them to himself. But we repress these emotional acids at our peril. They want out! And they always find a way. With the stutterer, that way is often stuttering.

These taboos against emotional release can be changed for some children by parental counseling, but some parents are themselves too inhibited or emotionally involved to make the necessary changes. As Sanders says, "When parents cooperate in a counseling program with insight and determination, the outlook for the young stutterer is most favorable."[14] But there are parents who do not cooperate, who cannot accept counseling. What do we do then?

Play Therapy   We can offer the child an opportunity through play to release his forbidden feelings. We can provide him with at least one situation in which he finds a loved and loving adult who understands and accepts his feelings, who actually rewards their expression whether the child expresses them verbally or through acting-out. A quotation from an excellent book by Murphy and Fitz-Simons helps us understand what takes place in play therapy.

> One of the clinician's prime tasks is to estimate how the child is perceiving self, parents, and the world as well as how much he is distorting, misperceiving, and misinterpreting. In order to do this the clinician must provide situations and materials which will give the child the opportunities to *externalize* and project his deeper feelings. Play's therapeutic value lies in giving the child a chance to communicate some aspects of his inner world to an understanding adult, to reevaluate his perceptions and confusions; in short, to integrate. The clinician enters the child's world by allowing him to speak his own language, often a highly nonverbal, symbolic esoteric one. The child will express his needs to be aggressive; to be infantile; to suck; to mess; to do what he wants and needs to do. The child's formerly sup-

---

[14] E. K. Sander, "Counseling Parents of Stuttering Children" *Journal of Speech and Hearing Disorders*, XXIV (1959), 262.

pressed and derogated behavior will be reacted to differently by the clinician whose role is one of "new parents." The clinician submits and resubmits the child's fears, desires, hostilities, condemned wants and wishes to the child's self or conscious awareness for relearning and resocialization, for differentiation and the integration of self.[15]

We have used play therapy with many of our young stutterers and not only with those in whom we suspect a primary neurosis. Where anxieties, guilts, and hostility play an important part in the child's stuttering problem and when their expression at home is denied or prevented by the parents, play therapy is absolutely essential. Not all young stutterers need it. There are some children who show no more than a normal amount of these feelings and in whose problems other factors are more important. With the neurotic stutterer it is the treatment of choice.

Creative Dramatics   Another method for relieving the pressures of anxiety, guilt, and hostility so that they do not contribute to the stuttering problem is that of creative dramatics. In this activity, the children, guided by an imaginative adult leader, improvise a play, take the various parts, and invent their own dialogue. Children frequently select and play parts which provide for the expression of their more intense feelings. Here is an account of an eight-year-old nonfluent child having this experience.

> He joined a creative dramatics group but took a relatively inactive part until one day when the children were playing the story of *King Midas and the Golden Touch.* Most of the children characterized King Midas as a grumpy man but not as a cruel one. Finally John said he wished to play King Midas. Suddenly the character of the king became completely different. Midas screamed at the servants, hit the table, ordered the impossible, ranted and raved and almost completely forgot the plot of the story. The children were impressed with the idea of the king, and a discussion followed. Several of the children thought that John had made King Midas too mean. Others thought maybe the previous attempts to play the king had been too mild. The children turned to John to get his opinion. "I think King Midas was a very cruel man. He's as mean as my teacher."[16]

[15] Albert T. Murphy and Ruth M. Fitz-Simons, *Stuttering and Personality Dynamics* (New York: The Ronald Press Company, 1960).

[16] B. M. McIntyre and B. J. McWilliams, "Creative Dramatics in Speech Correction," *Journal of Speech and Hearing Disorders,* XXIV (1959), 277.

We have found creative dramatics especially useful when much of the emotional conflict was due to sibling rivalry, fears of the local bully, or teasing by the child's playmates. In such instances, the child needs more than a permissive parent figure; he needs a permissive group. We find it very useful when play therapy fails because this particular child cannot come to have any trust in the clinician or any other adult. There are such children. There are also some children whose contact with reality is precariously slim. We do not use creative dramatics with these latter ones. Fantasy and role-playing have their dangers.

Parental Counseling   We have referred frequently to the counseling of parents in the reduction of all the factors that increase stuttering. Parents need education and information, but this is not all that counseling provides. They also need relief from their own anxieties, guilts, and hostilities. They need the opportunity to verbalize their own feelings in the presence of a permissive, understanding listener. They need to learn to view the stuttering child with strange eyes, objectively. Jointly with the clinician, they must explore all his problems, not just his stuttering. In so doing, they often realize their own perfectionistic strivings, their own childhood conflicts, their own present acting-out of relationships they had with their own parents long ago. There are many problems in counseling parents which produce difficulty. Some should be referred to the psychiatrist. With some, the conferences should be confined primarily to giving information. The depth of the counseling relationship should depend upon the clinician's own training and competence and on the severity of the interpersonal relationships which exist. There are Pandora's boxes no speech clinician should open.

Group Counseling   Often when the clinician can get a small group of parents together in the evening over coffee to discuss their mutual problem, the stuttering child, some real advantages are to be had. First of all, we are able to meet the fathers of these children, and often they play a most important role in the stuttering boy's difficulties. Secondly, through free discussion parents come to view their own children differently, more objectively. They get the opportunity to air and share their problems of parenthood. Each is a mirror for the other. Again the anxieties are verbalized, the guilt feelings explored, and the irritation exposed. Again the clinician plays the role of the catalyst. Group counseling can be very helpful.

Reducing the The final factor in the stuttering equation is communicative
Communicative stress. All stutterers at any stage show more stuttering when
Stress they are bedeviled by the fluency-disrupting influences we
now list. The beginning stutterer is especially vulnerable, and
we have been able to cure more early stutterers by reducing the fluency
disruptors in the speech environment than by any other means.

How to Prevent Hesitant speech (pauses, accessory vocalization, filibusters,
Hesitant Speech abortive speech attempts) occurs as the result of two opposing forces. First, there must be a strong need to communicate;
and second, this urge must be blocked by some counterpressure.
Some of the common counterpressures which oppose the desire for
utterance are:

1. *Inability to find or remember the appropriate words.* "I'm thinking of-of-
   of-of-uh that fellow who-uh—oh yes, Aaronson. That's his name." This
   is the adult form. In a child it might occur as: "Mummy, there's a birdy
   out there in the . . . in the . . . uh . . . he's . . . uh . . . he . . . he . . . he
   wash his bottom in the dirt." Similar sources of hesitant speech are
   found in bilingual conflicts, where vocabulary is deficient; in aphasia;
   and under emotional speech exhibition, as when children forget their
   "pieces."

2. *Inability to pronounce or doubt of ability to articulate.* Adult form: "I can
   never say sus-stus-susiss-stuh-stuhstiss-oh, you know what I mean,
   figures, statistics." The child's form could be illustrated by: "Mummy,
   we saw two poss-poss-uh-possumusses at the zoo. Huh? Yeah, two
   puh-pos-sums." Tongue twisters, unfamiliar sounds or words, too fast
   a rate of utterance, and articulation disorders can produce these sources
   of speech hesitancy.

3. *Fear of the unpleasant consequences of the communication.* "Y-yes I-I-I- uh
   I t-took the money." "W-wi-will y- you marry m-me?" "Duh-don't s-s-
   spank me, Mum-mummy." Some of the conflict may be due to uncertainty as to whether the content of the communication is acceptable or
   not. Contradicting, confessing, asking favors, refusing requests, shock-
   ing, tentative vulgarity, fear of exposing social inadequacy, fear of social penalty in school recitations or recitals.

4. *The communication itself is unpleasant, in that it recreates an unpleasant
   experience.* "I cu-cu-cut my f-f-finger . . . awful bi-big hole in it." "And
   then he said to me, 'You're f-f-fired.'" The narration of injuries, in-
   justices, penalties often produces speech hesitancy. Compulsory speech
   can also interrupt fluency.

5. *Presence, threat, or fear of interruption.* This is one of the most common
   of all the sources of speech hesitancy. Incomplete utterances are always
   frustrating, and the average speaker always tries to forestall or reject an
   approaching interruption. This he does by speeding up the rate, filling
   in the necessary pauses with repeated syllables or grunts or braying.
   This could be called "filibustering," since it is essentially a device to
   hold the floor. When speech becomes a battleground for competing

egos, this desire for dominance may become tremendous. More hesitations are always shown in attempting to interrupt another's speech as well as in refusing interruption.

6. *Loss of the listener's attention.* Communication involves both speaker and listener, and when the latter's attention wanders or is shifted to other concerns, a fundamental conflict occurs. ("Should I continue talking . . . even though she isn't listening? If I do, she'll miss what I just said . . . If I don't. I won't get it said. Probably never. . . . Shall I? . . . Shan't I?") The speaker often resolves this conflict by repeating or hesitating until the speech is very productive of speech hesitancy. "Mummy, I-I-I want a . . . Mummy, I . . . M . . . Mumm . . . Mummy, I . . . I . . . I want a cookie." Disturbing noises, the loss of the listener's eye contact, and many other similar disturbances can produce this type of fluency interrupter.

We must remember that the beginning stutterer is still learning to talk. His speech is not stabilized. But the mere fact that he has some fluency, and all stutterers do, indicates that, with a little less pressure, stabilization may occur. If, through counseling the mother and often by demonstrating better practices before her in play therapy, we can just ease his burden a little, the stuttering goes away. Often we are surprised to find how quickly these children respond to the reduction of any one of the precipitating factors. This is not so true of the children whose stuttering comes from constitutional or neurotic causes however, but it is true of the large proportion of garden variety stutterers. And even the others are helped thereby.

Lowering the Standards of Fluency   Communicative stress can also come from the need to talk like others do. If the parents or other children set standards of fluency far beyond the child's ability to imitate, he is almost certain to falter. Parents provide the models for all behavior whether they want to or not. It is not enough for parents to become better listeners; they must also provide models of fluency which are not too difficult for the child to follow. It is difficult for some parents to simplify their manner of talking to children, but most of them manage it once they understand why they should do so.

We observed that one of the beginning stutterers with whom we were working spoke in compound, complex sentences and used vocabulary which was not only that of the adult level but almost that of an English professor. We even heard him stutter on the word "innocuous," and this at six years of age. He was the only child and his parents were in their forties. They were voluble and precise in word choice. They read him to sleep each night, and the selections they chose were *good* literature. They italicized the word when they told us about it. They also played word games and lost no opportunity to teach the boy a new word.

The counseling was difficult, but finally they came to see that they were setting exorbitant standards of speech and they asked us for suggestions. We told them to stop reading any stories to the child. We told them to make up some tales instead about very little boys. We asked them to speak in simple sentences to the child as often as they could, to stop the wordplay and teaching, and to falter a bit in their own talking. We asked them to stop talking so much. We asked them at times to play games in which they pretended that the boy was a little baby and to encourage him to talk like one. They had kept him out of school because of his stuttering, and we insisted that he be placed in the kindergarten forthwith. We continued to counsel them. In two months the stuttering was gone.

Reducing the Communicative Demands Parents frequently report that the young child has more stuttering when he first comes back from school or from playing with the other children. They think it is because of the excitement or some baleful influence of the teacher. The better explanation often is that this is the time that parents give the child a cross-examination. "What did you do at school today?" No child remembers. He did lots of things, but he didn't memorize them. One question follows another when all he wants is a cookie and to go out to play.

Parents never seem to realize how much they question their children, nor that questioning always puts the child under communicative stress. The mother gets lonely. She needs someone to talk with; and her husband, when he does get home, hides behind the paper until after dinner. She also wants to keep her close umbilical relationship with the child. She wants to know what he's thinking and feeling and doing. We can understand and sympathize, but if her needs are making her child stutter, they've got to be satisfied in other ways.

Peter, aged five, never stuttered in school or on the playground, but he surely did so at home, especially when he talked to his mother (who illustrated the pattern outlined above). We did no counseling. Instead, with all the force and authority at our command, and enlisting her husband's aid in the matter, we insisted that from that moment she was to ask the boy *no* questions. None! Not another one for two months! She could answer his questions but she was not to demand, or wheedle any speech from him. She could talk all she wanted, but it had to be commentary, not questioning. We also got her to serve as a volunteer nurse's aid in the hospital each afternoon. The boy stopped stuttering and the father gave me a cigar (not a very good one).

Removing the Stimulus Value of the Stuttering A final, but very important, component of communicative stress is the unfavorable attention given to the stuttering by the parents. They call attention to the repetitive speech. They tell the child to "stop it," or to "stop stuttering." We know of no quicker way to throw a child into more severe stuttering than by such suggestions. They should be terminated immediately. Other parents interrupt the child when stuttering and ask him to relax or to stop and think over what he is about to say. When we tell them not to do so, they protest and say, "But it really works. If we stop him and tell him to relax or to stop stuttering he does stop stuttering. Why shouldn't we do this?" Advice again is not enough. Parents must understand how stuttering develops, how frustration and fear are born. We do point out that the child is still continuing to stutter, and is probably getting invisibly worse, that the policies they are using are frustrating in themselves, and that they are training him to fear and avoid. We help them to see that they should reduce the stimulus value of the stuttering, not make it more vivid.

Other parents do not nag their children when they hear them stuttering, but they respond to it by signals of alarm and distress, which are probably worse. They freeze in their conversational tracks. They hold their breath; they become jittery. Their faces suddenly become masks. Any little child will respond to such signals as though they were cannon shots. When the doe suddenly grows stiff with alarm, the fawn freezes. Quite as much as when the old buck snorts! We must reduce these signals. They add too much to communicative stress.

Usually, the only way to help parents change these attitudes is by providing counseling and information. Occasionally we actually train them out of their signaling behavior by being with them as they interact with their children and helping them to respond to what the child is saying rather than to how he is saying it. But we had one set of obstinate parents who would not accept our picture of the problem and its solution. Under their constant nagging, the boy was growing worse and worse, but they still felt they should "correct him" every time he had some repetitions. Finally, in desperation, we put them into a therapy room with a group of our very severe adult stutterers and locked the door. When we let them out they were a changed couple and from that time on followed our suggestions and the child became fluent.

Building Ego Strength   Ego strength is difficult to define, but we know when it's low and we know when it's high. It rises and falls in all of us depending upon our success-failure ratio, but its basic ingredients are love, faith, and opportunity. Some of our stuttering children are denied all three.

One of our beginning stutterers had a father who hated him, perhaps because he wanted the babying which the mother gave only to the child. He had not desired to have children. The boy's stuttering provided the excuse he needed for the expression of his hostility. At any rate, he made no bones about his feelings. Whenever the boy tried to talk to him, the father cut him short and showed his disgust and rejection. The mother's attempt at protection only redoubled the intensity of the father's dislike. He forbade the boy to play with other children, made him stay in the house or yard "so he wouldn't get hurt," refused to let him ride a tricycle, and in every way made the boy feel he was both unpleasant and inadequate. We had no success with this child despite some heroic efforts. He is now in high school, a lonely, frightened unhappy boy, barely passing in his school work despite a high IQ. His teachers say that he has no confidence in himself. In one of our recent interviews we asked him why it was so hard for him to work on his speech. He said, "I've been brainwashed all my life. Nobody thought I could do anything, and I can't. Every time I make a half-hearted attempt I hear my father saying what I've heard a hundred times: "My God, I'll have to support you all my life." He said that whenever I stuttered bad. I think he's right.

This parent was the exception, fortunately. We have come to have a great respect for parents, once they realize their child is in danger and know what to do. Some parents have to be taught to show their love. Some have to be shown how to put aside their own anxieties and to let the child run the risks of living in a dangerous world. Better to break a leg than break a spirit! We have found the overprotective mother to be one of our major problems in this regard. The child must have opportunity even to fail. Security does not come from success alone.

How do we build up ego strength, morale, self-confidence? It is difficult to generalize. Often the clinician must accept much of the responsibility for doing the job. We ourselves have done many things. We have taught a boy to box, another to swim, another to read, another to ride one of our horses. We once took a child to a cowboy movie every week for a whole semester. Each child has his own needs.

> One little girl stutterer, the next to the youngest in a family of six girls, had failed to show any improvement in her stuttering for almost a year despite all our attempts to reduce the denominator of her own particular stuttering equation. Then one of our student clinicians bought her a puppy, and she stopped stuttering. I asked the clinician, a girl, why she had bought the puppy. "It was obvious," she answered. "I have been out to Nancy's home several times, and it was clear that she had no status whatsoever. She's shy and quiet, and the other girls dominate her completely. I felt that she ought to have something she could dominate or feel superior to, someone to whom she could talk and not be interrupted, something to love. I had a puppy once and I remember."

We aren't sure that her analysis was correct, but we are sure that the stuttering disappeared. And we are certain that self-confidence, morale, and ego strength can be increased with love, faith, and opportunity.

Increasing Fluency   First of all, with the beginning stutterer, we should arrange things so that during the periods of more severe stuttering, he talks less. The converse is also true. Since early stuttering comes in waves, during the periods of excellent speech, the parents should provide him with every possible opportunity to exercise it. This simple policy has eliminated the disorder in many children.

Secondly, both in the play therapy sessions and in the home, self-talk should be encouraged. Parents should do it as they go about their ordinary activities, telling aloud what they are doing, perceiving, or feeling. In the sessions with the clinician she should provide the same models of commentary. Only a few children stutter in their self-talk. It should be facilitated.

We also institute games which might be called "speech play." No attention to the stuttering, of course, should be involved. The child should only know that he and the clinician or parent are having verbal fun. Some of these games involve speaking in unison, or echoing, or speech accompanied by rhythmic activities, or talking very slowly and lazily. Even babylike babbling seems to help. There are hundreds of variations, but the purpose of all of them is to increase the experience of fluency.

Desensitization Therapy   Any fluency under any conditions is to be sought, but fluency under conditions of communicative stress is especially to be prized. Most beginning stutterers respond favorably to a coordinated program of the type we have described, but there are some who become worse as the environmental pressures are removed, and there are many whose parents and teachers cannot be persuaded to change their unfortunate policies. What can we do with these children? Give up the case and blame the failure on the child's peculiar constitution or the parent's guilt? No, there is another alternative, if we can toughen the child, build up his tolerance to stress, and create callouses against the hecklings, rejections, or impatience. Human beings learn to adapt to extreme noise levels, to incredible heat and cold. Should we not try some desensitization, just as the physician gives the shots for hayfever? Instead of lowering the fluency disrupters at home while being unable to do anything about them on the school playground, should we not train our stuttering child to be able to tolerate them without breakdown? As we indicated earlier, some children lower their thresholds of speech breakdown as soon as the parents decrease their home pressures. This just makes such a child all the more helpless outside the home.

At any rate, this is what the speech clinician does. He first establishes a social relationship with the child in which the latter does not realize that he is doing any speech therapy. They may be setting up a toy railroad on the floor or participating in any other similar activity. The speech clinician then works to achieve a basal fluency level on the part of the child. This may in rare cases have to begin with grunts or interjections, but usually it consists of simple statements of fact, requests, observations, and so forth. The clinician, as he works, thinks aloud in snatches of self-talk, commenting on his activity. Soon the child will begin to do the same, and by appropriately altering the communicative conditions, and his own manner, the clinician gets the child to speak with complete fluency. In the young stutterer, this is not too difficult. Then, once the basal fluency level has been *felt* by the child, the clinician begins gradually to inject into the situation increasing amounts of those factors which tend to precipitate repetitions and nonfluency in that particular child. He may, for instance, begin gradually to hurry him, faster and faster. *But,* and this is vitally important, the clinician stops putting on the pressure and returns to the basal fluency level as soon as he sees the first sign of *impending* nonfluency. How can he tell? Experience and training will help, but we have found usually, that just before the nonfluencies appear, the child's mobility begins to decrease—he freezes, or his general body movements become jerkier, or the tempo of his speech changes. There are other signs peculiar to each child, and a little experimentation will help the clinician know when to stop putting on the pressure just before the stuttering appears.

As soon as the clinician returns to the basal fluency level, he again begins slowly to turn up the heat, to hurry the child a little faster, to avert his gaze more often, or whatever he happens to be trying to toughen the child against. Then an interesting thing occurs. The child can take more pressure the second time than he could the first. The increment is very marked. But again, the first signs of approaching stuttering appear, and again the clinician goes down to the original basal fluency level. Most children do not seem to profit from more than four of these cycles per therapy session, since the tolerance gain decreases somewhat with each subsequent "push." It should be made clear that throughout this training, the child never does stutter, if the clinician has been skillful. What he feels, probably, is that he is being fluent under pressure. Fluency becomes associated with the feeling of being hurried. Perhaps this is why there is a remarkable transfer. The effects of this toughening to stress are not confined to the speech sessions. The child seems to be able to stay fluent even when his father keeps interrupting him. This technique, for lack of a better term, we can call "desensitization therapy." We have found it very useful.

Prognosis If we can locate the child soon enough and initiate the type of therapy outlined above, the chances of a favorable outcome are excellent. Children in the early stages of the disorder usually seem to present no great difficulty if systematic treatment can be administered. For these children it seems as though all that is needed is the reduction of one or two of the factors that are precipitating the speech hesitancy so that homeostasis, self-healing, can take place. Indeed, many children seem to heal themselves without treatment. We are certain that many children who start stuttering are able to overcome it without professional therapy. Therefore the prognosis is favorable.

Treatment of the Stutterer Who Has Become Aware of His Stuttering [17]

Unfortunately, far too many children who begin to stutter do become aware of their disorder. From the rejecting reactions of their listeners or from their frustrations in not being able to communicate effectively, they come to recognize that there is something unacceptable in the way they talk. This is one of the real danger signs and it is marked by the beginnings of struggle. Every speech pathologist hates to see the appearance of facial contortions, pitch rises or tensions, and tremors in the speech musculartures of a young stutterer for they signal the beginning of the vicious spiral of self-reinforcement. Even though there is yet no evidence of fear, shame, or avoidance, the morbid growth of severe stuttering has begun. Fortunately, if the proper measures are taken at this critical period, that morbid growth can be reversed.

The treatment of children in this stage follows much the same course as that used in the treatment of primary stuttering. We must increase the essential emotional security, remove the environmental pressures that tend to disrupt speech, and increase the amount of fluent speech which he experiences. Every effort should be made to prevent traumatic experiences with other children or adults who might tend to penalize or label the disorders. By creating a permissive environment in which the nonfluency has little unpleasantness, much can be done to help the child regain his former automaticity of repetition. The wise parent will find ways of distracting the child so that the struggling will not be remembered with any vividness. Some parents have increased their own nonfluency, reacting to it with casualness and noncommittal acceptance. One of them used to pretend to stutter a little now and then, commenting, "I sure got tangled up on that, didn't I? What I meant to say was . . ." It is also wise to provide plenty of opportunity for release psychotherapy, for venti-

---

[17] For a description of the application of operant strategies to these children see the article by Bruce Ryan, "Operant Procedures Applied to Stuttering Therapy for Children," *Journal Speech Hearing Disorders*, XXXVI (1971), 264–80.

lation of the frustration. Let these children show their anger. Help them discharge it.

If teasing has reared its ugly head and the child does come home crying or unpleasantly puzzled by the rejecting behavior of his playmates, the situation should be faced rather than avoided. Here is a mother's report:

> Jack came home today at recess. He was crying and upset because some of the other kindergarten children had called him "stutter-box."And they had mocked him and laughed at him. He asked me what was a stutter-box and for a moment I was completely panicky, though I hope I hid the feelings from him. I comforted him, and then told him that everybody, including big people, sometimes got tangled up in their mouths when they tried to talk too fast or were mixed up about what they wanted to say. Stutter-box was just a way of kidding another person about getting tangled up in talking. I told him to listen for the same thing in the other kids and to tease them back. Later on that day he caught me once and called me a stutter-box. We laughed over it and I think he's forgotten all about it today. I hope I did right. I just didn't know what to do.

The Conspiracy of Silence Many parents have been told so often that they should always ignore the stuttering that they continue to do so even when it sticks out like a second nose. This is very unwise. When the child is struggling with his stuttering, when he is obviously reacting to it, no good is obtained by pretending that it doesn't exist. There is a time for ignoring it, for distracting the child's attention from it, but there also comes a time when we must confront it and share the child's problem with him. Otherwise, he will feel that his behavior is shameful, unspeakably evil. He will feel that his parents cannot bear even to mention it. This is the road to fear and avoidance. It is a dangerous road to travel alone and in the dark.

The desensitization therapy used with these stutterers varies in one respect from that used earlier. We do not use complete fluency as our basal level from which we start and to which we return after gradually increasing the stress. Instead, it is wiser to use the first appearance of tension in the repetitions or postural fixations as the cue to return to the basal level. As in early stuttering, we try to harden the child to the factors that precipitate his nonfluency, but in this third stage of stuttering we keep putting on the stress (the interruptions, impatience, hurry, etc.), even though the repetitions begin to appear. But we stop short and return to our basal fluency level just before the tension, forcing, or tremors show themselves. By this technique, it is possible to bring the child back to a condition where there may be many of the primary symptoms, but little or no struggle reactions.

Direct Therapy   Depending upon how far the child has entered this stage of frustration and struggle, there comes a moment when direct confrontation of the stuttering is necessary. There comes a time when the child needs some adult to show him that he need not struggle, that it is better to let his speech bounce and prolong easily, that this way "the words come out faster and easier."

This new direct attack on the problem should be done by the professional speech pathologist, but we have found it wise to do it in the presence of the parents so that they can feel the objective attitude employed and observe what we do. Here is a glimpse from the transcript of one such session:

Clinician: I understand that you've been having a lot of trouble talking lately, Peter.

Peter: Yea, I, I, I, I've been sssssss . . . stutt . . . stuttering." (*The boy squeezed his eyes shut and fast tremors appeared on his tightly closed lips. The word finally emerged after a surge of tension and a head jerk.*) "I've been stuttering bad."

Clinician: So I see. Let's try to help you. I know what you're doing wrong. You're fighting yourself. You're pushing too hard. Let me show you how you just stuttered and then show you how to do it easy. (*Clinician demonstrates.*)

Peter: Oh!

Clinician: Now I'm going to ask you a question, and if you stutter while answering it, I'll join you but show you how to let it come out easy. OK? All right, how close is the nearest drugstore to your house?

Peter: It's over on the next b . . . b . . . bbbbbbblock. (*While the boy is struggling, the clinician first duplicates what he is doing, and then slowly slides out of the fixation without tension. The child hears him, opens his eyes to watch him, and an expression of surprise is seen on the child's face.*)

Clinician: Yea, I told you was I going to stutter right along with you, but you'll have to watch me if you're to learn how to let the words come out easy. Let's try another. If I went through the front door of your house, how would I find your room?

> *Peter:* YYYYYYYYYYYou'd . . . *(The child joined the clinician in his grin.)* Yyyou'd have to gggggo upstairs.
>
> *Clinician:* That second time you didn't push it so hard, did you. Good. You went like this . . . *(Clinician demonstrates.)* Look, you've got to learn how to stutter my way, nice and easy, either like th-th-th-this or like th . . . is. *(Clinician prolongs the sound easily and without effort.)* Now let's play a speech game of follow the leader. You be my echo and say just what I say and stutter just like I do. Sometimes I'll stutter your way and sometimes my way, the better way, the way you've got to learn to do it.

The session continued along this line and, before the end of the half-hour, Peter was beginning to cease his struggling. It took four more meetings before he really learned how to stutter easily, but the parents reported a marked reduction not only in the severity but in frequency as well. We saw him again after four months and the only stuttering behavior he showed was that of the first stage. Within a year it was gone. Children learn quickly and forget their troubles quickly.

Treatment of the Young Confirmed Stutterer   In order to spell out exactly how we treat a confirmed stutterer, we have described our therapy as it would be administered to a person who is relatively adult. With slight modifications — especially those in which the therapy is done with the therapist in the safety of the speech room — these suggestions are also useful with the stutterer of high-school age. But there are confirmed stutterers in the elementary school as well. We have had to treat children as young as three and four years who showed all the overt and covert behavior characteristics of the terminal stage of the disorder though most of them come to the speech clinician later, when they are at least in school and in the third grade or above. How do we treat these children?

The general pattern of treatment is the same. It also follows *MIDVAS*. We begin by identifying with the child during his stuttering, sharing it, helping him confront it without shame. We teach him to watch it, feel it, try to change it so that when he does stutter he does not avoid or struggle. We give him models and have him imitate us directly as we show him how to ease out of his tremors, his hard contacts, his hypertensed mouth postures. "Watch me," we say. "Look!" Here's how you stuttered just now. Now see how I can start the way you do but ease out of it . . . like this. Try it again." Fortunately, in these younger children, the disorder is as yet not too

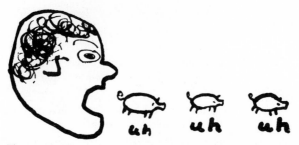

Figure 30 "Draw how you feel when you stutter." (*Speech in the Elementary School,* Harper & Row)

deeply rooted. They unlearn more easily. Once they put their trust and love in you, they will follow your demonstrations and directions most willingly. We almost always use play therapy along with the speech work to relieve the pressures. We provide situations in which there is little communicative stress. We do desensitization therapy often, as though the child were still in the earlier stages. We give him many experiences in being completely fluent through the use of echoing, unison speaking, rhythmic talking, and relaxation. We do our utmost to build his ego strength in every possible way. We use no speech assignments but, through parental counseling and home and school visits, we gradually incorporate his new ways of talking into his entire living space. We can help these children.

In concluding this chapter we wish to urge the student to do what he can to make the lot of the stutterers he meets a less miserable one. What they need most is understanding and hope, and surely by now you have the information to provide both. No one needs to go through life with a tangled tongue.

References

AINSWORTH, S. *Stuttering: What It Is and What to Do About It.* Lincoln, Nebr.: Cliffs Notes, Inc., 1975.

ANDREWS, G. and R. J. INGHAM. "Stuttering: An Evaluation of Follow-up Procedure for Syllable-timed Speech." *Journal Communication Disorders,* V (1972), 307–10.

BEECH, H. R. and F. FRANSELLA. *Research and Experiment in Stuttering.* London: Pergamon Press, 1968.

BERECZ, J. M. "The Treatment of Stuttering through Precision Punishment and Cognitive Arousal." *Journal Speech Hearing Disorders,* XXXVIII (1973), 256–67.

BLOODSTEIN, O. *A Handbook on Stuttering.* Chicago: National Easter Seal Society for Crippled Children and Adults, rev. ed., 1975.

BRUTTEN, G. J. and D. J. SHOEMAKER. "A Two-factor Theory of Stuttering." in

L. E. Travis (ed.) *Handbook of Speech Pathology and Audiology.* Englewood Cliffs, N.J.: Prentice-Hall, Inc., 1971.

BRUTTEN, E. J. and D. J. SHOEMAKER. *The Modification of Stuttering.* Englewood Cliffs, N.J.: Prentice-Hall, Inc., 1967.

COSTELLO, J. "The Establishment of Fluency with Time-out Procedures: Three Case Studies." *Journal Speech Hearing Disorders,* XL (1975), 216–31.

CURLEE, R. F. and W. H. PERKINS. "Conversational Rate Control Therapy for Stuttering." *Journal Speech Hearing Disorders,* XXXIV (1969), 245–50.

DEHIRSCH, K. "Cluttering and Stuttering." *Bulletin Orton Society,* XXV (1975), 57–68.

EGLAND, G. O. *Speech and Language Problems.* Englewood Cliffs, N.J.: Prentice-Hall, Inc., 1970.

EGOLF, D. B., G. H. SHAMES, and J. J. BLIND. "The Combined Use of Operant Procedures and Theoretical Concepts in the Treatment of an Adult Female Stutterer." *Journal Speech Hearing Disorders,* XXXVI (1971), 414–21.

EISENSON, J. "Stuttering as Perseverative Behavior." in Jon Eisenson (ed.) *Stuttering: A Second Symposium* (New York: Harper & Row, 1975).

FRIED, C. "Behavior Therapy and Psychoanalysis in the Treatment of a Severe Chronic Stutterer." *Journal Speech Hearing Disorders,* XXXVII (1972), 347–72.

GRUBER, L. "Sensory Feedback and Stuttering." *Journal Speech Hearing Disorders,* XXX (1965), 378–80.

HAROLDSON, S. K., R. R. MARTIN and C. D. STARR. "Time-out as a Punishment for Stuttering." *Journal Speech Hearing Research,* XI (1968), 560–66.

INGHAM, R. J. "Operant Methodology in Stuttering Therapy." in Jon Eisenson (ed.) *Stuttering: A Second Symposium* (New York: Harper & Row, 1975).

—— and G. ANDREWS. "Behavior Therapy and Stuttering." *Journal Speech Hearing Disorders,* XXXVIII (1973), 405–41.

LANYON, R. L. "Behavior Change in Stuttering Through Systematic Desensitization." *Journal Speech Hearing Disorders,* XXXIV (1969), 253–59.

LUPER, H. L. and R. L. MULDER. *Stuttering Therapy for Children.* Englewood Cliffs, N.J.: Prentice-Hall, Inc., 1964.

MCCABE, R. B. and J. D. MCCOLLUM. "The Personal Reactions of a Stuttering Adult to Delayed Auditory Feedback." *Journal Speech Hearing Disorders,* XXXVII (1972), 536–41.

MCINTYRE, B. M. and B. J. MCWILLIAMS. "Creative Dramatics in Speech Correction." *Journal Speech Hearing Disorders,* XXXIV (1959), 277.

MOWRER, D. "An Instructional Program to Increase Fluent Speech of Stutterers." *Journal Fluency Disorders,* I (1975), 25–35.

MURPHY, A. T. and RUTH FITZ-SIMONS. *Stuttering and Personality Dynamics.* New York: The Ronald Press Co., 1960.

PERKINS, W. H. "Replacement of Stuttering with Normal Speech. II. Clinical Procedures." *Journal Speech Hearing Disorders,* XXXVIII (1973), 295–303.

—— and R. F. CURLEE. "Clinical Impressions of Portable Masking Unit Effects in Stuttering." *Journal Speech Hearing Disorders,* XXXIV (1969), 360–62.

RYAN, B. P. "Operant Procedures Applied to Stuttering Therapy for Children." *Journal Speech Hearing Disorders,* XXXVI (1971), 264–80.

—— and B. VAN KIRK. "The Establishment, Transfer, and Maintenance of Fluent Speech in 50 Stutterers Using Delayed Auditory Feedback and Operant Procedures." *Journal Speech Hearing Disorders,* XXXIX (1974), 3–10.

SANDER, E. K. "Counseling Parents of Stuttering Children." *Journal Speech Hearing Disorders,* XXIV (1959), 262.

SCHWARTZ, M. F. *Stuttering Solved.* Philadelphia: J. B. Lippincott Company, 1976.

—— "The Core of the Stuttering Block." *Journal Speech Hearing Disorders,* XXXIX (1974), 169–77.

SHAMES, G. "Verbal Reinforcement During Therapy Interview with Stutterers." in B. Gray and G. England (eds.) *Stuttering and the Conditioning Therapies* (Monterey: Monterey Institute for Speech and Hearing, 1969), 99–114.

—— and D. EGOLF. *Operant Conditioning and the Management of Stuttering.* Englewood Cliffs, N.J.: Prentice-Hall, Inc., 1976.

SHAW, C. K. and W. F. SHAUM. "The Effects of Response—Contingent Reward on the Connected Speech of Children Who Stutter." *Journal Speech Hearing Disorders,* XXXVII (1972), 75–88.

SHEEHAN, J. G. "Conflict Theory of Stuttering." in J. Eisenson (ed.) *Stuttering: A Symposium.* (New York: Harper & Row, 1958).

—— *Stuttering: Research and Therapy.* New York: Harper & Row, 1970.

—— and M. M. MARTYN. "Stuttering and Its Disappearance." *Journal Speech Hearing Research,* XIII (1970), 279–89.

SPEECH FOUNDATION OF AMERICA. *Conditioning in Stuttering Therapy.* Memphis, Tenn.: Fraser, 1970.

TROTTER, W. D. and M. M. LESCH. "Personal Experience with a Stutter-Aid." *Journal Speech Hearing Disorders,* XXXII (1967), 270–72.

TYRE, TIMOTHY E., STEPHEN MAISTO, and PAUL COMPANIK. "The Use of Systematic Desensitization in the Treatment of Chronic Stuttering Behavior." *Journal Speech Hearing Disorders,* XXXVIII (1973), 514–19.

VAN RIPER, C. "A Clinical Success and a Clinical Failure." in M. Fraser (ed.) *Stuttering: Successes and Failures in Therapy.* (Memphis, Tenn.: Speech Foundation of America, 1968), 99–129.

—— "Stuttering: Where and Whither?" *Asha,* XVI (1974), 483–87.

—— *The Nature of Stuttering.* Englewood Cliffs, N.J.: Prentice-Hall, Inc., 1971.

—— *The Treatment of Stuttering.* Englewood Cliffs, N.J.: Prentice-Hall, Inc., 1973.

WEBSTER, R. L. *An Operant Response Shaping Program for the Establishment of Fluency in Stutterers: Final Report.* V.A.: Hollins College, 1972.

WEBSTER, L. M. and G. J. BRUTTEN. *The Modification of Stuttering and Associated Behavior.* in S. Dickson (ed.) *Communication Disorders* (Glenview, Ill.: Scott, Foresman and Company, 1974).

WEISS, D. *Cluttering.* Englewood Cliffs, N.J.: Prentice-Hall, Inc., 1964.

WILLIAMS, D. "A Point of View About Stuttering." *Jounal Speech Hearing Disorders,* XXII (1957), 390–97.

WILLIAMS, D.E. "Stuttering Therapy for Children." in L.E. Travis (ed.) *Handbook of Speech Pathology and Audiology* (New York: Appleton-Century-Croft, 1975).

YOUNG, M. A. "Onset, Prevalence, and Recovery from Stuttering." *Journal Speech Hearing Disorders,* XL (1975), 49–58.

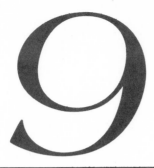

9

THE
ORGANIC
DISORDERS
OF
SPEECH

In this chapter we present four disorders which obviously have an organic basis. First, we shall consider the complete aphonia that occurs after laryngectomy (after the larynx has been surgically removed). Then we shall describe the problems associated with cleft palate, then those of aphasia, and finally those that characterize cerebral palsy.

Alaryngeal Aphonia

The term "alaryngeal" means that the person has no vocal mechanism, no larynx, to produce the phonation needed for speaking. The following account was written (for he could not speak at all) by a fifty-year-old client of ours.

> They told me I had cancer of the throat and that they would have to take out my voice box immediately. First I thought, "No, let me die!" I was scared to the marrow of my bones. How could I make a living? I could never talk again to my wife and children or to anyone. I thought of shooting myself and getting it over quick. That biopsy suddenly turned my whole existence upside down. What was I to do? My confusion and depression were so great that I just went along with the doctors. And so I found myself there in the hospital bed with my wife holding my hand; and I tried to tell her not to cry, but nothing came out of my mouth — just a rush of air out of the hole in my throat under the bandage. I could move my lips, but there was no sound. Then I cried — but silently. I was mute. I was not me.

> It is indeed a strange, lonely, threatening world for a person

who suddenly finds that he cannot utter a sound, cannot speak or laugh or cry aloud or even kiss. Deep depressions often occur and the speech pathologist often finds himself wrestling with many invisible demons of emotion when trying to convince the laryngectomee (the person whose larynx has been removed) that he need not remain mute, that he can learn to speak again.

But how can this be done? How can one possibly speak aloud when the only entrance and exit for the air in the lungs is a hole (stoma) in the neck? To preserve the person's life and because he knows how insidiously cancer can spread, the surgeon usually must remove the entire larynx, and then join the patient's windpipe (trachea) so that its upper opening is in the stoma through which inhalation and exhalation are now routed.[1] Nevertheless, it is possible for the laryngectomee to learn to speak again by using a different mechanism.

As illustrated in Figure 31 a *pseudoglottis* (a substitute vibrator for the vocal folds) can be developed by constricting the muscles along the upper edges of the esophagus, the tube that leads down to the stomach, and setting them into vibration by air that has been taken into the esophagus. It is the speech pathologist's job to teach the laryngectomee how to produce this new and different alaryngeal voice.

We are sure that you have more than once uttered sounds, if not speech, by using this substitute channel, usually after having eaten too well or having drunk too much beer. Certainly as a baby you were burped and those burps were very audible. The difference between those bottle burps and the esophageal (alaryngeal) phonation that we teach the laryngectomized is that the air does not come all the way up from the stomach, but instead it is trapped higher up in the esophagus before it is released. For those who have lost a larynx and are completely aphonic, the esophageal voice may be the way back to a fairly normal life. But it must be learned over the course of many sessions before sufficient control has been mastered to enable the client to communicate effectively.[2]

[1] In a few patients in whom the cancer has been caught early and appears to be localized, a partial laryngectomy may be performed so that the usual airway may be preserved. Also, as a result of a rather new form of surgery (called the Asai technique after its Japanese creator) a series of three operations provides the laryngectomee with a skin tube bypass so that when he closes the stoma with his finger the air from his lungs can go upward into the mouth. Even such a person, however, because the vocal folds are gone, must master a new way of producing sound. For a good review of the results of a tracheal-esophageal shunt surgical technique, see the reference by Zwitman and Calcaterre (1973).

[2] Did you ever hear the story of the man who put a frog in his mouth to develop alaryngeal speech? You'll find it in the old reference by Hauser (1947) in the bibliography at the end of this chapter.

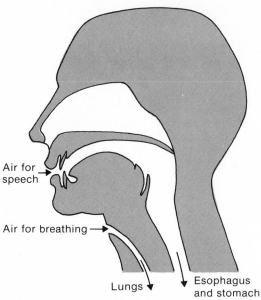

Air for speech

Air for breathing →

Lungs ↓   ↓ Esophagus
                and stomach

Figure 31   After laryngectomy. (Wilson, *Voice Articulation*)

The Artificial Larynx   Another method for producing vicarious voice involves the use of an artificial larynx, one of which is illustrated in Figure 32. The first such device we ever saw was a cumbersome instrument consisting of a bellows held under the arm, and a mouth-tube probe which contained a reed similar to that used in the ordinary harmonica. By inserting the tube into the corner of his mouth and pumping the bellows with his upper arm, the patient who owned it was able to talk intelligibly, though somewhat weakly. We now have much better artificial larynges, most of which can use an electrically activated diaphragm or reed as the sound source.[3] In the instrument illustrated below, one of those most commonly used, the battery is contained in the case; and the buzzing diaphragm at its end is held against the neck. By articulating carefully, the sound thus produced can be turned into usable speech. Other electrolarynges have the vibrating mechanism built into the bowl of a tobacco pipe, with the stem transmitting the sound into the mouth, or even into the upper plate of a denture. Some devices are held in the hand while a small plastic tube carries the sound into the corner of the mouth.

[3] The electrolarynx was evidently discovered by Gilbert Wright, who noted while shaving that when he pressed his buzzing electric razor against his throat and pantomimed talking while holding his breath, he could produce intelligible speech.

Comparison of Methods for Producing Vicarious Voice

Neither esophageal speech nor that produced by an external vibrator are ever as good as the voice which was lost. The esophageal voice, at its very best, is often low-pitched and hoarse. It is often difficult to master, and many laryngectomees give up before they achieve any real competence. Martin writes:

> Many esophageal voices, even though loud enough, are neither of such quality as to be adequate for practical needs, nor acceptable from the social standpoint. Other laryngectomees simply cannot achieve any usable esophageal speech, no matter how long or how hard they try. These unfortunates obviously should be urged to give up further public attempts at this form of artifical speech and rely entirely on the electrolarynx for all but family and other intimate contacts.[4]

Some of the features of esophageal speech which often appear during the learning process and which are regarded as objectionable by the laryngectomee are these: the gulping sound as air is taken into the eso-

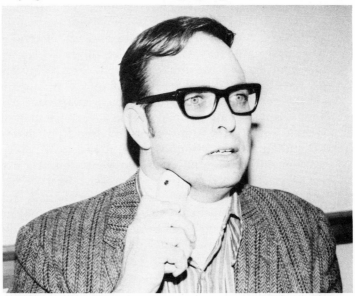

Figure 32 Artificial larynx: How the electrolarynx is used. (Reproduced by permission of the Western Electric Company.)

[4] H. Martin, "Rehabilitation of the Laryngectomee," *Cancer*, XVI (1963), 323–41.

phagus; the weakness of the sound produced; the very low pitch (often about an octave lower than the normal male voice); the hoarse quality; the contortions such as lip-squeezing or extending the neck with the head thrown back; the whoosh of air through the opening in the neck that accompanies the speech attempt and causes the little gauze apron covering the hole to flap; the feeling of abdominal distension when air is swallowed and collected in the stomach; the effort and carefulness required; and finally the flatulence or borborygmus that may occur. The latter refers to the abdominal noises which all of us experience at times when we have eaten too well. The old limerick says it best:

> I sat by the Duchess at tea
> She was haughty and proud as could be
> But her noises abdominal
> Were simply phenomenal
> And everyone thought it was me.

Nevertheless, despite these hurdles, some laryngectomees manage to acquire an esophageal speech so fluent and good that their listeners do not realize that they are speaking in a different way. They sound as though they have laryngitis, but they talk very well. One of our clients could make himself heard and understood in a large auditorium and could say Gilbert and Sullivan's classical definition of a falsehood on one air intake: "Merely corroborative detail intended to give verisimilitude to a bald and unconvincing narrative." William White, one of the instructors in our department of speech pathology and audiology for a time, was a laryngectomee whose esophageal speech was so fluent and clear and free from mannerisms that all of us, students and colleagues alike, found it difficult to realize that he was speaking differently than we were. The best esophageal speakers are very, very good, and they possess a sense of triumph over adversity which is very impressive. Some of them have better lives after the operation than they had before. We have met many of them who have dedicated their lives to helping speech pathologists teach other laryngectomees how to use the substitute voice. Some of them have organized Lost Cord or New Voice Clubs, where those who have just had surgery can find understanding and help. We once took a recording of sample communications from a local Lost Cord Club to a similar group in Melbourne, Australia, and we have never forgotten the way those Aussies closed their meeting with the same esophageal utterance of the Twenty-third Psalm ("Yea though I walk through the Valley of the Shadow of Death, I shall fear no evil."), that was used in our own group so far away. If any student can attend a meeting of some local chapter of the International Association of Laryngectomees (IAL), he will find it inspiring—and he will certainly quit smoking cigarettes.

Nevertheless, most of the evidence indicates that far too many laryngectomees fail to achieve good esophageal speech. Snidecor (1971) estimated that from 20 to 30 percent of them will either have to remain mute or use an artificial larynx. Others put the figure higher. We worked very hard with several who never got a decent esophageal tone. One was a refined elderly lady to whom a burp was an utter disgrace; another was too depressed to try; another was so tense the sphincter muscles of the cricopharyngeus at the upper end of the esophagus would clamp shut so hard no vibration was possible. Still another, a successful business executive, was so impatient that when he found that he could not immediately transform his first brief burst of esophageal sounds into long sentences, he left the clinic. More than half of our own patients have acquired fair to good esophageal voices and are able to speak in phrases and sentences loudly and clearly enough for ordinary communication. The others have had to learn to use the electrolarynx either as a supplemental aid when telephoning or trying to talk in a noisy environment, or they use it as their sole means of communicating. What is most important is that they are not aphonic and that they can speak. To be mute is to be touched by death.

The kind of voice and speech produced by the various electrolarynges is felt by most speech pathologists to be less satisfactory, and generally we recommend that the patient use the electrolarynx only when it becomes clear that he cannot learn esophageal speech. Some workers recommend that the electrolarynx be used immediately by the laryngectomee while he tries to master esophageal speech; but others protest that if this is done, he will tend to rely upon the easier mechanical aid and will never learn it. Our own practice has been to postpone its use until we are pretty certain that no adequate esophageal speech will be acquired. In its present form the artifical larynx has many shortcomings. It is conspicuous and immediately makes clear that the person is disabled. The buzzing noise that accompanies all speech detracts from communication. The sound produced seems very different in quality from normal speech, and although some speakers become highly proficient in varying the pitch of the buzz, the inflections leave much to be desired. It tends to be monotonous. As Greene writes:

> The voice artificially produced by means of the various types of electric vibrators available is a poor substitute for esophageal

voice and will never be mistaken for the normal voice which is hoarse from laryngitis. The voice generated artificially is always bizarre.[5]

Nevertheless, for many persons the electrolarynx has helped them return from alaryngeal muteness to a place in a communicating world.

Learning to Use *Esophageal Speech*   The clinician who seeks to help the laryngectomee acquire esophageal speech need not himself be able to produce it, though we have found our own ability to do so has contributed much to the patient's early progress. What is necessary is the provision of an adequate model such as that by some other skilled esophageal speaker or at the very least some tapes or films of such speakers. Also, the clinician must understand the basic principles for the intake of air into the upper esophagus and have some systematic sequence of subgoals such as the four basic skills listed by Berlin (1963): (1) ability to phonate reliably on demand; (2) ability to demonstrate short latency between inflation of the esophagus and vocalization; (3) ability to maintain an adequate duration of phonation on the vowel /æ/; (4) ability to sustain phonation during articulation of syllables, words, and phrases. Other clinicians prefer other sequences, but all of them start with the goal of being able to take air into the esophagus and to expel it in the production of tone.

In an introductory text such as this one, it would be unwise to go into too much detail; but there are at least three alleged methods for trapping enough air into the esophagus to permit vocalization. In the first, the inhalation method, the sphincters of the esophagus must be relaxed, and then, as the diaphragm descends, air is naturally gulped into the esophagus. Then the sphincters of the cricopharyngeus are tightened and vibrate as the diaphragm returns upward. The second procedure is termed the "injection procedure" or the "glossopharyngeal press."[6] In this method, the lips and soft palate are closed, and the cheeks are contracted simultaneously with an upward and backward bunching of the tongue. This forces or injects the air that was trapped within the mouth cavity down into the esophagus. Good esophageal speakers can use the concomitant con-

[5] M. C. L. Greene, *The Voice and Its Disorders* (Philadelphia: J. B. Lippincott, Co., 1964), p. 311.
[6] P. H. Damste and J. W. Lehrman, *An Introduction to Voice Pathology* (Springfield, Ill.: Charles C. Thomas), 1975.

striction of their plosive sounds to pump small amounts of air down into the esophagus, thus continually replenishing the supply, and so speak continuously. A third but less advisable method is based upon swallowing.

We have found our work with laryngectomees to be challenging and rewarding. It is challenging because there are many problems which must be solved: the need to provide motivation in the face of repeated failure, the need to relieve these patients of their emotional storms, the need for repeated restructuring of tasks and goals. With one of our patients, we discerned a deep resentment in him whenever we used a normal voice, but found that when we spoke esophageally or wrote out what we had to say, thereby sharing his problem, he could make real achievements. We kept some of these written records, and they run as follows:

Clinician: I'm getting tired of using my esophageal voice. Let's write for a while. You got a pretty good tone on both the *ah* and the *ee* just then, but I felt you waited too long after the air intake. Try to let it come out as soon as it comes in. Don't hold it. In and out, like this . . . (*demonstrates*).

Patient (writing): I get tired too, but that was better, wasn't it? Although I got tensed up too much.

Clinician: Yes, much better. Try letting your arms and shoulders go limp even if you press your lips and tongue to charge the esophagus with air. Like this . . . (*demonstrates*). It's like the old trick of patting your head and rubbing your stomach at the same time. We've got to squeeze the cheeks and mouth to inject the air, but we've also got to try to keep the esophagus from squeezing shut at the same time. Try it again.

Patient: It's so hard. I get discouraged.

Clinician: It *is* hard at first, but it'll get easier. Remember how impossible it seemed at first to get any sound at all. Now you can always get it but we have to find ways of lengthening it, letting it leak out, and not wasting it. I'll bet you can say "pie" (*patient does and is surprised and delighted*).

Patient: Look: I'll say "I" and "pie" with a pause in between, and you put in the word "want" so it makes "I want pie."

An understanding clinician can make the difference between success and failure and it is very good to know the joy of helping a fellow man to speak again.

Learning to Use the   It is much easier to learn to produce speech by the use of this
Artificial Larynx   instrument than to master intelligible esophageal phonation. One needs only to press the button on an electrolarynx and hold the diaphragm end of the device flush with the surface of the neck while articulating to be able to achieve some communicative ability. Many users have had no more training than that provided by the instruction booklet which comes with the instrument. The speech pathologist, however, can make the difference between inferior speech and highly intelligible speech by helping the patient to find the best areas of contact. He can show the patient how to turn on the apparatus intermittently rather than continuously and thereby prevent some of the droning buzz which often interferes with communication. The patient also needs training in mastering the pitch variations that enable him to produce the inflections required by questioning and other prosodic features of normal utterance. Phrasing can also be taught, but perhaps the major contribution a clinician can make is improving the intelligibility of the artificial speech. By helping the patient to articulate the consonants precisely and carefully, the clinician can improve the speech greatly. It is difficult for the user of an electrolarynx to achieve the full potential of this instrument by himself. He needs a clinician.

Cleft Palate Problems

Most babies look pretty good shortly after birth or at least after they have been washed and prettied up for that first inspection by the happy parents. But there are some, alas, who do not, because they have craniofacial (skull and face) anomalies due to some failure of the bones and tissues of the head to develop normally in the uterus. Some babies are even born without a tongue (aglossia), but here we shall be primarily concerned with the problems associated with clefts of the lip and palate.

Types of Clefts   Although classifications differ, there are three major problems involved: clefts of the lip only, clefts of the palate only, and clefts of both the lip and palate. Basically, each involves a failure of the two halves of the palate to grow together during the embryological period. As a result, when the baby is born it will show a cleft of the upper lip, the upper gum ridge, the hard palate, the soft palate, or combinations of the above. The clefts may be complete or incomplete, meaning that in some cases there was no fusion of the right and left halves of the structures, and in other cases, that the fusion had started but was disrupted before the structure was complete.

Clefts of the Lip   Clefts almost always involve the upper lip rather than the lower lip but they may be found in both the lip and the alveolar ridge (the upper gum ridge). They may be unilateral and affect only the left or only the right side, or they may be bilateral and affect both sides. If the cleft of the lip is complete, it will extend into the nostril; if the cleft is incomplete, the nostril will have been formed by the initial fusion of the structures but the lip will show a cleft below that area. These possibilities exist because of the way the upper lip is formed. Shortly after conception, one facial process called the frontonasal process joins with two other processes which grow towards the center from each side. These are the maxillary processes of the upper jaw. The frontonasal process eventually forms the middle part of the nose and the middle part of the upper lip, while the maxillary processes form the middle part of the cheeks and the sides of the upper lip. Unless these processes unite and fuse completely, a cleft of the lip will occur.

Clefts of the Palate   Both the hard and soft palates may be cleft, for the palate, like the lip, requires a fusion of three processes too. Somewhat later than the formation of the lip, a small triangular process (structure), which will eventually become the area behind the upper four front teeth, joins with the palatine plates to start the formation of the hard palate. As the processes continue to merge, the hard palate, the soft palate, and finally the uvula take shape. If the fusion of these processes is interrupted at any time, a cleft of the palate will result. If the processes never started to fuse, the cleft will be complete. Otherwise, an incomplete cleft will be apparent.

Clefts of Both the   Because the structures responsible for the formation of the lip
Lip and Palate   and palate are closely related, some children will have clefts of both the lip and palate. These babies are not pretty to look at because the center of their face is severely distorted. The middle part of their lip and the middle part of their palate may even swing freely if no attachment to either side is present.

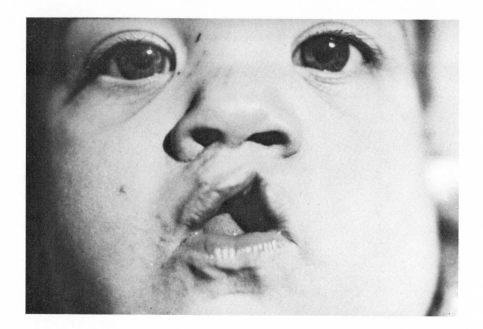

Cleft Lip

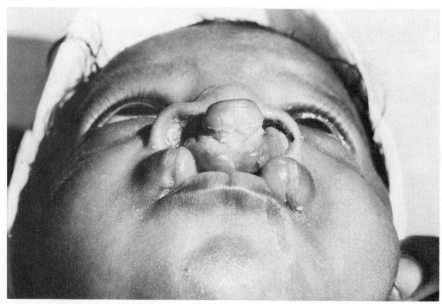

Before Surgery

Figure 33 Clefts of the lip and palate. (Courtesy Dr. Ralph Blocksma.)

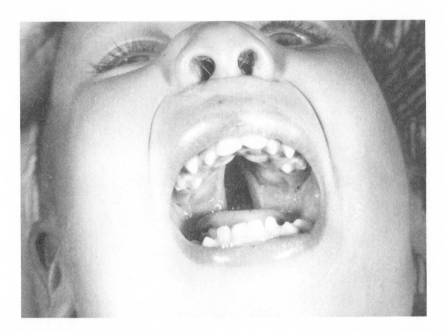

Cleft Palate

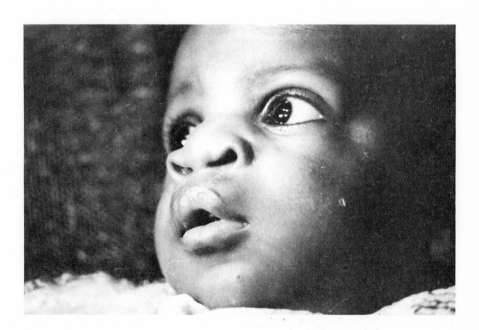

After Surgery

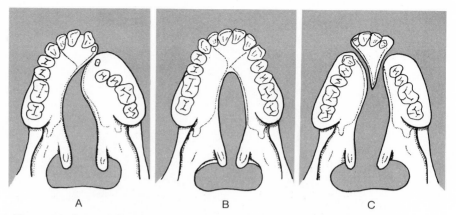

Figure 34 Some different types of clefts (A—Cleft of hard and soft palates; B—Unilateral cleft of palate and lip; C—Bilateral cleft of palate and lip).

Other Types of Clefts   Some clefts do not fit easily into any one of the classifications described above. For example, there are a few cases of median clefts with an absence of some of the tissue of the middle part of the face, and lateral clefts may also occur. In these cases, the division follows a line from the corner of the mouth toward the ear. This kind of cleft gives the appearance of a mouth that is far too wide.

Sub-Mucous Clefts   Some children show no apparent signs of clefts when their mouths are inspected visually, yet a cleft may exist under the mucous linings of the palate. You can feel them even if you can't see them. Clefts of this type are called sub-mucous clefts and may include several of the following: a bifid or split uvula, a notch in the back of the hard palate, a whitish translucent strip down the middle of the soft palate, or a deep pharyngeal vault. Hypernasal speech is usually a common result of these hidden sub-mucous clefts.

Congenital Palatal Insufficiency   Many authorities now recognize the classification of *congenital palatal insufficiency* (CPI) to describe the youngster who, usually after a tonsilectomy and adenoidectomy, suddenly develops hypernasal speech. It has been shown that many of these children have a congenitally short palate or an unusually deep throat (if we dare use the phrase) or both. While the adenoids are present, they act like a cushion against which the velum moves, but when they are removed by surgery, the gap is too great, a leak occurs, and the speech may become very nasal.

Causes of Clefts   The exact cause for a child's cleft is frequently unknown. We do know that failure of these structures to fuse occurs during the first trimester of pregnancy and when a full-term baby is born with a cleft, it has been in existence for over six months. During medieval times, it was believed that one of the causes of oral clefts was the exposure of expectant mothers to rabbits (who always have hare lips). There even were local laws prohibiting butchers' shops from displaying rabbits for fear that some unsuspecting pregnant woman might gaze upon the carcass, thereby increasing the likelihood that her child would be born with a cleft lip. Now we know that many of the oral clefts appear to have a genetic basis. Although the incidence of oral clefts in families with no previous occurrence of clefting is very small in live births, it increases significantly for families in which clefts have occurred.[7] Clefts of only the soft palate are more frequently inherited by females and clefts of only the lip are less likely to be inherited.

Effects of Clefts   When a baby is born with a cleft, special services are needed immediately. The first problem to be tackled is that of informing the new parent of the less than pleasant news for, unlike many other handicaps, the oral cleft is conspicuously apparent from the first. This task requires the skill and compassion of a specialist who knows a lot about the disorder and who understands the impact of the event. It is not an easy task and some physicians and nurses shirk their responsibility or perform poorly. For example, we have had mothers of cleft palate children tell us that they were kept under heavy anesthesia for hours after the birth of their child until someone was able to muster enough courage to talk with them. Fortunately, the situation is now improving. Most obstetricians now call in a specialist, probably a plastic surgeon, who will both inform and reassure the parents, and many hospitals now have a file of pre-operative and post-operative pictures to show the parents immediately that the children can be helped. Some progressive hospitals also have files of other parents who can be called in to assist the new parents to overcome their initial shock.

The Oral Cleft Team   During the last decade, the development of oral cleft teams has markedly improved the treatment of these children. The team approach saves the parents and the client time, money, and the

[7] According to Drillien, Ingram and Wilkinson (1966), 23 percent of their patients with cleft lip and/or palate had someone among the five nearest relatives who also had a cleft.

anguish of going from specialist to specialist and getting conflicting advice. The essential ingredients of a successful oral cleft team include the freedom for all professionals to give their points of view and freedom from domination by any one specialist. Speech pathologists become members of these teams and so those who work with cleft palate clients must have some detailed knowledge about the specialties of the other members. Here we are interested only in providing an overview of the professions involved and a little information about the kinds of responsibilities they have.

The *plastic surgeon* specializes in the modification of soft tissue. He is frequently the first specialist the parents meet, and often he coordinates the team approach to the entire treatment. The *otolaryngologist* (ENT specialist) is a physician who gives special attention to the ears, the nose, and the throat. He will evaluate and treat, if necessary, the tonsils and adenoids and will perform ear surgery, if indicated. The *orthodontist* is responsible for the positioning of the teeth. He may use devices to straighten teeth and to insure as normal an occlusion as possible. The *prosthodontist* designs and builds prostheses (artificial appliances) for the oral cleft client. These may include speech bulbs, palatal lifts, and obturators. The *radiologist,* also a physician, specializes in taking x-rays of the oral structures including still x-rays (lateral headplates), motion picture x-rays (cinefluoroscopy), and even can produce various images using ultrasound.

Because oral clefts are frequently accompanied by other anomalies, the general health of the child is also of major importance. The *pediatrician* oversees the general health of the child. Since both the client and the parents face many emotional problems associated with the cleft, a *psychologist* may also be called in to provide testing and treatment. Children with oral clefts have such a high incidence of hearing loss that routine hearing tests are essential, and so they are administered and interpreted by the *audiologist*. Finally, on these teams the *speech pathologist* not only seeks to improve the client's speech but also he is usually involved in evaluating, treating, and coordinating the efforts of the other members of the team. He must know not only his own field but be knowledgeable in all the other specialties.

Surgery for Clefts Surgical care for the oral cleft patient may be considered primary or secondary. Primary surgery for the cleft of the lip, for example, attempts to close the cleft. It is usually done early in the child's life with major consideration given to how the child is likely to look as an adult. Early lip surgery can almost always improve the facial appearance of the child greatly. The primary surgery on the palate is designed to close the cleft while leaving as little scar tissue as possible. Since scarring deters the growth of the facial bones, some plastic surgeons suggest that palatal surgery be postponed (Blocksma, 1975) or in some cases be eliminated altogether.

Secondary surgery on the palate usually involves some attempt to improve the speech of the client. Some of the procedures are designed to move the palate backward. These are called *push-back procedures.* More popular are the attempts to bring the back wall of the throat forward in some way. One of the more effective ways of doing this requires the creation of a flap of tissue which is left attached to the back wall of the throat but sutured to the soft palate in front, thus forming a bridge of tissue. This is called a *pharyngeal flap* and has several technical variations. Also, within the last decade the use of Teflon and other substances has gained some popularity. These substances may be injected or positioned surgically, again with the intent of bringing the back wall of the throat forward and making it easier for the velum to effect a closure.

Each year major advances in surgery seem to occur, and great strides have been made in providing the structures needed to shut off the nasal airway. We are not seeing nearly as many persons with cleft-palate speech as we did twenty years ago, and those we do see do not show the facial deformations and grossly deviant speech that were common at that time. Nevertheless, not even the best surgeon using the most modern techniques can help all these persons.

Prostheses   There are certain cases of cleft palate for whom surgery is not the wisest course. Certain clefts are so large or the tissue remaining so scant or poorly developed that the prognosis for good speech, easy swallowing, and a good facial appearance is very poor.

Essentially, prostheses are artificial substitutes for missing or deficient parts. In the case of oral prostheses, we have a substitute for one of the structures of the mouth, such as the teeth or the palate, or we may have a device that is designed to assist an existing structure in doing its job, such as in the case of a speech bulb or a palatal lift. Still other oral prostheses may be used temporarily to facilitate movement, as in the case of a palatal stimulator.

Prostheses have been made of many materials. There are accounts in ancient Greek literature of cleft-palate individuals filling their clefts of the hard palate with fruit rinds, cloth, leather, tar, and wax so that they could eat and drink. Passavant made a stud-shaped obturator which he inserted into a slit in the palate after it was sewed up, but it did not work too well. Others injected wax or inserted silver plate projections into the back wall of the pharynx. In the late 1800s artificial hard palates anchored to the teeth were provided with hinged gates, rubber bulbs, rubber tubes, silver balls, and other devices to plug or narrow the nasopharyngeal airway. All of these were very unsanitary, often prevented nasal breathing or interfered with it, and at times produced marked denasality on some sounds while failing to eliminate the nasality on others. Some of these devices were painful and caused gagging and choking. Ear infections were common.

Modern appliances use an acrylic resin that can be molded and worked by the designer so that it will fit any opening. They are highly sanitary, easily cleaned, and are very light in weight. Plastics opened the way for truly effective cleft-palate prostheses. They can even be modified without the need for new impressions to be taken or new casts made.

Types of Prostheses   The dental portion of a prosthesis may be designed to improve the cosmetic appearance as well as to improve speech. In addition to the obvious improvement that comes from having the teeth look better, a dental prosthesis may be so designed as to provide needed bulk to the upper lip portion of the face. This particular type of dental appliance is called an *onlay prosthesis* and compensates

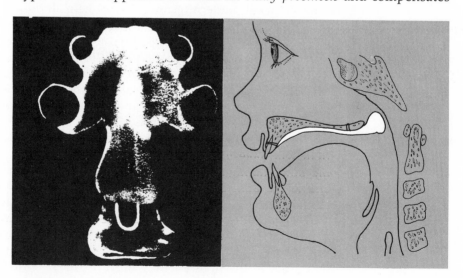

Figure 35 A velo-pharyngeal prosthesis and how it is fitted. (Westlake and Rutherford, *Cleft Palate*)

for the collapse of the middle third of the face that many cleft palate patients show. The portion of the appliance that is designed to plug or block the opening in an unrepaired palatal cleft is frequently referred to as an *obturator.* Obturators usually attach to existing teeth or may be attached to a dental prosthesis. We have known some infants fitted with such obturators who treat them much like pacifiers and become quite upset until they have been inserted by the parent.

When a device is needed to assist in velopharyngeal closure, the prosthodontist may design a speech bulb. This prosthesis extends from the palatal portion into the nasopharynx to fill the deficient velopharyngeal space. A speech bulb may be recommended when surgery is contraindicated or for health purposes or when previous surgery has failed. It is used, of course, to decrease the hypernasality. In the last few years, considerable attention has been given to the use of palatal lifts and palatal stimulators. A *palatal lift* is designed to elevate the middle section of the velum and is used in cases in which there is little evidence of enough muscular potential for velopharyngeal closure, even though the palate seems long enough. A *palatal stimulator* provides a mechanical resistance to the normal movement of the velum so that the client can strengthen the weak muscles in the velopharyngeal area.

Surgery vs. Prosthesis   A real controversy has raged for many years between the dentists and the surgeons about how these clefts should be treated. Surgeons claim that living tissue is always preferable to any artificial means of closing off the nasal chambers from the mouth cavity. They point to the unsanitariness, the inconvenience, the difficulty in fitting prostheses, and the expensiveness and duration of the treatment. Perhaps most important is the charge by the surgeons that prostheses often cause a gradual deterioration of the existing teeth and that eventually the patient is left without teeth, and therefore without a suitable anchor for the appliance, so that patient will have to resort to surgery anyway. The prosthodontists, on the other hand, point to the numerous instances of surgical failure and to the pain and the poor speech results which often occur after surgery. Also the dentists are especially concerned about the effect of surgery on the growth of the middle third of the face, and the major orthodontic and cosmetic problems that can be traced directly to the type of surgery the client had received. This argument still rages in many quarters, and although the development of oral cleft teams has improved the communication between the two professional groups, a suitable compromise has not yet been reached. Often the speech pathologist on the team is called upon to be the referee and he had better know enough about both points of view to play his part.

In general, the following principles should prevail: (1) Determination of treatment should be based on intensive evaluation by a team of specialists. There is no one approach that fits all clients; each patient's treatment must be custom designed. (2) Surgery, in order to fulfill its objectives, must conform to the following requirements: it should create no major risk to the patient's life; it should be designed to restore the basic functions without interfering with future growth; it should be based on clinical data that provide reasonable expectations for improved speech. (3) Prostheses should conform to these requirements: they should aid in restoring basic function without creating discomfort or damage to the surrounding or supporting structures; they should be shaped so that they allow other structures to function normally and efficiently; and they should be sturdy and designed with special attention given to retention, care, and cosmetic appearance. As these observations suggest, the speech pathologist on a cleft palate team must be really competent.

Speech Problems Associated with Cleft Palate

Clefts of the lip and palate affect speech in two major ways: the voice quality becomes deviant, and the articulation is impaired. With regard to the voice quality, the most prominent impression is that of excessive nasality. The person seems to be speaking through his nose, but this perception should not be confused with the nasal twang heard in certain dialects. Moreover, when closely analyzed, the voice quality differences shown by cleft-palate speakers are not confined entirely to excessive nasality.[8] Denasality also occurs, and the listener will often hear it first on the nasalized continuant sounds such as /m/, /n/, and /ŋ/ when these are spoken by persons with cleft palates. There are also other rather unique types of articulation errors present in cleft-palate speakers. They have more trouble with the plosives and fricative sounds since these require the storing up of air pressure behind the closure or the narrowed opening. Voiced sounds seem to be easier than the unvoiced ones, but the consonant blends present considerable difficulty. In contrast to the errors made by young normal children, young cleft-palate children (and often adults) tend to substitute glottal stops and pharyngeal fricatives for the stan-

---

[8] A good discussion of these voice quality differences is given in H. Westlake and D. Rutherford, *Cleft Palate* (Englewood Cliffs, N.J.: Prentice-Hall, Inc., 1966), pp. 34–44.

dard sounds. Their speech seems to be punctuated by the little "catches of the breath" they use instead of such sounds as /p/, /b/, /t/, /d/, /k/ and /g/, or clearing-of-the-throat noises which replace the fricatives. The distortion errors are almost unique to the cleft-palate speaker. They are primarily due to nasal emission, the person snorting the sounds out of his nose. One of our adults with a cleft palate who, despite surgery and prostheses, still showed very deviant speech summed it up this way when he heard himself on tape: "Jeez, that's terrible. I knew it was bad, but not that bad. I can hardly understand what I was saying with all that honking and snorting." In severe cases the intelligibility is very poor, and often one of the major tasks of the speech pathologist is to help the cleft-palate speaker to be understood. Fortunately, even without therapy, many cleft-palate speakers manage to discard some of their gross errors and improve their intelligibility somewhat as they grow older.

Evaluation of Velopharyngeal Competency
Surgery and prosthetic appliances unfortunately do not always guarantee that normal speech can be obtained even with the best of speech therapy. The person may come to us with a closure mechanism that will not close sufficiently to permit adequate speech no matter how long and hard we work. We may be able to improve the person's articulation and intelligibility, but he will still sound hypernasal and abnormal. We have known clinicians and clients who struggled for years to do the impossible, years which might better have been spent in designing a better prosthesis or in new surgery. How can we be sure that this client of ours can really close the rear passageway to the nose? How can we know that he has a competent velopharyngeal valve?

In the past, speech pathologists have used such simple tests as the ability to suck liquids through a straw or to blow out candles or to say a series of vowels to determine the client's capacity for velar closure. Or they have visually observed the uvular movement or the constriction of the posterior pharyngeal wall. Unfortunately, tests of this nature have proved inadequate. Participation on an oral cleft team requires that a speech pathologist have some familiarity with a growing number of much more sophisticated technique for evaluating velopharyngeal function.

Many of the newer techniques involve attempts to directly visualize the structures of the throat and palate. The radiologist may contribute any one of a number of x-ray techniques, including the motion picture x-rays called cinefluoroscopy. These are especially useful since they show the structures in motion during speech production.

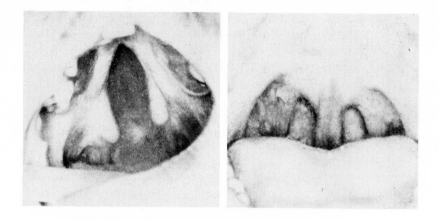

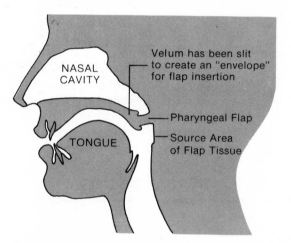

Figure 36   Pharyngeal flap. (Westlake and Rutherford, *Cleft Palate*)

Also recently, the traditional lateral views provided by these x-rays have been augmented by basal and frontal cineradiography and have added greatly to our ability to see all the structures involved in velopharyngeal activity. A few centers use ultrasound pictures to replace the x-ray techniques.

Other non-x-ray attempts to see what is happening have approached the structures from top and bottom. Nasendoscopy involves the insertion of a viewing scope up into and through the nasal cavity. Without interfering with the speech structures, one is thereby able to see clearly the muscles of the velum and throat during spontaneous speech. Even more useful to the speech pathologist are new techniques developed to view the palatal activity from the mouth itself. The oral panendoscope, for example, is a small tubular viewing instrument which can be used with adults and older children. It, like the nasendoscopic instruments, can be attached to videotape equipment, thereby allowing the image of the velopharyngeal area during speech to be displayed and replayed on a TV monitor. This permits the viewer to observe whether closure is occurring and it allows the examiner to share this important data with other members of the team.

Other indirect techniques for evaluating closure are gaining popularity and should be explored by the speech pathologist who specializes in working with cleft-palate patients. Some of these include TONAR (the oral nasal acoustic ratio), an instrument designed by Fletcher for comparing air emitted from the nose with air emitted from the mouth; *agnellography* and *oral manometry,* which record air pressure within the mouth.

However, we can also get some impression concerning the adequacy of the closure mechanism by analyzing the speech itself. First of all, we should check the articulation errors. If we find key words in which all of the defective sounds or most of them are used correctly, we can be pretty sure that enough closure is present. Again, if at times these errors are not accompanied by nose twitching or nasal emission of air, we can feel that the valve is all right. If the person

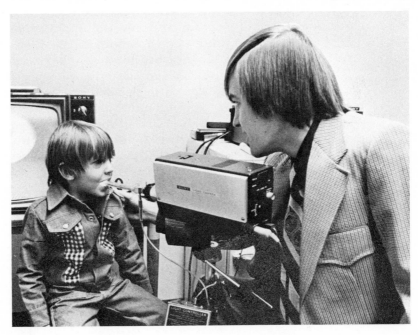

Figure 37   Panendoscopy.

can speak very well with his nostrils closed but has much nasal distortion when they are open, we would suspect inadequate closure. Finally, if the consonants that require extra mouth pressure *(p-b; t-d; k-g; s-z; ch-j)* are those which are nasally distorted, while the *r* and the *l* or *f* and *v* are quite adequate, we would feel that the closure was poor.

Speech Therapy   It is impossible to outline a program of speech therapy techniques which would be applicable to all cleft-palate clients, or even a majority, since the problems presented by the clients are so different. Individual diagnoses are absolutely essential. We deal with speech that reflects the personality of the client, with his concept of self. The basic attitude of a client who feels that, because he has an organic disability there is nothing which can be done to alter his speech, has a profound effect upon therapy. Often little speech therapy can be accomplished until psychotherapy has produced some reality testing, until some hope has been provoked, until the client can trust the clinician when he cannot trust his own parents or closest friends. Most of these clients know little about the nature of their problem or the possibilities for improving speech. They come as passively and as unenthusiastically as they go to the surgeon, the prosthodontist, or the orthodontist, because they have been told they should. Few of them feel any powerful urge to accept some of the responsibility for their speech improvement. Like the stutterer, the cleft-palate client has detached himself from his speech because it is too painful to confront. As in stuttering, we meet with strong resistance when we are forced to demand the active cooperation of the cleft-palate person in confronting his nasal emissions, his nasality, and his poor articulation. Without this control, without this monitoring, it is almost impossible to make any but perfunctory gains. Like the normal speaker, the cleft-palate person does not hear himself speaking; he hears his expressed thoughts. It is difficult for the normal speaker to concentrate on self-hearing. In the cleft-palate person, this self-hearing is not only burdensome, but also painful. Unless the speech clinician understands this basic psychology, he can hardly hope to be effective.

It is also necessary, quite apart from the individual's attitudes toward his speech and its therapy, to take into account the actual organic disability which may be present. Some cleft-palate persons with very defective speech may have complete closures and the potential for completely normal speech. Some of these are already using their closures in activities other than speech or on other speech sounds except those that are defective. Others of the same group may have the potential to use their soft palate or pharyngeal musculatures but have not learned to do so. But we must also recognize that there are some cleft-palate clients whose structures or prostheses are not adequate for normal speech, and for whom we may be able to do very little except in the improvement of intelligibility. Again, let us state our melioristic philosophy of speech therapy: We make the person's speech better and we make him a happier person. We do not have to make his speech perfect or make him a completely happy human. Within the limits of our time and energy and knowledge, and with an awareness of the limitations which the client also possesses, let us do our utmost and be content with that. They must learn to speak as well as they can, with as little interference to communication as possible and as little abnormality as possible.

Aims of Speech Therapy for Cleft-Palate Speech Our basic points of attack are these: We must decrease the nasal emission, the hypernasality, and the defective articulation. We must improve the oral air pressure and oral airflow.

We must eliminate abnormal foci of tension and abnormal nostril contractions. We must activate the tongue tip, lip, and jaws. We must improve the respiratory rhythms of speech and their rate and control. We must improve velar and pharyngeal contraction.

We once examined a person with a complete, unilateral cleft of both the hard and soft palates who had completely normal speech. How he managed this we were unable to tell, but he did use wide jaw movements, slow speech, short phrases, and dentalized most of his frontal sounds. All plosives were made with very loose contacts. He spoke softly and did become nasal when he spoke loudly. So far as we could ascertain, this person operated his speech with very little air pressure, and it flowed out of the larger mouth opening rather than the smaller nasal opening merely because it was larger. He was not tense, but very relaxed, and perhaps this accounted for his lack of hypernasality, since certain authorities feel that the characteristic tone of nasality is due to a *constricted* open-ended tube rather than to the open tube itself. At any rate, he demonstrated how much we might be able to do in speech therapy. This case also illustrates an important principle. We should work for altering the direction of airflow so that it flows outward toward the mouth rather than upward through the nose. And we should teach the cleft-palate person to articulate with a minimum of oral air pressure.

Air-Pressure   Air pressure within the mouth varies with the various speech
Controls   sounds. The plosives and the sibilants require the most air
pressure. Voiced sounds require less than do the unvoiced
sounds due to the increased audibility of the former. The /t/ and /d/
require less than /k/ and /g/. People vary widely one from another in
the degree of closure used in producing the plosives and the fricatives. Certain individuals use very tight closures and sudden releases;
others do not. Cleft-palate clients often use very tight closures and
sudden releases. This is very unwise since much more air pressure is
required for such plosives than for the loose-contact, slow-release
type. We experimented once by inserting a small air hose into the
corner of the lips and had the subjects, both normal and cleft-palate,
articulate a series of plosives and fricatives. They then held their
breath and pantomimed the various sounds both with tight contacts
and with loose ones. Less air pressure was required to produce clear
sounds when the loose contacts were used. In the cleft-palate clients
little air escaped from the nose when loose contacts were used; but it
was very evident when tight contacts were used. The cleft-palate person whose velum is functioning also reacts very characteristically to a
tight contact either of tongue tip or lips. These tight contacts almost
seem to act as triggers to cause a lowering of the palate and a relaxation of the superior constrictor in much the same way as they tend
to set off stuttering tremors in the stutterer.

This occurs not only with the plosives. The fricatives, which employ a narrow opening or channel for the airflow, are also produced
differently by different people. Certain ones use a very narrow channel; others a broader one. Cleft-palate individuals tend to use the
narrower ones that require a greater air pressure, and so nasal emission tends to occur. We therefore should teach them differently.

Much of the stimulus value of a sound can be increased by prolonging its duration. If cleft-palate persons are to soften their contacts
in order to make use of the lessened air pressure in the mouth due to
the palatal air leak, they must prolong these sounds somewhat, to
gain the same intelligibility. Weaker s sounds should be held longer.
A slightly prolonged /f/ in the word *fish* even if weaker in airflow
will be understood as readily as a quicker, stronger one.

Concentration in therapy upon these factors also emphasizes the
direction of airflow through the mouth rather than the nose. Cleft-palate people are nose-conscious as the contraction of their nostrils demonstrates. By concentrating on the longer, slower, looser contacts and the
shallower channels of articulation, the airflow tends to go mouthward.
This emphasis upon the mouth, rather than the nose as the major channel for speech and airflow, is among the major objectives of any speech

therapy. It is in large part a psychological problem as we have indicated. We have known cleft-palate children to speak much better as soon as they held a megaphone to their lips or thought that we were going to hold their noses. We have had several cases who were able to blow trumpets very well and yet could not manage a simple /p/ sound without having it come through their nose. For this reason, most speech clinicians do much lip and tongue training along with blowing exercises. We have given lip exercises with profit to cleft-palate persons who already had perfect lip control, primarily so that they would become mouth-conscious. We have had them talk through fringed holes in a sheet of paper, through various sizes of slits and blowing tubes, with their fingers in their mouths, with their mouths to ears, through fringed paper mustachios, into the vibrator mouthpiece of toy musical instruments, with their mouths held under water, into cones whose apex flickered a candle flame. One of our children spoke much better when he put on a clown's mask that had a monstrous big mouth which he watched in a mirror. He just became more mouth-conscious, and the air came out of that opening. We have improved the speech of cleft-palate clients by teaching them to read lips and to help in training deaf children in lipreading. One of our majors got better speech from a cleft-palate girl by putting lipstick on her mouth and having her watch it in the mirror. We have darkened a room and put a little flashlight focused on the outside of the mouth in a narrow beam, and also within the mouth, and improved the speech by having the client watch it in the mirror. Cleft-palate clients must think of speech as coming out of the mouth.

Many speech pathologists teach their cleft-palate clients to open the mouth widely in speech, as far as they can without appearing abnormal. This is often difficult to teach, and resistance is almost sure to be found; but when it can be used it does seem to improve speech markedly. It does this first because any larger opening attracts airflow. Air must take a tortuous course when it must go upstairs through the filters of the nasal caverns and then down and out through the narrow slits of our nostrils. It would much rather come out of a side door, especially if that side door is open. Moreover, larger mouth openings for the vowels tend to produce looser contacts of lips and tongue, and they certainly increase the consciousness of the mouth rather than the nose.

The source of the air pressure and airflow is, of course, in the contractions of the muscles that lower the chest and contract the abdomen and these muscles, with a relaxing diaphragm, create a condition of pressure upon the lungs. Many cleft-palate clients require training in breath control for speech. Their breathing records show many instances of air wastage, speaking on residual air, opposition, and staircase breathing. They often start speaking with a very strong pulse of air which goes up through the pharynx or cleft because of its pressure, and then creates the path for whatever air is left to follow. They often inhale too deeply prior to utterance (which causes tension all along the airway) to produce this initial strong blast or pulse. With much of the air wasted in the first few syllables, the person then must speak on residual air or opposition breathing, both of which increase tension everywhere. It is possible to improve the speech, the nasal emission, and the hypernasality by teaching the client to inhale a normal amount of air and to start his utterance gradually rather than suddenly and to monitor the amount of air used. Cleft-palate speakers must learn to watch their phrasing, which means their breathing.

Muscle Training   It is also possible of course, in many cases, to improve the state of air pressure within the mouth by shutting off the air leak, by improving velopharyngeal closure. Many of the muscles are weak and can be strengthened through appropriate exercises if surgery or prosthesis has been successful in creating the conditions for a possible closure. If the cleft-palate client can blow up a balloon or whistle, or if inspection with a dental mirror shows good occlusion of the nasopharynx, we should be able to help him use some closure in speech. Even when this is not possible but when, in phonation, yawning, or other activities, we can see the velum lift or the side walls of the pharynx contract or the rear wall come forward slightly, we must presume that we can improve this functioning until we find otherwise. (This last statement may not be true if the velum is too short or taut or the pharynx so enlarged that no closure seems possible.)

Such muscle training requires two major items besides devoted practice: location of the musculatures by the patient and perception of their movement. In physical therapy where comparable tasks are present, the physical therapist, through massage, positioning, and passive movement, is often able to get movement of muscles as inert as those of the cleft-palate patient's repaired velum. Unfortunately, a limb is easier to manipulate than is a palate. Nevertheless, speech pathologists have employed some of the same principles of physical therapy in activating the velar and pharyngeal muscles. Light massage with a finger cot (covering of rubber) first along one side of the uvula, then on the other, and then with two fingers straddling the midline, has helped to localize the area. The stroking must be done very lightly and both away from the midline in a horizontal direction, and anteroposteriorly. Care must be taken that the child does not gag or bite your fingers off. These exercises must also be done with caution lest tissues be injured; but when they are done lightly and the patient attempts to feel and predict the location and direction of movement, they can be very effective. Only a little of this can be done at a time since the patient tires quickly. Another procedure involves the tapping of these structures in the same areas, the patient being requested to tell the numbers of taps and their intensity. We also may slightly depress the surface of the palate or tickle it or the pharyngeal wall if the gag reflex is not present or is weak. These techniques all involve the location of the structures by the tactual sense.

We may also use the visual sense. Many cleft-palate clients have no visual imagery of their palates with which to correlate movement. They should study and describe the action of the clinician's palate in action. They should watch both their own and their clinician's palate in mirrors. They can be shown large pictures of the palate on charts and be taught to point to the area which the clinician touches. When there is residual movement, it should be viewed visually, and then imagined. A very clear picture should be possessed by every cleft-palate patient of the nature of his problem. Even little children can be given this in imaginative terms: "the little red gate or door."

Since most repaired cleft-palate clients have some movement of the levator and tensor muscles as well as of the constrictor muscles in certain activities, they must be taught to isolate and to identify the experience. Certain key words should be conditioned to palatal activity: "up . . . down . . . squeeze . . . let go . . . open . . . shut." These must be used by the clinician only when the activity actually occurs. They should first be used by the client when observing the clinician's palatal movements, then when observing his own, then with intermittent eye-closing with attention to kinesthesia.

It is also possible to become aware of palatal movement by other sensations. With the mouth open, try to get the case to feel some air pressure in his middle ear, to feel it click or pop. This must be done while holding the breath. The palatal tensor, when it contracts, has some effect upon opening the Eustachian tube. Also in yawning, the palatal muscles tend to contract and can be felt in action. Closed-mouth yawning is especially effective in developing kinesthesia, and it can be combined with the middle-ear pressure cues. Also use different mouth openings.

Some of the tactual sensations can also be achieved with a syringe by blowing a stream of air or "warm water" against certain parts of the soft palate. The child may also explore his own mouth with his own finger, using the fingers cut from sterilized rubber gloves. Loud snoring (with the nose held so that all inhalations are made through the mouth) will vibrate the uvula, and research has shown that in this snoring the palate is raised. It is possible to snore on the various vowels and with different tongue positions or lip postures. Tight closures of the tongue and velum in silence as in the position for a /k/ sound will, if the release is very sudden, provoke some upward movement of the palate at the same time that the tongue is jerked downward. The sound-play known as "gibbega-dong" is also effective when the client can do it, since it is based upon the last-mentioned principle.

Weak palatal movements, when present, can be made more effective in closure by having the patient lie on a cot with his head held far backward so that the force of gravity aids rather than resists the palatal movement. When there is asymmetrical pull on the palate, turning the head or the jaw to one side seems to be of some assistance.

Dry swallowing, when repeated, often helps the patient to activate and localize the velopharyngeal contractions. Often a state of localized strain or fatigue may help the client to become aware that he has such muscles. Very slow chewing may also produce certain muscular contractions of the pharynx and velum. Sudden sucking of air through various sizes of tubes will also initiate velar activity. Tubes of different sizes and shapes will produce more palatal contraction than others, but the sucking must be sudden.[9]

Blowing Exercises   Perhaps blowing exercises have been used more frequently than any other single device for strengthening the palate. Blowing takes air pressure, and if the air is to come out of the mouth, a velopharyngeal opening will reduce that pressure enough to reduce the airflow through the mouth to a considerable degree. We must be certain, however, that we are having an increasingly greater ratio of mouth airflow to nasal airflow if we can hope that the palate is being strengthened. Various devices have been employed to demonstrate this ratio: double shelves to be placed under nose and mouth openings with feathers or fringes to indicate airflow, tubes from the nose to the ear, contact microphones, the phonodeik and phonoscope, polygraphic recording, candle flame affected by tubes from the nose

[9] An interesting device for improving velopharyngeal closure is a palatal exerciser invented by E. C. Lubit and R. E. Larsen. See their article "The Lubit Palatal Exerciser: A Preliminary Report" in *Cleft Palate Journal*, VI (1969), 120–33.

and mouth, clouded mirrors, and many others. Usually it is necessary that the patient become familiar with the two air channels by sucking air in through the nose, then through the mouth, then exhaling alternately through each channel. By using different mouth openings and palpating the nostrils during the blowing or interrupting the oral airflow with vibrating palms across the orifice, the client can come to have a clear idea of these channels. We must not expect him to already have such a concept. Also by having the client alternate nasal and oral airflow while he holds his fingers in his ears, he can hear a difference in the pitch of the two blowings. The oral airflow can be made to vary markedly in pitch by changing the lip protrusion or mouth opening; the nasal airflow is pretty well fixed in pitch. By attending to the different palatal and pharyngeal sensations during the different airflows, a more adequate control of the velopharyngeal musculatures can be achieved.

We should emphasize that blowing exercises performed with great tension and the constriction of the nostrils are most unwise. They merely inform the client that palatal contraction is too laborious to be used in speech. Besides, they often can cause ear infections. We also doubt the efficacy of blowing air out of the mouth while holding the nose shut, since we may raise the air pressure too high in the middle ear and make the client too nose-conscious and in any event, closure of the nostrils does not help the velopharyngeal valve to shut. Indeed, there seems to be a sort of inverse reciprocal reaction in the action of the nares (nostrils) and the velar musculatures. Even in normal speakers, voluntary contraction of the nares often produces an increase in nasality. As the front door shuts, the back door opens. Often there is very little transfer of training from blowing to speech. This is especially true if the blowing is too strained, if air pressures far exceeding those used in normal speech are used, and if set mouth openings and passive tongue postures are employed. We could hardly expect much transfer with so many variables in the training. Nevertheless, others have shown that the palatal and pharyngeal activity in blowing (especially in soft blowing) is more like that used in speech than is shown in such activities as yawning, swallowing, and so on. We must not throw the baby out with the bath. Blowing exercises can help the client to become mouth-conscious; they can help him discriminate the two airflow channels; they can help him to increase the amount of oral air pressure needed for good articulation; and they can improve the contraction of the velar and pharyngeal muscles. But they must be used wisely rather than indiscriminately.

We conclude this section on velopharyngeal closure training by mentioning two other techniques which we have used with some success with adults. In the first, a large balloon is blown up (preferably by the client while holding his nose) and then held shut by the clinician's fingers on the stem as the client holds a tube leading from the stem with his lips. The clinician gradually releases his grip and allows some of the air to escape into the client's mouth. The latter tries, while holding his breath, to keep from letting the balloon collapse; this requires velar closure or the air will leak out of the nostrils. Another variation of this technique has the outlet to the balloon enter a Y-tube, the arms of which are attached to nasal olives inserted into the client's nostrils. He tries to retard the collapse of the balloon as he produces various vowels or merely contracts his palate in silence.

Articulation Problems   The backward playing of samples of speech of various degrees of nasality has demonstrated that the listener judges a given sample as being more nasal if it has poorer articulation. The voice quality itself seems more nasal when it is played forward than when it is played backward. Thus, the improvement of articulation can produce a decrease in perceived nasality. We have also seen that the majority of cleft-palate speakers have speech sounds which are defective.

The basic problems in articulation are three: lalling, the substitution of glottal stops and fricatives for the standard stops and fricatives, and the nasalization or nasal emission of most of the consonants.

Lalling   The treatment for lalling requires training in increasing the mobility of the tongue tip; in raising the points of anterior contact for the /t/, /d/, /l/, and /tʃ/, and /dʒ/ sounds; and the differentiation of tongue-lifting from simultaneous jaw movement.

Exercises for increasing the mobility of the tongue include sensitization of the tongue tip—curling, grooving, lifting, lowering, thrusting, arching, tapping, sustaining postures, pressing, scraping, fluttering, and many others. These should not be practiced while holding the breath but while blowing gently both voiced and unvoiced air if the training is to generalize to speech. Undue tension is to be avoided. Speed gains should be made in terms of rhythmic patterns. Different sizes of mouth opening and lip postures should also be practiced with the tongue-training. Many of these clients have never explored the many possibilities of tongue movement or action. It is wise to use these exercises as warm-up periods for consonant practice. Often the production of certain consonants is sandwiched between two tongue-training exercises.

The localizing of the focal articulation points higher and more forward in the mouth can be done only by identifying those ordinarily used and searching for higher points while continuously articulating the sounds. This "stretching" of the phonemes in terms of height of contact will at first seem unpleasant and will seldom be used at their extremes, but practice will cause the necessary compromise. Most cleft-palate persons also have certain scar tissue, indentations, or bulges on the alveolar ridge that can be used as landmarks; but they must be found and localized. Tactual feedbacks must be sharpened. The teeth, especially the lower teeth, must come to lose their functions as the basic contact point. Silent practice in touching these new focal articulation points should be done. With one of our clients, we inserted a bit of toothpick or dental floss between the upper incisors and used this as the guide. An immediate improvement in speech occurred.

The differentiation of tongue movement from the accompanying jaw movements can be done by immobilizing the jaw with various heights of tooth props until enough independence is achieved to permit the activity without this aid. Frequent checking is necessary. Visual feedback from a mirror is also useful. Lateral movements of the mandible during tongue-tapping and consonant production will also be useful. The use of the first two fingers forked to monitor the location of both lips will help. Also, if the client will place one finger on his nose and his thumb under his chin, any accompanying movement of the jaw will be noticed immediately. Ventriloquism often provides an interesting motivation for these clients, and aids in the freeing of the tongue.

Eliminating Glottal Stop Errors   The use of the glottal stop or fricative substitutions requires a state of localized tension in the larynx, and therefore we try to create some relaxation in this area. The use of slight coughs to teach a /k/ sound is very unwise. Instead, the back of the tongue must be raised, and this can be accomplished more easily on the /k/ and /g/ sounds by pressing hard with the tongue tip against the lower teeth and closing the jaws partially. Ear training is essential. We have also been able to eliminate this difficult error by having the client produce the consonants on inhalation, a procedure which improves much of the articulation of cleft-palate clients. The subsequent use of donkey breathing (inhaled, then exhaled) in the production of the sounds often solves the glottal problem.

Decreasing Nasality   While much of the success of articulating the consonant
and Nasal Emission   sounds without nasality or nasal emission will depend upon
the success of establishing oral airflow and better velopharyngeal closure, we find that by teaching the plosives with very loose
contacts, great improvement can be made. Too hard contacts seem to
trigger off a lowering of the velum and a relaxation of the superior
constrictor.

For the fricatives, the use of wider mouth openings on the following or preceding vowels tends to decrease the nasality. We also
suggest the prolongation of these sounds with decreasing air pressure, thus using the duration rather than the clear quality of the
fricative as the message-carrying feature.

It is important, of course, to use the usual ear training to identify the defectiveness of a given sound and to contrast it with the
correct sound. Then we must teach the proper production of the isolated sound, strengthening and stabilizing it. We have mentioned before that cleft-palate clients often speak very rapidly so as to conserve
the breath pressure. Slowing down the speed of utterance with
proper phrasing and breathing often produces immediate improvement in all of the articulation even when little attention is paid to the
isolated sounds.

Perhaps the most pronounced of all the ticlike mannerisms
which characterize cleft-palate speech is the nostril contraction or
flaring. This often serves as an equivalent for velar contraction, and
often prevents the latter from taking place. It is cosmetically unattractive, often interferes with the utterance of the labial plosives, and
helps to produce the snorting-snuffling which is so unpleasant in
these persons. It has no effect upon nasality or nasal emission except
to make them worse. We therefore always do as much as we can to
eliminate this habit. We first attempt to bring this nostril tic up to
consciousness, to help the client become aware of its unpleasant
stimulus value, and then through negative practice, canceling, pull-
outs, and preparatory sets to eliminate it. Usually it is responsive to
this treatment, especially when mirror work is used. In the more severe cases a nucleus of nonnostril-contraction speech can be achieved
by contracting the lips in a wide tight smile, stretching them so far
that the upper teeth are bared. The clinician must be sure that he
does not penalize contraction and thus suppress it before it is
weakened.

Many cleft-palate clients have as poor eye contact as do stutterers, a behavior which makes the speech and condition more noticeable. They also may have unusual head postures and lip bitings,

or they may cover their mouths in speaking. All these should be reduced.

Speech therapy with cleft-palate clients is usually long-term
therapy. Few of these persons show any dramatic improvement in a
short time. There are many problems to be solved and many avenues
to be explored. The work is time-consuming and often difficult. Nevertheless, we can do much to help the persons with cleft-palates
speak better.

Aphasia

Speech pathologists who work in hospital speech and hearing clinics,
or community speech and hearing centers, or in private practice find
that many of their clients come to them with the disorder called
aphasia (or more accurately, *dysphasia*). Most generally, these individuals are adults of fifty years or older (Sarno, 1969) who have suffered
a stroke or cerebral vascular accident (CVA). Some are younger persons who have been in automobile or other accidents that caused
brain damage. It has been estimated that approximately two million
Americans are handicapped to some degree as the result of strokes.
While many of those who survive this common hazard of aging
(about 200,000 die from strokes each year) they often are disastrously
handicapped as we shall see, and one of the major features of that
handicap is an impairment in the ability to use language.

The Disorder   Aphasia is the general term used for disorders of symbolization. The aphasic has difficulty in (1) formulating, (2)
comprehending, or (3) expressing *meanings*. Often there is some impairment in all of these functions. Along with these difficulties there
may be associated problems of defective articulation, inability to produce voice, and broken fluency; but the basic problem in aphasia lies
in handling *symbolic* behavior. Aphasics not only have difficulty in
speaking, they also find it difficult to read silently, to write, to comprehend the speech of others, to calculate mathematically, or even to
gesture. Let us illustrate some of this behavior in a severe case of
aphasia.

Mr. A. was fifty-five when he had his "stroke." Some blood
vessels in his brain had ruptured. As a result of this injury, his
right arm and leg became paralyzed, his face pulled to one side

a little, and he had many symptoms of aphasia. For example, he was unable to tell time even when he looked at his watch. He was still able to speak a little, but often he spoke a gibberish or his meanings were very difficult to understand. Here is how he asked for a cigarette: "Me me my . . . ah . . . go come . . . no . . . me go . . . no no no . . . um . . . suck now . . . suck, smuck, smoker . . . scum . . . oh my . . . smoker me smoker . . . oh dear . . . goddamm . . ."

And this is how he wrote to his wife. We found that this was the best of his methods for communicating, although the script was very poor because he had to use his left hand. "I want you you come now see mmy. Butter I am. (He meant "better.") I love tell John. I come well sssssn."

But Mr. A. could not write his name, not even in his checkbook, not even from copy. He could print from copy, but the letters were often reversed. He seemed unable to read and had no interest in doing so, but he spent much time looking at the pictures of an illustrated magazine and enjoyed the television. Most of the gestures, and he gestured a lot, were fairly easy to understand, but at times he would shake his head vertically when he really meant "No!"

We had known Mr. A. before his stroke and knew him as an extrovert, a pleasant, highly verbal person. He was a crack salesman for a life insurance agency. When we saw him six months after the stroke, he seemed markedly different. He cried frequently and did not seem to be able to stop crying once he had begun. Often he was profoundly depressed, confused, and withdrawn. Occasional bursts of profanity and vile language appeared in many inappropriate situations, and this behavior was very unlike his former manner.

There are some terms which are commonly used to describe some of this behavior. Mr. A.'s inability to write is termed "agraphia"; his inability to read, "alexia"; his inability to handle mathematics, "acalculia"; his jumbled sentences, "paraphasia." The inability to stop crying, the repetition of words in speaking or letters in writing is called "perseveration." His inability to remember or find a necessary word is called "anomia." Recovered aphasics tell us that often they can see the letters but that they appear to have no meaning, or they see the picture of an object but cannot tell what it is. This is termed a "visual agnosia." Or they can hear someone talking to them but cannot comprehend. The speech sounds "jumbled." This is called an "auditory agnosia." There is one other major term we must, reluctantly, provide you: "apraxia." This refers to an inability to command a part of the body to make a willed movement. An aphasic who may understand perfectly what you mean when you ask him to protrude his tongue or to pick up a pencil may not be able to command his tongue or hand to do so. Perhaps he lacks the inner speech that determines voluntary movement. At any rate, this inability to make a voluntary movement is termed "apraxia." There are many other technical words, but these are the most common.

Different aphasics show different patterns of impairment. The case we cited, Mr. A., was severely affected not only in the *expressive* and *receptive* aspects of handling meaningful symbols but also in their *formulation*. Most aphasics show some general loss in language ability, and it becomes more marked under fatigue or stress. However, certain aphasics may show their difficulty *primarily* in only one area. One of our clients after an automobile accident could speak fairly well but she could not read even a child's primer. Another could read magazines and newspapers readily but had much paraphasia in speaking.

This difficulty in comprehension is one of the major features of aphasia; and some impairment is usually present in one or another of the sense modalities, though in some patients it appears only under stress. A clear picture of this receptive disability is provided by Boone (1965):

> One man who recovered fully from aphasia described his inability to understand spoken language in this way: he knew that his wife was talking to him as he could hear her voice, but all the words she said were meaningless. When she asked him if he wanted a cup of coffee, he said it sounded like "ba boo la cakka somma ba boo?" It was without sense. When she finally poured him a cup of coffee and pointed to it, he knew immediately what she meant. The same thing was true when he tried to read the morning paper. He remembered the name "Johnson," which was the only word he could recognize. He could see the various letters and even the grouping of the letters into words, but the words didn't mean anything to him. It was like trying to read a foreign language. As he improved, he was able to understand a spoken command if it were simply stated. Then, if his wife said, "Have a cup of coffee?" he could understand it. But had she said something more complex like "The coffee pot's on the stove; why don't you let me pour you a cup?" he would not have been able to understand all that she had said.(p. 18)

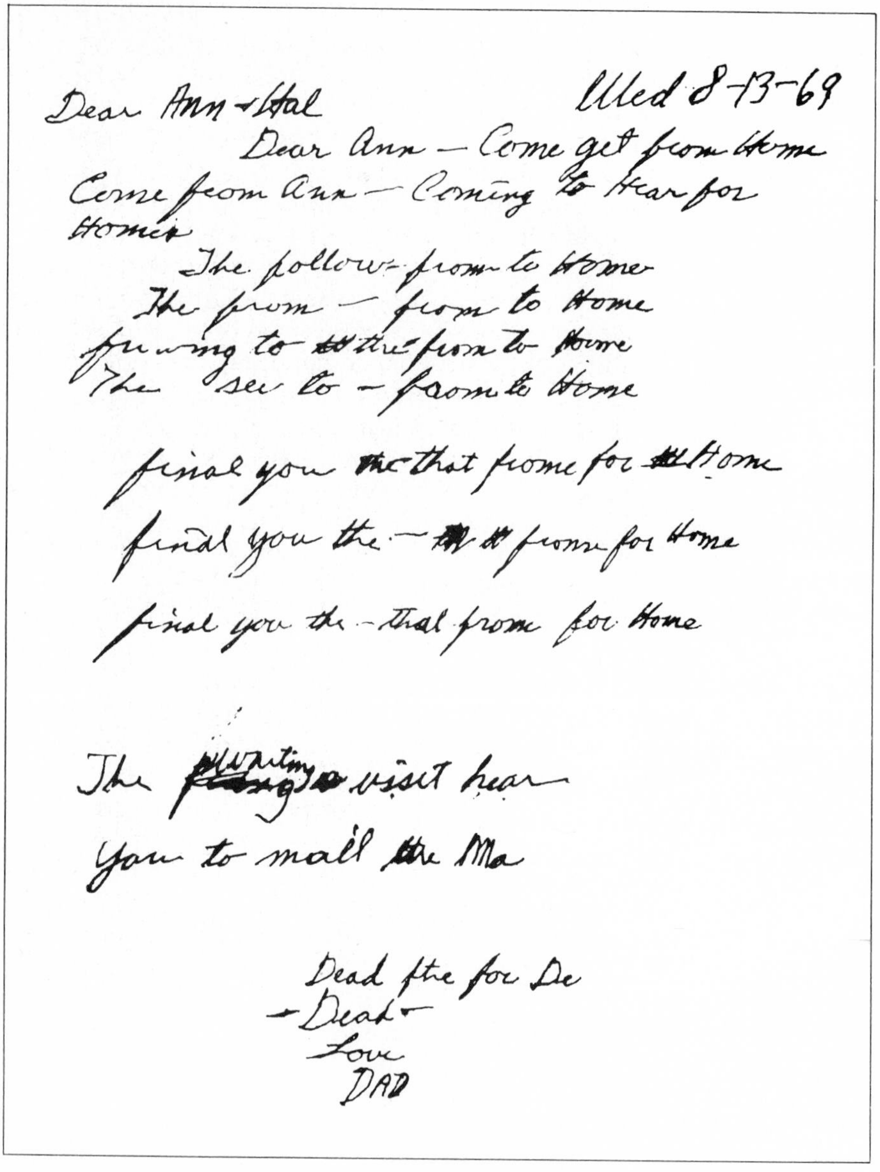
Dear Ann + Hal Wed 8-13-69

Dear Ann — Come get from Home
Come from Ann — Coming to Hear for
Home
The follow — from to Home
The from — from to Home
fruwing to the from to Home
The see to — from to Home

final you that frome for Home

final you the — from for Home

final you the — thal from for Home

The writing visit hear
you to mail the Ma

Dead the for De
— Dead —
Love
DAD

Figure 38 Letter from an aphasic father to his children.

Causes As we have said, one of the most common causes of aphasia is a cerebral vascular accident (CVA) or "stroke" that results in damage to the brain. This damage, however, may be due not only to an impairment in the blood supply to the brain, but also to tumors or to traumatic injuries that destroy brain tissue. When brain damage occurs as the result of a CVA the restricted or blocked blood flow may be due to (1) a *thrombosis* in which a blood clot forms in one of the blood vessels within the brain, or (2) an *embolism* in which a blood clot arising in some other area of the body (such as an injured limb) travels upward and lodges in one of the brain's blood vessels; or (3) a *hemorrhage* in which an essential blood vessel breaks. Most of the aphasias produced by direct head injuries result from automobile or motorcycle accidents, gunshot wounds, brain surgery, or certain diseases.

Tests for Aphasia   The first task of the speech clinician who seeks to help the person with aphasia is to determine the extent of his disability. Among the many tests that can be used to assess the language deficits are the screening tests such as Eisenson's *Examining for Aphasia* or the *Halstead-Wepman Test*. These may be used to get some general impressions of the aphasic's problem behavior. However, most clinicians agree that more comprehensive tests are necessary if an effective treatment plan is to be designed. Four of the most frequently used diagnostic tests are the *Porch Index of Communicative Ability* (PICA) (1967), Schuell's *Minnesota Test for Differential Diagnosis of Aphasia* (1965), Wepman and Jones' *The Language Modalities Test for Aphasia* (1961), and the *Boston Diagnostic Aphasia Examination* by Goodglass and Kaplan (1972).

The Porch or PICA test is a popular test that stresses a systematic presentation of ten stimuli. There are eighteen subtests designed to evaluate verbal, gestural, and graphic skills, but the major innovation is a multidimensional scoring system that replaces the more traditional right-wrong method of scoring. Thus Porch's system is based on a clinical evaluation of : *Accuracy* (the degree of correctness or rightness of a response); *Responsiveness* (the ease with which the response is elicited, especially in terms of how much information the patient requires in order to complete the task); *Completeness* (the degree to which the patient carries out the task in its entirety); *Promptness* (the presence or absence of significant delay in making a response); and *Efficiency* (the degree of facility the patient demonstrates in performing the motoric aspects of the response).

The Schuell test evaluates the aphasic's performance in five major areas: auditory disturbances; visual and reading difficulties; speech and language difficulties; visuomotor and writing disturbances, and deficits in handling mathematical concepts. A brief and incomplete outline of the subtests in each area may be illustrative.

Auditory Disturbances: The examiner evaluates the patient's abilities in recognizing common words; understanding sentences; following directions; repeating digits and sentences.

Visual and Reading Difficulties: This part examines the patient's ability to match forms, letters, pictures, and words with visual symbols, and checks for comprehension of silent and oral reading passages.

Speech and Language Difficulties: This section of the test explores the aphasic's difficulties in expressing himself in oral language. Speech movements and articulation patterns are checked, and the presence or absence of dysarthria and dyspraxia are confirmed.

Visual and Writing Difficulties: This section requires writing numbers, spelling, copying, and other such activities.

Mathematical Deficits: The testing here examines the patient's ability to handle the simple mathematical skills, knowledge of coin values, ability to tell time, and other similar skills.

The Eisenson test is less structured and is designed primarily to assess the aphasic's difficulties in reception and expression. It is primarily a screening test consisting of two parts. The first part tests auditory and visual comprehension and seeks to determine what auditory, visual, and tactile agnosias exist. In the second part of the test we find tasks that reveal nonverbal and verbal apraxias. The patient is asked to write numbers, letters, and words from dictation, to spell, to do arithmetic problems, oral reading, and clock-setting.

The *Language Modalities Test for Aphasia* (LMTA) by Wepman and Jones uses film strips to present the stimulus materials, though they are also supplemented by words spoken by the examiner. It was based upon extensive research and explores the patient's deficiencies in being able to translate from visual to oral symbols, aural to oral, aural to graphic, and visual to graphic. The test also explores the ability to do arithmetic and to comprehend language symbols. By analyzing the responses, the examiner is able to place the patient in one or another of the following types of aphasic categories: syntactic, semantic, jargon, paradigmatic, and global aphasia. A brief description of the essential characteristics of these "types" of aphasia would run as follows:

Syntactic aphasia: The person speaks telegraphically, omitting many of the function words. Often has a moderate receptive loss.

Semantic aphasia: The patient has difficulty finding or recalling the words he needs. He seems to be searching, often frantically, for these words. Some difficulty in understanding spoken messages, especially when they are long or complex.

Paradigmatic aphasia: The patient has moderate to severe problems in comprehension and thus cannot respond appropriately.

Jargon aphasia: The patient has great difficulties in auditory reception, not only for the speech of others but also for his own speech. His utterances are garbled often to such a degree that communication is impossible, and yet he does not seem to be aware of what he is saying. He thinks he's making sense.

Global aphasia: Both receptive and expressive language are so greatly impaired that the handicap is almost total. Despite this, the person often seems alert and tries to understand and to speak.

The Boston Diagnostic Aphasia Examination includes a five-factor analysis of the patient's performance on the examination. Factor I relates to reading and writing; Factor II concerns performance on spatial-quantitative-body parts tests; Factor III appears to be highly related to speech fluency; Factor IV is related to auditory comprehension; and Factor V to the presence of paraphasia. The authors, Goodglass and Kaplan, suggest that these factors are useful in identifying major types of aphasia, including Broca's aphasia, Wernick's aphasia, anomic aphasia, conduction aphasia, and transcortical aphasia. To some extent, this test is based on research in psycholinguistics.

There are other tests besides these six for diagnosing and appraising the extent of the aphasic involvement, but these are representative. Our brief description of their content should be sufficient to indicate the kinds of impairment shown by aphasics. What the tests do not show are the frustrations, anxiety, and helplessness experienced by people who have suffered a loss in the ability to handle symbols. They are lost souls. Speech pathologists must also explore these areas if they hope to help the aphasic person. The text by McKenzie Buck entitled *Dysphasia* can provide much of the needed understanding.[10]

[10] M. Buck, *Dysphasia* (Englewood Cliffs, N.J.: Prentice-Hall, Inc., 1968).

Most aphasics also show a one-sided paralysis (hemiplegia) or weakness of one arm and leg on the side opposite the brain injury, usually the right side. This may persist in some patients, but usually the patient regains the use of the leg enough to permit walking. Aphasics sometimes show *hemianopia,* a visual disturbance that makes it impossible for them to see more than half of the field of vision. Some of them have convulsions. For these reasons, no speech pathologist will work with aphasics without consultation with the physician. Some patients show personality changes, an outgoing happy person becoming despondent and moody, while others become aggressive and controlling; but usually the basic personality traits persist despite the tremendous frustration and change in self-concepts which take place. Some laugh or cry without reason. They all fatigue very easily, find it difficult to concentrate, and tend to perseverate.

> Not long ago a wife of an aphasic patient said that it was not the situation or the familiarity of the words which would determine if her husband could understand, but rather that he might fail because sudden fatigue occurred. Surely we see many of the aphasic adults performing well, and then with a sudden clogging of the circuits they are deprived of the ability to understand or to express an idea. The aphasic seems to experience sudden momentary disorganization.[11]

Prognosis　Immediately after the injury, the patient often shows a picture of extreme helplessness, but much of the impairment may subside within three or four months when what is known as "spontaneous recovery" occurs, though it is seldom complete and residual signs of aphasic disturbance can usually be found even in those who apparently have become well. Most authorities feel that spontaneous recovery seldom can be expected after six months and any improvement thereafter must be viewed as due to the relearning efforts of the patient himself or the teaching efforts of his clinicians. The younger and the more intelligent and the more motivated the person is, the better are his chances for regaining his place in a communicative world. Wise handling of these patients immediately after the injury is absolutely essential if the terrific frustration that pro-

[11] J. Simonson, "Associated Social Problems of the Aphasic Patient . . .," in C. R. Willis, (ed.) *The Vocational Rehabilitation Problems of the Patient with Aphasia* (Washington, D.C.: U. S. Dept. of Health, Education and Welfare, 1967), p. 43.

duces depression and defeatism is to be avoided. Often the attitudes of the members of the family, doctors, and nurses can create unfavorable prognoses. With professional speech therapy and the cooperation of all those who tend the patient, many individuals suffering from the milder forms of aphasia can regain much of their ability to communicate.

Treatment   In the section of this chapter devoted to diagnostic testing, the various deficits and impairments in reception, formulation, and expression were explored. In therapy we begin with those functions that have remained comparatively unaffected—we begin with what the patient can do. If he can gesture but not talk, we would start by strengthening that gesture language, then seek to attach simple verbalizations to the gestures. If he cannot write but has less difficulty in reading simple material, we would begin with reading and then later have him start copying. If there is a pronounced difficulty in word-finding, we may instead have him identify pictures or words by pointing. Or we may start with the automatic speech that remains—"How are you?" "Good morning," "bread and butter," or counting or naming the days of the week. If he has difficulties in comprehension, as most aphasics do, we make sure that we speak simply and slowly, though naturally. Aphasics are very susceptible to time pressure. We make sure that we make silence comfortable so that he has time to search. Often he may get only one or two words of a sentence we say to him, and he must have time to guess how they are related. When we repeat what we say, we wait, and then repeat it exactly so that he will not have to decode a new message when he's just beginning to comprehend the old one. We avoid abstractions as much as we can. We talk about the things related to his major interests. Discovering one day that one of our patients had been a racing buff—a fact that had not appeared in our case history or family interviews, we procured some racing forms and had him help us select the horses to win, place, and show. At first he could only point, but from this nucleus we were eventually able to help him recapture some of the speech and mathematical skills he had lost.

Aphasic therapy consists of building bridges from the things the patient can do to those he cannot do. One of the surprising features of aphasic therapy is that when the patient begins to progress in one area of his language-handling, that progress often spreads to other areas. We do not have to teach these people new skills of symbolic processing; we have to help them *find* the ones that they have lost. We have to teach them to search without becoming frantic and frustrated. Our role is that of an immensely patient guide and companion to one lost in a wilderness not of his own making.

Although it is often difficult to get the person with aphasia, so overwhelmed is he by the catastrophe of the sudden change, to accept some responsibility for his own recovery of language, it is of paramount importance that this be done. As soon as we can, therefore, we try to encourage him to do his homework, setting up the tasks which he can perform by himself or with the help of his family: copying, writing, memorizing, naming pictures in a catalog, describing, echoing — whatever is within his capacity and can be reinforced. The Language Master, which uses pre-recorded drill material, is a useful tool for this purpose, but the daily newspaper and television have been used by some of our aphasics in their determined effort to regain some of their speech and comprehension. In achieving this self-therapy, the speech pathologist must work closely with the family of the patient. As McKenzie Buck says, "Aphasia is a family illness as well as a family catastrophe." By helping the members of the family understand the nature of the problem, by helping them make the necessary adjustments, they can aid the aphasic greatly in his self-therapy.

It is very difficult to describe the treatment for aphasia in general terms because the patterns of disability vary so much from case to case. As we have said, most of our early work with these patients consists of strengthening and improving the symbolic skills which are least impaired so that they can feel that they are not helpless and hopeless but beginning to improve. But we also work hard on the whole general language disability, building foundations for improvements in all areas; and it is this that we wish to consider next.

Stimulation   The world of an aphasic must be a most confusing place. Depending upon the particular functions affected, he may hear sounds or people talking to him but be unable to comprehend them; he may pick up the morning paper and see only meaningless squiggles running across the page. He may try to write his name in his checkbook and be unable to do so. He tries to ask for a cigarette and either he cannot remember its name or he speaks gibberish. He looks at the clock and cannot tell the time. He puts his hand in his pocket and feels something but does not know that what he feels is a coin. It is a blooming, buzzing confusion without rhyme, reason, or meaning. Here and there are moments of clarity, but they flit by too swiftly or are lost in frustration and depression.

One of the major tasks of the speech pathologist is to provide islands of consistency in this sea of uncertainty. Patiently she explores her patient to determine the things he can do. Perhaps he can copy letters from the alphabet; or if he cannot, perhaps he can trace over those she provides. Very well, she begins with this activity and continues with it until he knows that this function at least is within his powers. Then she stimulates him with other things. She may have him echo her words, animal noises, or gestures. They may put their spoons in their coffee cups in unison and stir the sugar and cream. She may ask him to point predictively to which one of the objects—knife, fork, or spoon—she will use in a moment to spread his bread. She may ask him to read her lips as she stimulates him with the number "three" for the three peanuts in her hand, then help him count them aloud. She may guide his hand in writing a few sentences to his wife. She will take his hand and touch it to his nose, his ears, his mouth, his feet, saying these names as she does so. Always she uses self-talk and parallel talk in very simple words, phrases, or sentences, providing the spoken symbols for every experience, for every activity. Day after day, she reviews this patient stimulation, tolerant of failure and happy when success comes. For success will come as the confusion subsides and the aphasic begins to find the functions he has lost.

Inhibition   Brain injury makes it hard to inhibit oneself. The lower centers of the brain miss their old brakes, as we see in the frequent overflow of emotion in the form of crying and laughing spells or catastrophic responses. Perseveration continues too long. One of our aphasics, once he had begun a sentence with "I think" could not stop saying these two words, over and over, over and over, over and over. Another was unable to speak what he desired to utter because all speech attempts began with "Yes, yes, yes," and the broken record went round and round on that single word. Accordingly we train our aphasics to inhibit themselves, to stop doing what they are doing, first upon our command, and then upon their own. We train them to inhibit any attempt to speak until we give the signal, or until they tap their foot five times. We teach them to wait, to pause, to say "No more that." We give them time to reorganize. We have them wait until we smile before they try again. We ask them to rehearse silently or in a mirror or in pantomime what they are about to do or say. We have them duplicate on purpose their crying or laughing jags and to stop them when the second hand of the watch points down. For the aphasic who can read, we provide "inhibition cards" which might, for example, read as follows: "Stop laughing!" "Wait!" "Whisper first!" We have them confess and cancel the perseveration which does occur.

Translation   The aphasic often gets blocked in formulating, receiving, or sending messages because he keeps going up the same blind alley over and over again. We must teach him to shift when he meets these dead ends, to try another tack. Basic to this is translation training. By this we mean that we train the aphasic to shift from one type of symbolization to another. We may ask him to spell aloud, then print the name of the animal he hears meowing on the tape recorder. We have him count to three by the taps, again by drawing vertical lines, again by clapping hands, again by tracing the numeral, and finally by saying it. We say "Sit down!" and he must try to point to the appropriate picture, then to pantomime it with his lips silently, then to act it out, then to find the phrase on a card. We don't overwhelm him with too many translations at first; we let him lead us; but we always work to give him experiences in shifting from one set of symbolic meanings to another.

Memorization   One of the best ways of creating islands of consistency in the hurly-burly world of the aphasic is to teach him to memorize. Often we begin by having them memorize sequences of movements as in a calisthenic exercise or a sequence of lines to be drawn or the selection of a set of objects in a definite order. We demonstrate such sequences as opening the window, then closing the door, then saying "Too hot!" and then ask them to duplicate our performance. We have them find us three desired objects in a catalogue in the order in which we write them on the board. We arrange wood block letters in a row on the table so that they spell his name. We have him memorize the cards of different sizes and shapes which have written upon them such phrases as "Good morning," "Nice day," "How are you?" "Goodbye," so that he can show them to us appropriately long before he can say these things. We have him write from memory, draw from memory, using flash cards to stimulate him and varying the exposure and delay time so he succeeds more than he fails. Finally, we ask him to learn by rote such passages as this:

> I have been sick. I had a stroke. I must learn to read and write and speak again. Getting better. Takes time. Must work hard. No use feeling sorry. Get to work now.

Later on, we have the aphasic memorize poems and prose passages of increasing complexity. These not only help to provide associations between words, but also help in relearning the basic syntax of language.

Parallel Talking We emphasize stimulation with simple materials, not complex ones. We speak simply and clearly, supplementing with gesture or written or pictured materials when needed. We do a great amount of parallel talking in this stimulation, telling him, simply and in short phrases or sentences, what he is doing, feeling, or perceiving. We use not only this sort of commentary but also prediction and recall. Often, as we do this parallel talk, we find the patient will almost unconsciously join in and say a word for us on which we fumble or postpone the utterance. This technique we have come to make the basic part of our therapy. It is a bit difficult to learn to do this well, for the clinician must make sure that he does the appropriate verbalization and hesitates at exactly the moment when the patient is experiencing the thought expressed. It is also necessary to keep from making too much of the client's spontaneous utterance when it does occur under these conditions. We merely say yes, and then restimulate him with what he has spoken in the context of the entire utterance. This is especially effective with the *expressive* aphasic, but we have also used a whispered or pantomimed form of parallel talking to help those who have trouble understanding spoken speech to read our lips. Often these individuals, if they learn to pantomime the speech they *see,* can then comprehend it, and some of the auditory agnosia subsides. The wife and other associates of the patient can be taught to do much of this parallel talking. We have found it most useful.

Scanning and The aphasic is like a man who suddenly finds himself in a
Concentrating strange country. He is overwhelmed by strange sights and
sounds. He may hear people talking and be unable to understand what they are saying. He cannot write their language. He does not know what purposes some of the objects about him serve. Even a spoon is something strange. What he must do, in such a situation, is learn to observe and scan for meanings and consistencies. He must come to concentrate on things that look alike or on meaningless words which always seem to appear in the same context. Only in this way can such a person, suddenly transported to a strange land, come to find a place in it. But it is difficult for him to concentrate and diffi-

cult for him to observe closely. He needs help in scanning and concentration.

Accordingly, the clinician assists him to create order out of his
chaos by training him in sorting out things that look alike, feel alike,
sound alike. She may give him a magazine and ask him to find all
the pictures in which shoes are portrayed, to tear them out, and to
put them under one of his own shoes. She may say some words for
him and ask him to signal every time he hears one that begins with
an /s/ sound. She may have him feel a series of objects with his eyes
closed and select those which are smooth to the touch. She may work
with opposites: big things and little things; hot foods and cold foods.
She asks him to choose, to match, to classify. He needs categories.
She helps him acquire them again.

Organization   The aphasic needs order in his disordered cosmos. He needs
definite routines of daily living, consistent schedules of
events. When we come to our daily sessions with an aphasic, we use
the same greeting each time and begin our therapy with the same
sort of activity before we try something new. The other people about
him must help in this same ordering of his life so that a portion of it
will become familiar and organized rather than confused.

But he must also learn to organize his own life, his own
thoughts, and outward behaviors. He needs help in patterning his
consciousness. Accordingly we train him to make patterns of all
types. We may begin by merely asking him or showing him how to
set the table, or to turn the pages of a magazine left to right, or to arrange a few scrambled numbers in the proper order. We may have
him raise his arm in a series of gradual steps. We may ask him to
count the number of windows in the room, to draw a house, to roll a
clay model of the cigarette he cannot ask for. We give him form
boards to assemble. We give him some cards, each with a word on it,
and ask him to place them serially so they make a sentence which
commands us to do something. We get him to sing some old tunes.
We ask him to read aloud a sentence through the window of a shield
which exposes only one word at a time. We ask him to correct our
mispronunciations, our use of wrong words, his own mistakes. All
these activities require scanning and concentration. The clinician
helps, always using her self-talk and parallel talk to provide a running commentary for his thinking.

Formulation   The aphasic often has trouble not only in sending his messages or in receiving them; he also cannot formulate them
with precision. Sometimes he cannot find the exact word he needs;

and instead of searching for another almost as good, or revising the whole utterance, he stops right there, helplessly, fixed on the thorn of his frustration. Basically, what he needs is the freedom to make new wholes, to try it again in a different way, so that this different way also makes sense.[12]

Although, as we have indicated, we use self-talk and parallel talking constantly throughout all of these various approaches to therapy with the aphasic, we use these techniques with greatest effectiveness in helping him to formulate. Here is a brief excerpt from such a therapy session:

Clinician: All right, John. Let's begin. Talk to yourself. Say what you do. Like this. (*Clinician opens her purse, takes out pencil, writes his name. As she does so, she speaks in unison with her activity.*) Open purse, . . . here pencil . . . write name. (*She hands him the purse and signals him to repeat her behavior.*)

Aphasic (opens purse): Open puss . . . no . . . poos . . . no . . . oh dear oh my . . . (*gives up*).

Clinician: OK. You got mixed up on "purse" . . . Purrrrrse . . . Never mind. Say the whole thing. (*She repeats action.*)

Aphasic: Open puss . . .

Clinician: And here pencil . . .

Aphasic: Pencil . . . and now I write mame . . . no . . . mama . . . no . . .

Clinician: Write name . . . name . . . like this. (*Demonstrates.*)

Aphasic: Write name like . . . (*writes John*) . . . John . . . John . . . Write no good . . .

Clinician: Fine! You did it. Now let's do it again. Talk to yourself. Say what you're doing.

A thousand experiences of this sort, based on the experiences of daily living, cannot help but aid the patient to improve in formulation. His wife and children can easily learn to do these things. They should use simple self-talk whenever he can hear them so he knows what they are doing, perceiving, or feeling. Through parallel talking, they can put the words in his ears at the moment he needs them, thus reauditorizing his thinking and giving them the verbal symbols that have become lost or scrambled. Sooner or later, the aphasic will begin to talk to himself as he does things, sees things, or feels things. This should be highly rewarded by all about him. He may even begin

---

[12] For some aphasias, the use of melodic intonation therapy (MIT) is effective. This approach involves the use of specified melody patterns in attempts to get aphasics to encode phrases and sentences (Sparks and Holland, 1976) that include humming the sentence, tapping the rhythm, or intoning the desired response.

to use parallel talk as he views the behavior of others. We have found no difficulty in having this vocalized thinking persist in appropriate situations because later, as he becomes facile in their use, we have him learn to do his self-talk and parallel talking in a whisper or in pantomime.

We may also help him to formulate in other ways. We ask him to complete unfinished figures, to assemble toys, to repair a broken electric cord, to weave a rug, to complete the writing of unfinished sentences, to prewrite what he is about to say, or to rehearse it in pantomime. We have him do simple description and exposition on paper or aloud. We teach him to fill in the hands of a series of blank clock faces to indicate the hours. We teach him to make change; to do mental arithmetic, or if he cannot do so, to do the operations on paper. We give him simple problems to solve. We teach him to paraphrase, to tell us what he has read in the paper or heard on the radio. The fascinating thing about all of this is to discover how each new achievement seems to unlock the doors to new achievements. If this clinician could begin over again, he would specialize in aphasia.

Body Image Integration   It is not only the outside world which is strange to the aphasic. He also is a stranger to himself. He has changed. He is not the person he used to be. The various members of his family often show this by their reactions. They treat him like a child or as a nuisance or as though he were an imbecile. Good counseling can prevent much of this, but it is difficult for a family to become adjusted to a handicapped stranger in the house.

We have said that the aphasic is also a stranger to himself. Often there is paralysis of the arm or leg. A part of him will not obey his bidding; he has suddenly sprouted a dead limb. Any one of us who has lain too long on an arm in bed and awakes to find it "gone to sleep," a strange and inert thing there in bed with him, will vaguely understand how important this experience must be. But there are a thousand other changes in the person too. He has trouble reading, writing, talking, telling time, comprehending, counting. Who is this person who suddenly has come to inhabit his skin? It is the clinician's job to help him become acquainted, to introduce him to his new self and to get him to like this new person. It isn't easy but it can be done.

We begin by introducing him to his body. We massage his feet and name them as we do so. We lift his arm and tell him what we are doing. We have him stroke his face and find his eyes and ears and mouth. We get him to move his lips and his tongue as we do. We do much of our work with the body image in front of the mirror. We command the helpless hand to squeeze on the exercise ball, and we squeeze it. We take his picture in all sorts of therapeutic activities and show them to him. We look together in old albums at the snapshots of his childhood and youth. Perhaps all the king's horses couldn't do it, but a good clinician can put Humpty Dumpty together again.

Psychotherapy   It should be obvious by now that these patients need psycho-
therapy. They meet many penalties, experience frustrations so intense they would break up almost any physically normal person. They find their cups overflowing with anxiety, guilt, and hostility. They worry about the hospital bills, about the paycheck that is no more, about their possible future in a nursing home. They become furious with anger, often over trifles. And yet, fortunately, the same brain injury that creates these storms of emotion also makes them transient. They do not last, do not reverberate. Furious one moment, the next moment he is laughing.

Such an outline of therapeutic activities is far from being comprehensive, but it may provide a starting platform. It does not indicate how the clinician works especially on the functions of one area in which progress seems most likely to occur. And it does not show, except by implication, the need for ingenuity and, above all, the patient perseverance needed to rehabilitate these persons. Personally, we have found our work with aphasics to be more fascinating and rewarding than that with many other communicative disabilities. This is true not only with children with aphasia but also with the many adults who have been brought to us for help. To see a person who has been stricken down at the entrance to the valley of death rejoin the human race, and to feel that perhaps you have had a humble part in that rejoining, is reward enough for all the failures and frustrations aphasia therapy brings.

Cerebral Palsy

All those who work with physically handicapped children or adults will encounter the disorder of cerebral palsy. Certainly the speech pathologist will meet them often, for many persons with this handicap show some difficulty in speaking. All of the dimensions of speech, articulation, language, voice, and fluency may present abnormalities of greater or lesser degrees. A few individuals, less involved, may be able to speak fairly normally but those whose ability to communicate is markedly impaired are in urgent need of the kind of services speech pathologists can offer. Seldom do they work alone. Although cerebral palsy is basically a motor disorder, it may be accompanied by perceptual, learning, social, and other disabilities requiring a team approach. As a member of the rehabilitation team, the speech pathologist therefore finds himself working closely with special education teachers, physical and occupational therapists, pediatricians, orthopedists, and many other specialists. Therefore, it is important that he understand the nature of the group of disorders that are classified under the general label of cerebral palsy.

Varieties of Cerebral Palsy Disorders Although the term *spastic paralysis* has come to be used as the popular designation for all types of cerebral-palsy cases, there seem to be four major varieties: the athetoid, the ataxic, the myasthenic, and the spastic. Usually more than one of these four symptom complexes are found in the same case. According to Phelps the athetoid and spastic varieties make up more than 80 percent of all cases.

Spasticity itself has been defined as the paralysis due to simultaneous contraction of antagonistic or reciprocal muscle groups accompanied by a definite degree of hypertension or hypertonicity. It is due to a lesion or injury in the pyramidal nerve tracts. The muscles overcontract; they pull too hard and too suddenly. Slight stimuli will set off major contractions. The spastic who tries to move his little finger may jerk not only the hand, but the arm or trunk as well. The spastic may have a characteristic manner of walking—the typical "scissors gait." The hands may be clenched and curled up along the wrists in their extreme contraction, or the whole arm may be drawn upward and backward along the neck. The spastic tends to contract his chest muscles and thus enlarge the thoracic cavity during the act of speaking, which compels him in turn to compress the abdomen excessively in order to force out some air. He thus may be said to inhale with the thorax at the same time that he exhales with the abdomen. Great tension is thereby produced and this reflects itself in muscular abnormality all over the body. It also shows up in speech in the form of unnatural pauses and gasping and weak or aphonic voice. Many of the "breaks" in the spastic's speech are due to this form of faulty breathing.

Since it is difficult for the spastic to make gradual and smooth movements, the speech is often explosive and blurting. Often the extreme tension that characterizes spasticity will produce articulatory contacts so hard as to resemble or engender stuttering symptoms. The sounds involving complex coordinations are, of course, usually defective; and the tongue tip sounds which make contact with the upper-gum ridge are very difficult. Where there is some facial paralysis, the labial sounds are much more difficult than might be expected. In cases where there are both symptoms of spasticity and athetosis, the articulation is prone to be more distorted than if spasticity alone is present. Finally, the diadochokinetic rate of tongue-lifting is a pretty good indication of the number of articulation errors to be found in any one case.

Cerebral-palsy cases are also classified in terms of how much of the body is affected. If one limb is spastic or athetoid, the term *monoplegia* is used; if half the body (right or left) is affected, the word *hemiplegia* designates the condition. *Diplegia* refers to involvement of both upper *or* both lower limbs; *quadriplegia* to spasticity or athetosis in all four limbs. The greatest number of articulatory errors are shown in quadriplegia involving combined athetosis and spasticity, and the fewest errors are evidenced in spastic diplegia.

By *athetosis* we refer to the cerebral-palsy cases with marked tremors. Athetosis may be described as a series of involuntary contractions that affect one muscle after another. These contractions may be fast or slow, large or small. The head may swing from side to side. The arm may shake rhythmically. The jaw and facial muscles may show a rhythmic contortion or repetitive grimaces but in some athetoids, these movements disappear in sleep or under the influence of alcohol. There seem to be two major types of athetoids, the nontension type and the tension athetoid, who is often mistaken for a true spastic. The tension athetoids are those who have tried to hold their trembling arms and legs still by using so much tension that it has become habitual. The latter may be distinguished from true spastics by moving their arms against their resistance. The tension athetoid's arm tends to yield gradually; the spastic's releases with a jerk.

Athetoid speech often becomes weak in volume. The final sounds of words and final words of phrases are often whispered. A marked tremulo is heard. Monotones are very common, and in the tension athetoids the habitual pitch is near the upper limit of the range. Falsetto voice qualities are not unusual. Another common voice quality is that of hoarseness, especially in the males. Like the true spastics, athetoids make many articulation errors; and the finer the coordination involved in producing the sound, the more it is likely to be distorted. Tongue-tip sounds are especially difficult. Breathing disturbances are common.

Other Varieties of Cerebral Palsy   The other subvarieties of cerebral palsy are encountered only rarely. *Ataxia* manifests itself mainly in a lack of ability to balance oneself or to coordinate the muscles and these appear to have a low tonicity. Ataxic speech is slurred and arhythmical. This condition seems to be due to a lesion in the cerebellum. In myasthenia or flaccid paralysis we find the same weakness of the muscles but no primary loss of balance. Also, a variety of cerebral palsy which is marked most conspicuously by sustained tremor is occasionally seen. The student should understand that many of these features may appear in any one individual and that few pure types exist, although the spastic variety tends to show more consistency.

Causes of Cerebral Cerebral palsy is due to a brain injury occurring before birth
Palsy Disorders (prenatal), at the time of birth (paranatal), or at any time after birth (postnatal). The prenatal injuries may be due to the mother's suffering from rubella (measles), toxemia, or physical trauma. Paranatal causes may include difficult or prolonged labor, anoxia, instrument injuries, among others. Later in life certain diseases marked by very high fever such as pneumonia and meningitis can also result in cerebral palsy, and every war produces its share of such victims due to gunshot wounds in the head. We also find instances of cerebral palsy resulting from severe automobile accidents or from adult neurological disorders such as Huntington's Disease.

Intelligent cerebral-palsied individuals meet so many frustrations during their daily lives that they tend to build emotional handicaps as great as their physical disabilities. Fears develop about walking, talking, eating, going downstairs, carrying a tray, holding a pencil, and a hundred other daily activities. These often become so intense that they create more tensions and hence more spasticity or athetosis. Thus one girl so feared to lift a coffee cup to her lips that she could not do so without spilling and breaking it, yet she was able to etch delicate tracings on a copper dish.

Many of these children are so pampered and protected by their parents that they never have an opportunity to learn the skills required of them for social living. Their parents are constantly afraid that they will hurt themselves, but as one adult tension athetoid said to us, "My parents never let me try to ride a bicycle and now at last I've done it. Better to break your neck than your spirit." Many spastics come to a fatalistic attitude of passive acceptance of whatever blows, kindnesses, or pity society may give them. Others put up a gallant battle and succeed in creating useful and satisfying lives for themselves.

Speech Therapy Very often the cerebral-palsied child is first presented as a case of delayed speech. These children often do not begin to talk until five or six, but many of them could learn earlier with proper parental teaching. In general, the same procedures used on other delayed-speech cases and in teaching the baby to talk are employed.[13] Imitation must be taught. Sounds must come to have meaning and identity. Words must be taught in terms of their sound sequences and associations. Babbling games using puppets are especially effective in getting a young spastic child to talk. It is especially necessary that the child be praised for all vocalization, since he is likely to fall into a whispered or mere lip-moving type of speech. When possible, the first speech teaching should be done when the child is lying on his back in bed. Phonograph records with singing and speech games are very useful in stimulating these children.

In most cases of cerebral palsy the physiotherapist and occupational therapist will have done a great deal of work with the child before the speech pathologist is called in. Many of the activities used in physiotherapy can be made more interesting to the child if vocalization is used in conjunction with them. Thus one child whose very spastic left leg was being passively rotated in a whirlpool bath was taught to say "round and round; round and round" as the leg moved. He was unable to say these words at first under any other condition; but soon he had attained the ability to say them anywhere, and the distraction seemed to ease some of the spasticity. In some programs, general relaxation of the whole body forms a large part of the treatment of the spastic and tension athetoid, and even these exercises may be combined with sighing or yawning on the various vowels. Relaxation of the articulatory or the throat muscles seems to be very difficult for these cases, and we often indirectly attain decreases in the tension of these structures by teaching the child to speak while chewing.

Among several interesting new approaches to the treatment of the cerebral palsy is that advocated by the Bobaths. Instead of using the traditional methods to induce general relaxation, the Bobath method, essentially a physical therapy approach, seeks first to inhibit the pathological reflex activity by holding the child firmly in a posture that prevents the usual abnormal motor activity. Then the primitive but normal reflexes are stimulated and facilitated, and finally, voluntary motor control is evoked. Some very surprising changes occur when this sequence is successfully carried out. We have seen young cerebral-palsied children who were thrashing around and unable to produce anything but strangled bursts of tortured vocalization become quiet and relaxed and able to babble normally when treated by a skillful Bobath practitioner.[14]

[13] The urgent need to give the cerebral-palsied child some useful language as early as possible is well described by T. Trombly, "Linguistic Concepts and the Cerebral Palsied Child." *Cerebral Palsy Journal*, XXIX (1968), 7–8.
[14] The book by Marie Crickmay, *Speech Therapy and the Bobath Approach to Cerebral Palsy* (Springfield, Ill.: Charles C. Thomas, 1966) presents a clear picture of this kind of treatment.

SUPINE POSITIONS DESIGNED TO BREAK UP REFLEX PATTERNS OF EXTENSION

PRONE POSITIONS DESIGNED TO BREAK UP REFLEX PATTERNS OF FLEXION

➡ = force applied to counteract reflex.

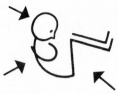

1. A position of total flexion—diametrically opposed to reflex patterns of extension.

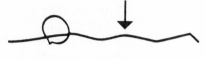

1. A position of total extension—diametrically opposed to reflex patterns of flexion.

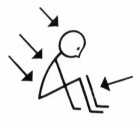

2. A position introducing some extension (of spine and arms) but flexion of neck, hips and knees.

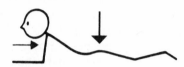

2. A position introducing some flexion (of elbows) but with spine and hips still extended.

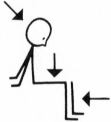

3. A position introducing greater extension, but controlled so as not to provoke former reflex pattern of total extension.

3. A position introducing greater flexion of hips and knees, but with spine and arms extended.

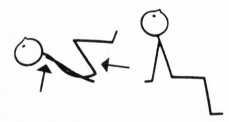

BEST POSITIONS IN WHICH TO REACH THE SOUNDS OF "K" AND "G"

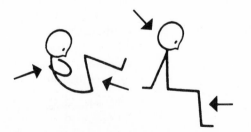

BEST POSITIONS IN WHICH TO REACH THE SOUNDS OF "T" "D" "L" "S" "Z"

Figure 39 Reflex-inhibiting patterns for cerebral palsy. (Bobath)

Some speech pathologists work closely with physical therapists using the Rood technique. This involves a systematic sequence of stimulation and relaxation of the muscular groups required for more effective coordination. By using such tools as ice, brushes, and other surface stimulators to stimulate or relax certain muscles, patterns of more normal motor behaviors can be developed. We have witnessed some remarkable improvement when these are introduced and reinforced. Articulation and voice changes resulting from the joint efforts of the speech pathologist and physical therapist working together in the application of these techniques are often very impressive.

Rhythms of all kinds seem to provide especially favorable media for speech practice, if the rhythms are given at a speed which suits the particular case. In following these rhythms it is not wise to combine speech with muscular movements because of the nature of the disability. Visual stimuli such as the rhythmic swinging of a flashlight beam on a wall are very effective in producing more fluent speech. Tonal stimuli of all kinds are also used. Many cerebral-palsied children can utter polysyllabic words in unison with a recurrent melody whether they sing them or not.

In general, the spastic's articulation disorder is of the lalling type. Most of the sounds that require lifting of the tongue tip are defective. When the /t/, /d/, and /n/ sounds are adequate, it will be observed that they are dentalized. The tongue does not make contact with the upper-gum ridge but with the back surface of the teeth or it may be protruded. Several of these cases were able to acquire good /l/ and /r/ sounds without any direct teaching. Instead, we taught them to make the /t/, /d/, and /n/ sounds against the upper-gum ridge, and the tongue-tip lifting carried over into the /l/ and /r/ sounds immediately.

In most of these cases, the essential task is to free the tongue from its tendency to move only in conjunction with the lower jaw. The old traditional tongue exercises have little value, but those that involve the emergence of a finer movement from a gross one are very useful. Just as we have been able to teach spastics to pick up a pin by beginning with trunk, arm, and wrist movements, so we can finally teach him to move his tongue tip without closing his mouth.

Phonetic placement methods in the teaching of new sounds are seldom successful. The auditory stimulation and modification of known sounds are much better. Babbling practice has great value in making the new sounds habitual. We have found that it is wise to make a set of tape recordings for each case that provides him with material appropriate to his level and with which he can speak in unison when alone.

It should be obvious that no speech pathologist can hope to solve the many problems of giving the cerebral-palsied child usable speech unless the parents and other professional members help in the process. Much of the work of the speech clinician will involve demonstration and consultation. We cannot simply tell others how to facilitate speech. We must show them. In turn, in our work we also must reinforce the treatment being provided by other members of the team.

At times one of the major obstacles in achieving useful speech in the cerebral-palsied person is the inability to produce voice without great struggle. When he tries to talk, he may exert great physical effort; and this may induce closures of both the true and false vocal folds. So we rarely work directly on voice production for this reason. Instead, we try to combine sounds and movements, or we vibrate the child's chest with our hands as he is vocally exhaling and as we stimulate him with pleasant sounds. We do a lot of singing and humming in our early speech therapy with these children, making speech pleasant, making sound production desirable. Often the breathing of the cerebral-palsied child shows great abnormality, especially when he tries to produce speech. He may inhale far too deeply, then exhale most of this air prior to speech attempt or in the utterance of just one syllable, and then strain from that time onward. He may even try to speak while inhaling, an activity which will evoke strain even in a normal speaker. These persons must be trained to eliminate these faulty procedures.

The breaks in fluency which are so characteristic of the spastic are often eliminated by this training but it is usually wise to teach these children a type of phrasing that will not place too much demand upon them for sustained utterance. The pauses must be much more frequent than those of the normal individual, and they should be slightly longer. Thus the sentence: "Practice about thirty words involving the /s/ blends according to the following models" might be spoken as a single unit by an adult normal speaker, but the adult cerebral-palsy case should pause for a new breath at least three or four times during its course. If he trains himself to speak short phrases on one breath, his fluency will improve. Moreover, since no untimely gasps for breath will occur, his voice will be less likely to rise in pitch, or to be strained, and the final sounds of the words will be better articulated.

Fluency may be improved also by giving the child training in making smooth transitions between vowels or consecutive consonants. Thus, he is asked to practice shifting gradually rather than suddenly from a prolonged /u/ to a prolonged /i/ sound to produce the word *we*. At first, breaks are likely to occur, but they can be greatly improved through practice; and the child's general speech reflects the improvement. Again the plosives often cause breaks in rhythm because the contacts are made too hard and consequently set up tremors. We have had marked success in treating these errors with the same methods we use for the stutterer's hard contacts. In one case, who always "stuck" on his /p/, /t/, and /k/ sounds and showed breaks in his speech, we were able to solve the problem by simply asking him "to keep his mouth in motion" whenever he said a word beginning with these sounds.

It is, of course, necessary to supplement this speech therapy with a great deal of informal psychotherapy, especially in adult cerebral-palsied individuals. They must be taught an objective attitude toward their disorder. They must whittle down the emotional fraction of their total handicap; they must increase their assets in every way. As fear and shame diminish, the tensions will decrease. In many cases, greater improvement in speech and muscular coordination will come from psychotherapy than from the speech therapy itself.

The Severely Impaired   There are some clients with such severe cerebral palsy or other motor disabilities such as those due to paralysis that the acquisition of intelligible speech is virtually impossible. Despite years of competent professional help, they lack the motor control needed for effective oral communication. In such cases, it is both appropriate and defensible for the speech clinician to help the speechless client communicate through nonverbal means. Several approaches have been devised for this purpose and the advanced form of one of them is illustrated in Figure 40. Sometimes the person can only point to the appropriate picture on the language board by flailing at it with his fists. At other times, for this pointing he may be able to use a headstick such as that illustrated on the right of the figure. Many other ingenious devices and techniques have been invented to help these speechless individuals communicate. The basic requirement, of course, is the handicapped person's ability to indicate a picture, letter, word, or symbol that codes the meaning of his message. The signalling can be done through the use of electronic switches coupled to breathing or head, eye, arm, or trunk movements, even to the slight tensing of a muscle that doesn't move. It is only necessary that the handicapped individual has one movement or signal that he can use *consistently* to indicate yes or no.

Communication boards of various types have been designed to aid in the communicative process. For those who cannot even point, the desired picture symbol or word may be located by scanning first the horizontal and then the vertical columns, the client indicating by his yes or no signal which one contains the item needed. Very simple boards are used at first and more complicated ones later. One of those which has gained acceptance uses the Bliss symbols rather than pictures. Although the symbols at first appear rather abstract, they seem to be easily learned and can be combined together to express more exact meanings. Moreover, since the word represented by the symbol is printed underneath it, many severely handicapped children learn to read this way, and other people who do not know the system can use the printed words to communicate with them.[15]

All members of the healing professions will encounter these clients sooner or later. Certainly the speech pathologist will, and when he does he must remember that effective communication is his goal, not simply better speech.

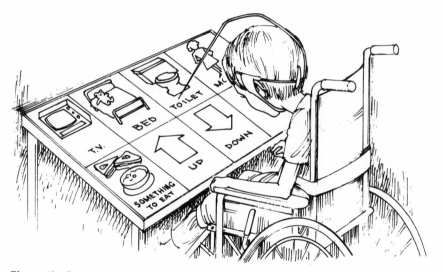

Figure 40 Communication aids for the severely handicapped.

[15] For further information concerning communication therapy for the severely handicapped see the references by Lloyd (1976), Dixon and Curry (1973), McDonald and Schultz (1973), and the very useful book by E. T. McDonald, S. McNaughton, D. Harris-Vanderheiden, and G. C. Vander-Reiden, *Non-vocal Communication Techniques and Aids for the Severely Handicapped,* (Baltimore: University Park Press, 1976). This last text describes the Bliss symbols.

References (Laryngectomy)

BERLIN, C. I. "Clinical Measurement During the Acquisition of Esophageal Speech." *Journal Speech and Hearing Disorders,* XXVIII (1963), 42–51.

DABRIEL, B. *The Laryngectomee.* Danville, Ill.: Interstate, 1973.

DAMSTE, P. H. and J. W. LEHRMAN. *An Introduction to Voice Pathology.* Springfield, Ill.: Charles C. Thomas, 1975.

DIEDRICH, W. and K. YOUNGSTROM. *Alaryngeal Speech.* Springfield, Ill.: Charles C. Thomas, 1966.

GARDNER, W. H. *Laryngectomee Speech and Rehabilitation.* Springfield, Ill.: Charles C. Thomas, 1971.

GATELY, G. "A Technique for Teaching the Laryngectomized to Trap Air for the Production of Esophageal Speech." *Journal Speech Hearing Disorders,* XXXVI (1971), 486–95.

HAUSER, P. "The Talking Frog of Marion County." *Journal of Speech Disorders,* XII (1947), 8–10.

KEITH, R. L. *A Handbook for the Laryngectomee.* Danville, Ill.: Interstate, 1974.

——, J. C. EWERT, and C. R. FLOWERS. "Factors Influencing the Learning of Esophageal Speech." *British Journal Disorders Communication,* IX (1974), 110–16.

LAUDER, E. "The Laryngectomee and the Artificial Larynx: A Second Look." *Journal Speech Hearing Disorders,* XXXV (1970), 62–65.

MARSHALL, R. C. "Conversion from Asai to Esophageal Speech." *Journal Speech Hearing Disorders,* XXXVII (1972), 262–66.

MARTIN, H. "Rehabilitation of the Laryngectomee." *Cancer,* XVI (1963), 323–41.

McCROSKEY, R. L. and M. MULLIGAN. "The Relative Intelligibility of Esophageal Speech and Artificial Larynx." *Journal Speech and Hearing Disorders,* XXVIII (1963), 37–41.

PALMER, J. M. "Clinical Expectations in Esophageal Speech." *Journal Speech Hearing Disorders,* XXXV (1970), 160–69.

PETERSON, H. A. "A Case Report of Speech and Language Training for a Two-Year-Old Laryngectomized Child." *Journal Speech and Hearing Disorders,* XXXVIII (1973), 275–78.

SNIDECOR, J. (ed.) *Speech Rehabilitation of the Laryngectomized.* (2nd ed.) Springfield, Ill.: C. C. Thomas, 1969.

SNIDECOR, J. C. "Speech Without a Larynx." in L. E. Travis (ed.) *Handbook of Speech Pathology and Audiology.* Englewood Cliffs, N.J.: Prentice-Hall, Inc., 1971.

WEINBERG, B. and J. WESTERHOUSE. "A Study of Pharyngeal Speech." *Journal Speech Hearing Disorders,* XXXVIII (1973), 111–18.

ZWITMAN, D. H. and T. C. CALCATERRA. "Phonation Using the Tracheo-Esophageal Shant After Total Laryngectomy." *Journal Speech Hearing Disorders,* XXXVIII (1973), 369–73.

References (Cleft Palate)

ARAMANY, M. A. "A History of Prosthetic Management of Cleft Palate: Pare to Suersen." *Cleft Palate Journal,* VIII (1971), 415–30.

399

BLAKELY, R. W. "The Complementary Use of Speech Prostheses and Pharyngeal Flaps in Palatal Insufficiency." *Cleft Palate Journal*, I (1964), 194–98.

BLOCKSMA, R., C. A. LEUZ, and J. H. BEERMINK. "A Study of Deformity Following Cleft Palate Repair in Patients with Normal Lip and Alveolus." *Cleft Palate Journal*, XIII (1973), 390–99.

BZOCH, K. R. (ed.) *Communicative Disorders Related to Cleft Lip and Palate*. Boston: Little, Brown & Co., 1972.

CHASE, R. A. and R. P. JOBE. "Rehabilitation Literature of the Forgotten Cleft Child." *Rehabilitation Record*, X (1969), 10–14.

COCCARO, P. J. "Orthodontics in Cleft-Palate Children: A Continuing Process." *Cleft Palate Journal*, VI (1969), 495–505.

DENES, P. B. and E. N. PINSON. *The Speech Chain*. Baltimore: Bell Telephone Laboratories, 1966.

DRILLIAN, C. M., T. T. S. INGRAM, and E. M. WILKINSON. *The Causes and Natural History of Cleft Lip and Palate*. Baltimore: Williams and Wilkins Co., 1966.

FALK, M. L. (ed.) *A Cleft Palate Team Addresses the Speech Clinician*. Springfield, Ill.: Charles C. Thomas, 1971.

GRABB, W. C., S. W. ROSENSTEIN, and K. R. BZOCH. (eds.) *Cleft Lip and Palate: Surgical, Dental and Speech Aspects*. Boston: Little, Brown & Co., 1971.

IRWIN, E. C. and B. J. McWILLIAMS. "Play Therapy for Children with Cleft Palates." *Children Today*, III (1974), 18–22.

KERMAN, P. C., L. SOSNOW, and A. DAVIDOFF. "Palatal Lift and Speech Therapy for Velopharyngeal Incompetence." *Archives of Physical Medicine*, LIV (1973), 271–76.

LUBIT, E. C. and R. E. LARSEN. "A Speech Aid for Velopharyngeal Incompetency." *Journal Speech Hearing Disorders*, XXXVI (1971), 61–70.

McDONALD, E. T. *Bright Promise*. Chicago: National Society for Crippled Children and Adults, 1959.

MIRZA, F. D. "Treatment of Velopharyngeal Incompetence by Prosthesis and Speech Therapy." *Journal Indian Dental Association*, XLIV (1972), 51–56.

MORLEY, M. *Cleft Palate and Speech*. (6th ed.) Baltimore: Williams and Wilkins, 1967.

SHELTON, RALPH, A. PAESANI, KEENER McCLELLAND, and SHARI BRADFIELD. "Panendoscopic Feedback in the Study of Voluntary Velpharyngeal Movements." *Journal Speech Hearing Disorders*, XL (1975), 232–44.

SMITH, J. K. "Contraindications for Speech Therapy for Cleft-Palate Speakers." *Cleft Palate Journal*, VI (1969), 202–4.

SPRIESTERSBACH, D. C. and D. SHERMAN. (eds.) *Cleft Palate and Communication*. New York: Academic Press, 1968.

STARK, R. B. (ed.) *Cleft Palate: A Multidisciplinary Approach*. New York: Harper & Row, 1968.

WEISS, C. E. "The Speech Pathologists Role in Dealing with Obturator-Wearing School Children." *Journal Speech Hearing Disorders*, XXXIX (1974), 153–62.

WELLS, C. *Cleft Palate and Its Associated Speech Disorders*. New York: McGraw-Hill Book Company, 1971.

WESTLAKE, H. and D. RUTHERFORD. *Cleft Palate*. Englewood Cliffs, N.J.: Prentice-Hall, Inc., 1966.

WILLIS, C. R. and M. L. STUTZ. "The Clinical Use of the Taub Panendoscope in the Observation of Velopharyngeal Function." *Journal Speech Hearing Disorders,* XXXVII (1972), 495–502.

YULES, R. B. and R. D. CHASE. "Pharyngeal Flap Surgery: A Review of the Literature." *Cleft Palate Journal,* VI (1969), 303–8.

References (Aphasia)

AURELIA, J. C. *Aphasia Therapy Manual.* Danville, Ill.: Interstate, 1974.

BANNATYNE, A. "Speech and Language Rehabilitation: A Workbook for the Neurologically Impaired." *Journal Learning Disabilities,* VII (1974), 269–70.

BELT, L. H. "Working with Dysphasic Patients." *American Journal Nursing,* LXXIV (1974), 1320–22.

BIXBY, L. "Comeback from a Brain Operation." *Harper's Magazine,* Nov. 1952, 69–73.

BOONE, D. R. *An Adult Has Aphasia.* Danville, Ill.: Interstate, 1965.

BUCK, M. *Dysphasia.* Englewood Cliffs, N.J.: Prentice-Hall, Inc., 1968.

CULTON, G. L. "Spontaneous Recovery from Aphasia." *Journal Speech Hearing Research,* XII (1969), 825–32.

DARLEY, F. L. "The Effect of Language Rehabilitation on Aphasia." *Journal Speech Hearing Disorders,* XXXVII (1972), 3–21.

DUBNER, H. "The Role of the Speech Pathologist in the Early Treatment of the Aphasic Patient." *Rehabilitation Literature,* XXXIII (1972), 330–31, 338.

EISENSON, J. *Adult Aphasia: Assessment and Treatment.* Englewood Cliffs, N.J.: Prentice-Hall, Inc., 1973.

—— *Aphasia in Children.* New York: Harper & Row, 1972.

—— *Examining for Aphasia.* New York: Psychological Corporation, 1954.

FRANK, S. "Patricia Neal: Suddenly I Wanted to Live." *Good Housekeeping,* July, 1967, 70.

GARGAN, W. *Why Me?* New York: Doubleday & Co. Inc., 1969.

GOODGLASS, N. and E. KAPLAN. *The Assessment of Aphasia and Related Disorders.* Philadelphia: Lee and Febiger, 1972.

HALL, W. A. "Return from Silence—A Personal Experience." *Journal Speech Hearing Disorders,* XXVI (1961), 174–77.

HALSTEAD, W. C. and J. M. WEPMAN. *Manual for the Halstead-Wepman Screening Test for Aphasia.* Chicago: University of Chicago Clinics, 1949.

HODGINS, E. *Episode: Report on the Accident Inside My Skull.* New York: Atheneum, 1964.

HOLLAND, A. L. "Some Current Trends in Aphasia Rehabilitation." *Asha,* (1969) 3–7.

—— "Case Studies in Aphasia Rehabilitation Using Programmed Instruction." *Journal Speech Hearing Disorders,* XXXV (1970), 377–90.

KEENAN, J. S. *A Procedure Manual In Speech Pathology with Brain-damaged Adults.* Danville, Ill.: Interstate, 1975.

KEENAN, J. and E. BRASSELL. "A Study of Factors Related to Prognosis for Individual Aphasic Patients." *Journal Speech Hearing Disorders,* XXXIX (1974), 257–69.

KNOX, D. R. *Portrait of Aphasia.* Detroit: Wayne State University Press, 1971.

LECHE, P. "Speech Therapy with Adult Brain-damaged Patients." *Occupational Therapy,* XXXI (1968), 20–21.

LURIA, A. *The Man with a Shattered World.* New York: Basic Books, 1972.

MALONE, R. L. "Expressed Attitudes of Families of Aphasics." *Journal Speech Hearing Disorders,* XXXIV (1969), 146–51.

McBRIDE, C. *Silent Victory.* Chicago: Nelson-Hall, 1969.

MONTGOMERY, J. "The Importance of Seeing Red; Self-Teaching Techniques for Adult Aphasia." *Journal Speech Hearing Disorders,* XXXVI (1971), 250–1.

MORLEY, M. E. "Receptive/Expressive Developmental Aphasia." *British Journal Disorders Communication,* VIII (1973), 47–53.

PORCH, B. *Porch Index of Communicative Ability.* Palo Alto, Calif.: Consulting Psychologists, 1967.

ROLNICK, M. and H. R. HOOPS. "Aphasia as Seen by the Aphasic." *Journal Speech Hearing Disorders,* XXXIV (1969), 48–53.

RONSENBEK, JOHN C., MARGARET LEMME, MARGERY AHERN, ELIZABETH HARRIS, and ROBERT WERTZ. "A Treatment for Apraxia of Speech in Adults." *Journal Speech Hearing Disorders,* XXXVIII (1973), 462–72.

ROSE, R. "A Physician's Account of His Own Aphasia." *Journal Speech Hearing Disorders,* XIII (1948), 294–305.

SARNO, J. E. and M. T. SARNO. *Stroke: The Condition and the Patient.* New York: McGraw-Hill Book Company, 1969.

SARNO, M. T. *Aphasia: Selected Readings.* Englewood Cliffs, N.J.: Prentice-Hall, Inc., 1972.

SCHUELL, H. *The Minnesota Test for Differential Diagnosis of Aphasia.* (rev. ed.). Minneapolis: University of Minnesota Press, 1965.

SEFER, J. and H. SCHUELL. "A Year of Aphasia Therapy: A Case Study." *British Journal of Disorders of Communication,* IV (1969), 73–82.

SIES, L. F. and R. BUTLER. "Personal Account of Dysphasia." *Journal Speech Hearing Disorders,* XXVIII (1963), 261–66.

SMITH, A. "Objective Indices of Severity of Chronic Aphasia in Stroke Patients." *Journal Speech Hearing Disorders,* XXXVI (1971), 167–207.

SPARKS, R. W. and A. L. HOLLAND. "Method: Melodic Intonation Therapy for Aphasia." *Journal Speech Hearing Disorders,* 41 (1976), 287–97.

SPARKS, R., N. HELM, and M. ALBERT. "Aphasia Rehabilitation Resulting from Melodic Intonation Therapy." *Cortex,* X (1974), 303–16.

STRYKER, S. *Speech After Stroke.* Springfield, Ill.: Charles C. Thomas, 1975.

ULALOWSKA, H. A., S. MACALUSO-HAYNES, and S. MENDEL-RICHARDSON. "The Assessment of Functional Communication in Aphasia," *Asha,* XVIII (1976), 619.

VAN RIPER, C. "Case Study of an Aphasic." in I. A. Berg and L. A. Pennington. *An Introduction to Clinical Psychology* (3d ed.) New York: The Ronald Press Co., 1966, 344–54.

WEPMAN, J. M. "Aphasia Therapy: A New Look." *Journal Speech Hearing Disorders,* XXXVII (1972), 203–14.

——and L. V. JONES. *Studies in Aphasia; An Approach to Testing: Manual of Administration and Scoring for the Language Modalities Test of Aphasia.* Chicago: Education Industry Service, 1961.

WULF, H. H. *Aphasia: My World Alone.* Detroit: Wayne State University Press, 1973.

References (Cerebral Palsy)

ANONYMOUS, "Facts About Cerebral Palsy." *Special Children,* I (1974), 29–30.

BLISS, C. *Semantography.* Sydney, Australia: Semantography Publications, 1968.

BOONE, D. R. *Cerebral Palsy.* Indianapolis, Ind.: Bobbs-Merrill, 1972.

CRICKMAY, M. C. *Speech Therapy and the Bobath Approach to Cerebral Palsy.* Springfield, Ill.: Charles C. Thomas, 1966.

DARLEY, F. L., A. E. ARONSON, AND J. R. BROWN. *Motor Speech Disorders.* Philadelphia: W. B. Saunders Co., 1975.

DIXON, C. C. and B. CURRY. "Some Thoughts on the Communication Board." *Journal Speech Hearing Disorders,* XXXVIII (1973), 73–88.

FITZ, J. L. "Treatment of a Case of Cerebral Palsy with Hearing Impairment." *Journal Speech and Hearing Disorders,* XXXVII (1972), 373–78.

KEATS, S. *Cerebral Palsy.* Springfield, Ill.: Charles C. Thomas, 1968.

LENCIONE, R. M. "Speech and Language Problems in Cerebral Palsy." in W. M. Cruikshank (ed.) *Cerebral Palsy* (2d ed.) Syracuse: Syracuse University Press, 1966.

LLOYD, R. (ed.) *Communication Assessment and Intervention Strategies.* Baltimore: University Park Press, 1976.

McDONALD, E. and B. CHANCE. *Cerebral Palsy.* Englewood Cliffs, N.J.: Prentice-Hall, 1964.

McDONALD, E. T. and A. R. SCHULTZ. "Communication Boards for Cerebral-Palsied Children." *Journal Speech Hearing Disorders,* XXXVIII (1973), 73–88.

——,S. McNAUGHTON, D. HARRIS-VANDERHEIDEN, and G. C. VANDERHEIDEN. *Non-vocal Communication Techniques and Aids for the Severely Handicapped.* Baltimore: University Park Press, 1976.

MYERS, P. "A Study of Language Disabilities in Cerebral-Palsied Individuals." *Journal Speech Hearing Research,* VIII (1965), 129–36.

10

HEARING PROBLEMS

Thus far we have been considering the communicative problems associated with the formulation and sending of messages. But communication is a two-way street; messages must also be received, be heard. We have seen that some children with language difficulties have a history of hearing loss and that clients with voice or articulation problems or organic disorders may also have hearing difficulties that contribute to their disabilities. So it would seem wise to include in this introductory text in speech pathology some basic information concerning the problems that have been created by defective hearing. If you plan to become a speech pathologist, you will have to take several courses in audiology, but even if you do not, you need at least to have a cursory acquaintance with this information in order to be able to serve the many persons who will come to you with some kind of hearing impairment.

The Hearing Mechanism

Although we shall not describe the hearing mechanism in detail, we must at least present its three major parts: the outer ear, the middle ear, and the inner ear.

The Auricle   When we ordinarily think of the ear we think of its visible portion, the *auricle* or *pinna*. Some of us can wiggle our auricles or pinnae. A few persons are born without them and yet may have adequate hearing because the ear you see makes only a minor contribution to hearing in humans. In some animals, however, the external ears can be raised and pointed to help in the location of sounds. Human auricles vary widely in size and shape so much that some European police regularly use ear prints as well as fingerprints

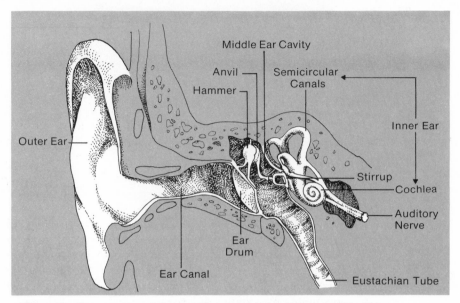

Figure 41   Cross-section of the ear. (Courtesy Michigan Board of Health)

for identification. But even if your ears were cut off, their removal would result in a loss of hearing sensitivity of only about five or six decibels[1], not enough to make any real difference, and cupping your hand to your ear increases your hearing sensitivity by the same negligible amount. Turning your head toward the sound source helps somewhat in locating it because of the head shadow effect.

Besides the auricle, the outer ear includes the *external auditory canal*, a short passageway leading to the ear drum (*tympanic membrane*). When sound waves are conveyed down this short funnel they cause the tympanic membrane to vibrate in synchronization with the sound. On the inner surface of the canal there are small hairs, called *cilia*, and the cerumenous glands which secrete the yellow wax you doubtless have noticed from time to time. Both the cilia and the wax help to protect the tympanic membrane from the dirt, insects, and foreign objects that far too often find their way into the canal.[2] The inner portion of the canal is bony and becomes narrowed just in front of the ear drum and it is there that foreign objects tend to lodge. Help your children learn to keep things out of their ears.

---

[1] A decibel is the unit of sound intensity. The abbreviated symbol is *dB*.

[2] The family doctor's advice that you should never put anything except your elbow into your ear has merit. And in this connection, we hope your education has not deprived you of the old drinking song that goes: "God bless the human elbow. God bless it where it bends. If it bends too short, I'll be dry I fear; if it bends too long, I'll be drinking through my ear. . . ."

The Middle Ear   The second major part of our auditory mechanism is called the middle ear or tympanic cavity. Imagine it as a tiny irregularly-shaped room or chamber about the size of a garden pea with a ceiling, a floor and walls. The tympanic membrane is situated on the side wall of this chamber and it separates the outer ear from the middle ear. It is conical in shape, not flat, the tip of the shallow cone facing inward. When the otologist (the physican who specializes in diseases of the ear) inspects the ear, he sees only the outer surface of this tympanic membrane, and if normal, it appears pearly gray and tightly drawn and without perforations or other abnormalities. The rear surface of the tympanic membrane is attached to one of a set of three tiny bones, the malleus (hammer), which with the incus (anvil), and stapes (stirrup), forms an *ossicular chain* which transforms the acoustic energy in the airborne sound waves as reflected by the vibration of the ear drum into a mechanical type of energy. This energy is transmitted across the tympanic cavity by the movements of the ossicular chain to the membrane of the oval window of the inner ear. There it is transformed into liquid waves which trigger the nervous impulses that go to the brain.

Another important structure that we find within the middle ear is the opening to the *eustachian tube.* The eustachian tube forms a back-door connection between the middle ear and the nasopharynx. Its function is to aerate the middle ear so that the air pressure behind the drum equals that in front of it, an arrangement which lets it vibrate freely. We experience a feeling of fullness in our ears when we climb a mountain or make a rapid plane descent. This condition is due to differences in outside and inside air pressure and is relieved by yawning or swallowing, since during these activities the eustachian tube is then opened allowing air to pass into the middle ear.

Although the eustachian tube performs this useful function, it is also the avenue for many infections which travel upward from the throat into the middle ear cavity and result in ear aches. Finally, in the middle ear there are two muscles, the tensor tympani and the stapedius, which tighten the ear drum immediately when very loud sounds occur, thus protecting our hearing from damage.

The Inner Ear   The third major part of the auditory mechanism is called the inner ear, also known as the labyrinth because of its complexity. It contains three *semicircular canals* which help us balance ourselves, a snailshell-shaped structure called the *cochlea* which contains the nerve endings of the eighth cranial nerve essential for the transmission of auditory information to the brain, and the *vestibule* which connects the cochlea with the semicircular canals. Since one of the tiny bones of the ossicular chain within the middle ear fits into an opening of the vestibule known as the *oval window,* its vibration excites the nerve endings in the cochlea; and the nervous impulses so produced then travel to the auditory cortex via the eighth (VIII) cranial nerve to produce the sensations we call hearing.

The Determination of Hearing Loss

The amount and nature of hearing loss is determined by two major testing procedures, pure tone audiometry and speech audiometry. In both types certain stimuli (tones of various frequency or test words and phrases) are systematically presented to one or both ears of the client at varying intensity levels so that the threshold of hearing can be ascertained. In other words, the examiner seeks to discover how much the test stimuli must be amplified before the client can hear or recognize them.

Pure Tone Audiometry   The pure tone audiometer is a carefully calibrated instrument which can generate and amplify a tone of fixed frequency. Since hearing sensitivity varies over the range of audible frequencies, the audiometer can produce test tones ranging from the very low-pitched frequency level of 125 Hz[3] through the 250 (Middle C), 500, 1000, 2000, 3000, 6000 frequency levels to a final testing at the high-pitched sound of 8000 Hz. Using just one tone at a time, and feeding it into only one ear, the audiologist gradually increases its intensity in small steps until the client signals (usually by turning on a light) that he can hear it.

The following instructions to a client whose hearing is being tested by pure tone audiometry may make the procedure clearer.

"We are now going to test your hearing. I am going to place an earphone over each ear, but we shall test only one ear at a time. The object of the test is to find the point where you can just barely detect the presence of the tone. We shall start each time with the tone off. Then I shall gradually introduce the tone until you can just hear it. As soon as you first hear the tone, signal me. Then I'll make the tone louder so you can hear it well. I shall next make the tone softer until you signal me that you can no longer hear it. Then I'll make it louder and softer and turn it on and off while you tell me whether or not you can hear the

[3] Hz is an abbreviation of Hertz. It refers to cycles per second.

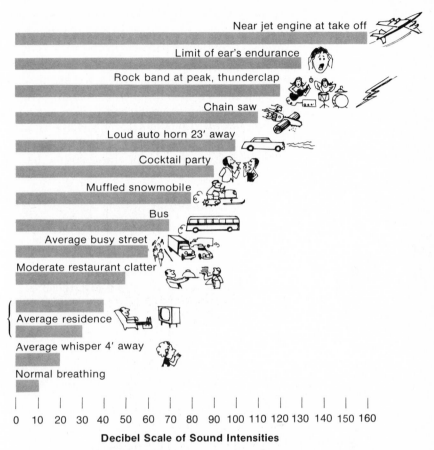

Near jet engine at take off
Limit of ear's endurance
Rock band at peak, thunderclap
Chain saw
Loud auto horn 23' away
Cocktail party
Muffled snowmobile
Bus
Average busy street
Moderate restaurant clatter
Average residence
Average whisper 4' away
Normal breathing

| | | | | | | | | | | | | | | | |
0 10 20 30 40 50 60 70 80 90 100 110 120 130 140 150 160

Decibel Scale of Sound Intensities

Figure 42   Noise levels in decibels.

tone each time, until I am satisfied that we have the point
where you can just detect the presence of the tone. Then we'll
shift to a different tone and start the process all over. You can
signal that you hear the tone by pressing the button on the end
of this cord, which will cause a light on the audiometer to turn
on. Keep the button depressed as long as you hear the tone at
all. When you no longer hear the tone, do not push the button.
Do you hear any better with one ear than with the other? If so,
we'll test the better ear first; if not, we'll begin with the right
ear. Are you ready? Signal when you hear the tone by pushing
the button, and hold it down until you cease to hear the tone.
Here we go." . . . (Newby, 1972), p. 75.

Normally we hear other people talking by means of air conduction, whereby the sound travels through the outer and middle ear

and into the inner ear. When *we* speak, we hear ourselves by air conduction and also by bone conduction. In bone-conduction hearing, the stimulus is conveyed directly to the inner ear by the vibrations of the bones of the skull. It is because we normally hear ourselves by both air and bone conduction when we speak that many people are quite amazed to hear how their voices sound the first time they hear a tape recording of themselves. The reason they sound so different is because they are hearing themselves strictly by air conduction for the first time.

In examining hearing, the audiologist tests both by air conduction and by bone conduction. The air-conduction testing is accomplished through earphones, whereas bone conduction is tested by bypassing the outer and middle ears and testing directly with a bone vibrator placed at some point on the skull. Formerly, the mastoid was the usual choice, but other placements, such as the forehead and teeth, are becoming more popular as the site for the vibrator.

The results obtained from this testing are expressed as an audiogram such as that shown in Figure 43. The upper horizontal line represents normal hearing at each of the frequency levels that were being tested. The horizontal lines below it show the intensity (loudness) levels of the test tones as expressed in decibels. The client's hearing loss in each ear is charted across this grid in terms of both air conduction and bone conduction. By inspecting this audiogram we can determine how much of a hearing loss the client shows for each of the frequencies being tested.

Speech Audiometry Although the pure tone audiometer can provide a fairly accurate evaluation of hearing loss, the hearing handicapped individual's main disability lies in his comprehension of speech. Accordingly, speech audiometers and testing procedures have been devised to determine how loud simple speech must be before the person can understand it. Speech audiometry, therefore, uses standardized sets of test words for this purpose. Among these are the lists of two-syllable words called *spondee* words. They are used to determine the *SRT* or *Speech Reception Threshold*, defined as the hearing level at which the client can repeat half of the series of words correctly. The more hard-of-hearing the person is, the more the words must be amplified before he gets half of them correct. These test words may come from the live voice of the audiologist in another soundproof room or from a recording. Either way they are delivered via earphones or through a loud speaker.

Besides determining the speech reception threshold, speech

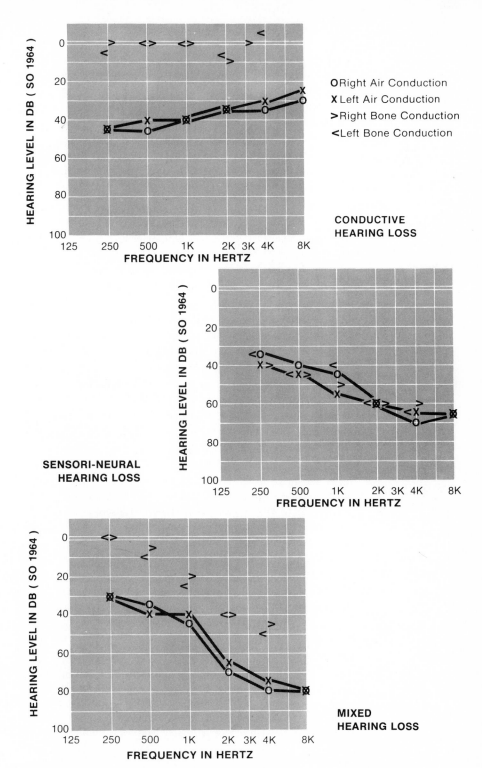

Figure 43 Some audiograms showing hearing losses.

411

audiometry may include other testing procedures to discover, for example, the person's tolerance of amplified speech. In other words, the audiologist tries to find the intensity level at which the client feels too much discomfort, a factor important in the fitting of hearing aids. Again, since the hard-of-hearing person can often hear speech without understanding it because of the interference of the hearing loss with intelligibility, speech discrimination testing is also administered to some clients. The stimuli used in discrimination testing consist of lists of phonetically balanced *(PB)* monosyllabic words and are scored in terms of the percentage of words heard correctly as shown by the client's ability to write them out on a test sheet.

Types of Hearing Loss

When testing reveals a loss of hearing sensitivity by air conduction and the bone-conduction thresholds are normal, then the hearing loss is classified as *conductive.* A typical audiogram for a conductive hearing loss is shown in Figure 43. In a conductive type loss, the inner ear is normal and the breakdown lies in either the outer or middle ear. The problem is with the "conduction" of the sound to the inner ear.

When a loss of hearing is found by both air conduction and bone conduction and the bone-conduction thresholds are essentially at the same level as the air-conduction thresholds, the loss is classified as *sensori-neural.* A typical audiogram for a sensori-neural hearing loss is shown in Figure 43. In this instance, the outer and middle ears are normal and the breakdown is in the cochlear sense organ itself, or in the auditory nerve. The problem is with the "perception" of sound in the inner ear or beyond.

A third major classification of hearing loss is termed a *mixed type* of loss. As the term implies, this type of loss is a combination of a conductive and a sensori-neural type loss.There is a loss of hearing by both air conduction and bone conduction, but the loss by bone conduction is not as great as the loss by air conduction, thus producing what is termed an "air-bone gap" at certain test frequencies. A typical audiogram for a mixed type hearing loss is also shown in Figure 43. With this type of loss the bone-conduction thresholds show the presence of a sensori-neural loss, but, since air-conduction thresholds are much worse, there is also a conductive component to the hearing loss. This type of loss could result from any number of factors.

Conductive   Hearing loss can, of course, occur at any time. Losses occur-
Impairments ring before birth are said to be congenital. One kind of congenital hearing loss involving the outer ear is atresia of the
external ear canal. Atresia means that a natural canal has been
blocked. When this blocking occurs in the ear canal, it results in a
conductive type hearing loss. Atresia of the ear canal is usually not
found as an isolated defect, but usually in conjunction with a small
or deformed auricle or with middle-ear abnormalities. The following
case illustrates the classic symptoms of this kind of conductive hearing impairment:

> Judy, age six, had a hearing loss due to congenital bilateral mi-
> crotia of the auricle and bilateral atresia of the external auditory
> canal. She had a moderate, bilateral, conductive hearing loss.
> At the time of the audiological evaluation, the extent of middle-
> ear involvement had not been determined, and she had under-
> gone several operations for restoration of the auricles. Her
> speech was quite good, and she had only a few minor articula-
> tion errors.
>
> Since surgery to correct her hearing loss would entail several
> years, steps had to be taken to insure that she would not be
> handicapped educationally, as well as having a hearing handi-
> cap. Further testing revealed speech reception thresholds of 52
> dB in the right ear and 50 dB in the left ear. Her ability to un-
> derstand speech was normal when speech was presented at an
> intensity level sufficient to overcome the conductive barrier.
>
> Persons with conductive losses are generally excellent candi-
> dates for hearing aids. Judy was no exception, and a hearing-aid
> evaluation with a body-type hearing aid employing a bone-
> conduction receiver yielded a speech reception threshold of 8
> dB—she had normal understanding of speech.
>
> Because of her excellent performance with a hearing aid, provi-
> sions were made for her to remain in the regular classroom and
> to obtain instructions from a homebound teacher during the
> times she had to miss school following an opperaration on her
> ears. Judy was placed in a regular second grade in her commu-
> nity, and the follow-up report indicated that she was a "good
> student, attentive and in the best reading group."

Another congenital defect resulting in a conductive hearing loss is

the *Treacher–Collins Syndrome*. This syndrome is marked by deformities of the facial bones resulting in a small receding lower jaw and
eyes that are slanted downward in an antimongoloid fashion at the
lateral corners. The auricles are deformed, and usually both external
auditory canals and eardrums are missing bilaterally, along with ossicular chain deformities.

> Vivian, age five, was born with Treacher–Collins Syndrome.
> There was malformation of both auricles, along with complete
> atresia of the left ear canal and marked stenosis (narrowing or
> stricture) of the right ear canal. Audiological evaluation revealed
> normal, bilateral inner-ear function with a moderate to severe
> loss by air conduction in the right ear. The left ear was not
> tested by air conduction due to the complete absence of an ear
> canal. A sound field (loudspeaker) speech reception threshold of
> 55 dB was obtained, and understanding of speech was normal
> when it was presented at a sufficient loudness level to overcome
> the conductive barrier. Further testing revealed that Vivian was
> considerably retarded in her language development and had
> markedly defective articulation.

> Remedial procedures included an air-conduction hearing aid fit-
> ted to her right ear by a special earmold. In addition, Vivian
> was placed in a special school where she could receive an in-
> tensive program of academic instruction and remedial assistance
> in speech, language, and auditory training. Later, corrective sur-
> gery would be performed in an attempt to alleviate her con-
> ductive hearing loss.

Acquired Hearing   Hearing losses occurring at any time after birth are referred
Losses   to as acquired losses. One of the most common acquired
losses involving the outer ear is that of simple blockage of the
ear canal by foreign objects or impacted wax. Children have been
known to put into their ears such things as beans, color crayons,
small ball bearings, wads of paper, and just about anything else small
enough to fit into their ear canals. Foreign objects cause a mild conductive loss if the blockage is complete. They are readily visible on
otoscopic examination and should be extracted by the otologist.

The most common blockage is a result of impacted wax. Well-
meaning mothers can cause this type of loss by cleaning their children's ears with cotton swabs. Since the cotton tip just fits the ear canal, it cannot get behind the wax and instead forces it back and may

impact it against the tympanic membrane. One otologist, an acquaintance of the author, is very vehement in his objection to mothers using cotton swabs to clean their children's ears. If he had his
way, cotton swabs would be taken off the market. He maintains that
it is unnecessary to clean wax from the ears, since old accumulations
will dry up and fall out naturally if left alone.

Impacted wax should be removed by the otologist since there is
always danger of perforating the tympanic membrane unless it is
done by a skilled person and with proper instruments such as a ceru-
men spoon. Often it is necessary to soften the wax with some type of
softening agent before the wax can be removed. After the wax is softened the ear is syringed and the wax flushed out. Syringing of the
ear must also be done carefully, since a forceful stream of water directed at the tympanic membrane could rupture it. For this reason,
the water is usually directed at the canal walls, so that only reflected
water hits the membrane. Although impacted wax results in only a
mild hearing loss, it often enough causes a youngster to have difficulty in school. This is the child who often becomes what the teachers refer to as a "behavior problem." Any child who does not seem
to pay attention in school or suddenly changes in alertness should be
suspected of having a hearing loss.

There are a number of other problems involving the outer ear
which come under the broad title of *external otitis*. These would include erysipelas, seborrheic dermatitis, eczema, and other inflamma-
tory conditions. The hearing loss resulting from these conditions resembles the loss from simple blockage of the ear canal. These
conditions result in a swelling of the external ear canal so that it is
closed or nearly closed, or the collection of scaly debris in the canal.
These types of conditions are treated medically and may involve
other areas of the body as well as the ear canal and auricle.

A common type of otitis externa is called otomycosis or "swim-
mers ears," since it is often found in people who are habitual swim-
mers. It consists of a fungus growth in the external canal which results in irritation and itching. Secondary infection can be set up by
scratching in attempts to relieve the itching. The following case is an
example of this type of ear problem:

Mr. J. V., age forty-three, was seen for an audiological evaluation. Although he complained of some loss of hearing, his
chief complaint was the itching in his left ear canal. He at-
tributed the itching to an accumulation of wax. (The average
person tends to lay the blame for all hearing problems or ear
conditions on excessive amounts of wax.) In attempts to rid his

left ear canal of what he thought was an accumulation of wax, Mr. J. V. poured hydrogen peroxide into it since this can be used to soften wax. This procedure resulted in a pain deep in the left ear and left him dizzy and nauseous.

Audiological evaluation showed evidence of air-bone gaps in the low frequencies, indicating the presence of a conductive hearing loss. In addition, a mild high-frequency sensori-neural hearing loss was present bilaterally. Physical examination of the left ear revealed a fungoid external otitis and a perforated tympanic membrane. Thus, the pain experienced upon application of the hydrogen peroxide was due to the fact that the peroxide was getting into the middle ear through the perforated tympanic membrane. By carrying the bacteria from the ear canal with it, a middle-ear infection could have resulted. Mr. J. V. was referred for otologic treatment, and medication was prescribed to eliminate the fungus and to relieve the itching in his ear canal.

The foregoing case points up the danger of self-treatment combined with ignorance. Since Mr. J. V.'s hearing loss in the high frequencies was mild, further rehabilitation was deemed unnecessary.

Middle Ear Abnormalities and Problems Congenital malformations can also be found in the middle ear. These take the form of deformed ossicular chains, missing ossicles, replacement of the tympanic membrane by a primitive bony plate, fixation of the stapes in the oval window, and breaks in the ossicular chain. As indicated earlier, these abnormalities are usually found with congenital atresia of the outer ear, but they can also be restricted to the middle ear itself. The following is a case of congenital middle-ear deformities resulting in a conductive type hearing loss:

Miss T. W., a university student eighteen-years-old, was seen for an audiological evaluation, which showed the presence of a severe, bilateral, conductive hearing loss. Case history information revealed that Miss T. W. had a bilateral, congenital middle-ear problem for which surgery was being contemplated. Both outer ears were normal, and she wore a binaural hearing aid built into glasses. With this type of amplification, speech reception thresholds and understanding of speech were well within the normal range. The left corner of her mouth was pulled to the side slightly, indicating a possible paralysis of the facial nerve. She had a distorted /s/ sound.

Subsequent surgery on the left ear revealed a normal tympanic membrane but a defective ossicular chain consisting of a deformed incus and a rudimentary stapes. In addition, the oval window could not be identified. The operation was not successful from the audiologic standpoint because air-conduction thresholds in the left ear were not improved.

Since she was already wearing a binaural hearing aid, from which she appeared to obtain substantial benefit, Miss T. W. was enrolled in therapy for correction of her defective /s/ sound and strengthening of muscular control around the mouth area. Within two semesters she was dismissed from therapy, but she continued to receive periodic hearing evaluations. She is scheduled for further ear surgery, which hopefully will prove to be more successful.

Acquired middle-ear problems resulting in conductive hearing loss can result from many causes. One very common problem associated with this type of hearing loss is caused by a ruptured eardrum. The tympanic membrane can be penetrated by any number of sharp objects. In attempts to relieve itching or to dig out the wax from the ear canal people use hairpins or paper clips, and any slip can result in the penetration of the tympanic membrane. The tympanic membrane can also be ruptured by a sharp blow across the ears and is one of many very good reasons why children should not be struck on or about the head. Nature has provided a much lower and safer target for such disciplinary measures. Sharp objects should never be introduced into the external ear canal.

The eardrum can also be perforated from within by the building up of fluid in the middle ear. The size and location of the perforation will indicate how serious the problem is. Fortunately, small perforations will tend to heal spontaneously once the middle-ear infection has been removed. Other persistent perforations may indicate the presence of a more serious problem.

Otitis Media   Otitis media is an inflammation or infection of the middle ear. There are a number of types, the most common cause of conductive hearing loss in children being due to eustachian tube malfunction. Most often the tube is swollen so that it can no longer open properly. This swelling may be due to allergies or upper respiratory infection or to the growth of a large amount of adenoidal tissue around the opening. This excessive growth of adenoidal tissue is probably the most common cause of otitis media. Since the middle ear is aerated through the eustachian tube, blockage of the latter results in the eardrum bulging inwards and secretion of a clear, watery fluid from the mucous lining of the middle ear. As a result of this retraction of the eardrum, the ossicular chain is impeded and a conductive hearing loss results. This condition is then known as *serous otitis media*. The term serous refers to the fluid or serum that may partially or completey fill the middle-ear cavity.

Treatment of serous otitis media consists of ridding the ear of fluid by *myringotomy* (in which the eardrum is cut to allow the fluid to drain or to be pumped out,) and by tonsillectomy and adenoidectomy (T & A). If the condition persists after adenoidectomy, small polyethylene tubes may have to be inserted in the eardrums in order to aerate the middle ear until further growth restores the proper functioning of the eustachian tube. The following is a case of serous otitis media in need of medical attention:

David, age seven, had been enrolled in speech therapy for correction of an articulation problem. After about two months of therapy, it was decided to have his hearing evaluated. It was readily apparent that David was a mouth breather, and when asked to close his mouth and breath through his nose, he was unable to do so because of the congestion. Oral examination revealed such extremely large tonsils we wondered how the child was able to swallow his food.

Audiological evaluation showed a mild, bilateral, conductive type of hearing loss. The child, however, did not complain of pain in his ears which would be the case with serous otitis media. Treatment called for a T & A and myringotomy as well as investigation of a possible allergic condition that might account for the chronic nasal congestion.

Following the T & A the child's congestion diminished, and he actually became much more understandable, since the denasality in his speech disappeared. Hearing returned to the normal range. Further speech therapy could then be expected to correct his misarticulations.

Acute otitis media is the problem which is usually experienced by a child or adult as a result of an upper respiratory infection such as a cold or an allergy attack. Coughing, sneezing, or blowing the nose forces secretions containing bacteria through the eustachian tube into the middle ear. Infants and children are particularly susceptible to this type of infection because their eustachian tubes tend to lie on a horizontal plane. In the adult this relationship changes, the tube becoming more vertical, and thus it is more difficult for infected material to be forced into the middle ear. Acute otitis media is accompanied by the earache familiar to all of us. The fluid in the ear may initially be clear but it soon changes to pus and the pressure of this fluid causes the eardrum to bulge outwardly to produce pain.

If the condition is caught in time, medical treatment with antibiotics may be all that is needed. Once the infection has cleared up, the debris will be absorbed. However, it is interesting to note that some otologists feel that their work has increased because of antibiotics. The drug clears up the infection, but the fluid is left in the middle ear. If left there over a period of time, the fluid will turn into a thick, mucous, sludgelike material resulting in even greater loss of hearing. This condition is often referred to as "glue ear."

Chronic otitis media is a condition in which there is a continuous infection of the middle ear over a long period of time. It is not a recurring infection, but one that is never completely cleared up. In it we usually find a perforated eardrum and an accumulation of fluid in the middle ear which gradually erodes the ossicular chain. The combination of these factors may result in a severe conductive hearing loss. If the mastoid process becomes infected and the infection is allowed to persist, it could result in an infection of the brain.

G. O., age forty-nine, suffered from chronic otitis media for years. The infection was not properly controlled and resulted in infection of the mastoid bones. Eventually the infection travelled to the brain and resulted in some tissue damage. G. O. is now subject to epileptic-like seizures and is under constant medication for control of them. In addition, he has a severe conductive hearing loss due to the erosion of his middle-ear structures.

Discharge from the ear or complaints of earaches from children should never be ignored. The speech pathologist in the public schools can do much to help the teachers understand conductive type hearing losses, refer children for proper medical treatment, help the otologist with follow-up, and provide the child with the extra help he may need until an infection can be cleared up.

Otosclerosis Another disease of the middle ear that accounts for a great number of conductive-type hearing losses is *otosclerosis*. In it, the hearing loss is the result of a formation of spongy bone which fixates the footplate of the stapes in the oval window. The cause of this type of growth is unknown. There are, however, some interesting aspects of this disease. It is more common in females than males and is usually first noticed during the late teens or early twenties. The hearing loss is usually accompanied by tinnitus (ringing in the ears) and increases during pregnancy. Evidently the hormonal changes which take place in the body during pregnancy enhance the spongy bone growth.

There are no effective drugs for otosclerosis, and the medical treatment consists of a number of surgical procedures. One of the most popular and successful of these is called a *stapedectomy*. In this procedure the fixated stapes is removed and replaced by a prosthetic device. Speech pathologists should know that there is a high percentage of success with this procedure and that hearing thresholds can be returned to within the normal range or at least be markedly improved.

Mr. D. G., age twenty-seven, has had otosclerosis since the age of sixteen. He underwent surgery on his right ear on two different occasions without any apparent success. He has worn several binaural hearing aids for a number of years, but complained that his present aid was not giving him satisfactory service.

Audiological evaluation revealed the audiogram shown in Figure 44. As shown by the audiogram, Mr. G. has had a moderate conductive type hearing loss in his right ear. The surgical procedures performed on the right ear were not successful and had apparently resulted in some inner-ear damage.

Hearing-aid evaluation procedures indicated that Mr. G. was unable to use amplification in his right ear to any advantage because of the depressed speech reception threshold and poor understanding of speech in that ear. Since a hearing aid on the right ear was not feasible and a hearing aid on the left ear brought his hearing to within the normal range, he was fitted with a glasses type hearing aid in a Bi–CROS arrangement. With this type of aid a pickup microphone is located in each bow of the glasses, but the output of the one on the poorer ear is fed into the better ear. The abbreviation CROS stands for the contra-lateral routing of signals and is a fairly recent concept in amplification for the hearing impaired.

Sensori-Neural Congenital sensori-neural hearing losses can result from he-
Impairments reditary factors or be caused by conditions affecting the
mother during pregnancy. Relatively little is known about
hearing loss suspected to be the result of a genetic defect. We do
know that hearing loss tends to run in certain families and that deaf
parents are more likely to have deaf children although the exact genetic mechanism for many of these losses is as yet undiscovered. The
following family history of hearing loss illustrates a kind of loss that
has no apparent etiology other than a possible genetic problem:

> Patty, age twelve, Lois, age eleven, and Vanessa, age seven, are
> sisters who, as far as could be determined, were probably born
> with mild, bilateral, sensori-neural hearing losses. The hearing
> losses of the two older girls were discovered just before they en-
> tered school, whereas Vanessa's loss was known quite early,
> since hearing testing was carried out at a much younger age due
> to the family history of hearing loss.
>
> This type of progressive hearing loss can be very challenging in
> terms of therapy and educational placement. The two oldest
> girls progressed from mild-gain hearing aids worn on the head
> to high-gain body aids. Their gradually deteriorating hearing
> caused them to go through a series of educational placements
> from the regular classroom with the use of amplification, to
> regular classroom with extra help, to placement in a special class
> for the severely hard of hearing. In addition, because of educa-
> tional considerations, these children needed remedial proce-
> dures to develop their speech and language skills.
>
> A most interesting twist to this family's history is the fact that a
> fourth child, a boy, has completely normal hearing. This poses
> the possibility that the hearing losses experienced by the girls
> are due to some sex-linked genetic factor. The problem is fur-
> ther complicated by the fact that both parents have normal hear-
> ing, and there is no history of significant hearing loss on either
> side.

Congenital hearing loss can also occur as a result of illnesses,
drugs, and accidents sustained by the mother during pregnancy. At
one time it was thought that the placental barrier shielded the fetus
to a great extent from infections of the mother, but it is now realized
that a great many diseases are transmitted directly from the mother.
This is also true of drugs taken by the mother. Such drugs as streptomycin and kanomycin are especially dangerous during pregnancy.
Quinine and aspirin may also affect hearing, and alcohol and smok-

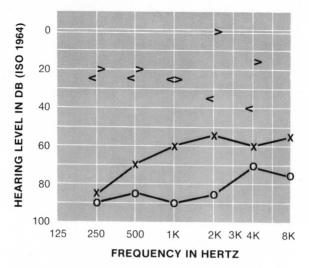

Figure 44   Bilateral Otosclerosis.

ing are also suspect, especially if used excessively. It is probably a good rule for a woman not to take any type of drug during pregnancy that is not specifically prescribed by her physician and even then reluctantly.

One of the greatest causes of congenital hearing losses is maternal *rubella*. This is the name given to German measles occurring during pregnancy. Rubella is usually a rather mild disease in the child or adult, but it is extremely dangerous to the fetus. The greatest danger comes during the first three months of pregnancy, though there is evidence that defects can also be caused during the second three months.[4] In addition to hearing loss and deafness, rubella can also cause other defects such as blindness and heart problems. The disease is rather insidious since the symptoms are so very mild in the adult and a rash may not appear. Fortunately, a rubella vaccine has been developed, and a program to immunize all children in the lower grades in school was started in early 1970. Since children are the carriers of this disease, by immunizing them it can be stamped out. The following case is typical of the so-called "rubella babies."

Doug, age four, is the youngest of four children. His two older brothers and a sister are normal in all respects. Doug's mother's

_____

[4] "Investigators Reveal Greater Rubella Risks During Pregnancy," *Washington Sounds*, III (1969), 3.

pregnancy was uneventful, except that she contracted rubella during the early months. Doug appeared normal at birth; but as he developed, a slight heart murmur and an eye problem were discovered. He was also subject to occasional dizzy spells. His hearing loss was first noticed when he was two and a half years old. Later audiological evaluation showed a moderate to severe sensori-neural hearing loss in the left ear and a severe loss in the right ear.

Rehabilitation procedures consisted of fitting him with a body-type hearing aid and enrollment in a preschool nursery program for children with hearing impairments. Doug was fortunate that such a program was available in the area since usually there is a considerable lack of help for many preschool youngsters like him. He adjusted well to the program, and he has been able to make good use of his residual hearing and is now able to do some lipreading. His articulation skills are fairly good, and the speech he does use is intelligible. However, his vocabulary and language skills are below normal for children of his age. The preschool program appears to have been of significant value to Doug, and he will be entering special classes for the hard-of-hearing in a short time.

Unfortunately some children who have had rubella sustain much greater losses, and the prognosis is not as favorable as for the case just cited.

Having survived intrauterine life and birth trauma, the human being is still subject to a great many events that can cause hearing loss. Accidents, drugs, and diseases all take their toll and a complete discussion of all the possible causes of acquired hearing loss is beyond the scope of this chapter. However, there are some common causes which we can mention.

Effects of Drugs on Hearing Just as drugs taken by the mother can be harmful to the fetus, so too can drugs taken by the individual be ototoxic to him. Some people, of course, are allergic to them. For instance, some people cannot take penicillin, since they are prone to allergic reactions that might prove fatal. Drugs such as dihydrostreptomycin, streptomycin, neomycin, and kanomycin are extremely ototoxic and must be given with great care. Usually the hearing should be monitored while a person is on these drugs, and any changes in thresholds should signal that the drug must be stopped. Even such drugs as quinine and aspirin may prove to be ototoxic in susceptible individuals. The hearing loss caused by drugs is usually bilateral and usually permanent, but not progressive. Ototoxic drugs are especially dangerous when used in conjunction with any kidney disease. The following is a case of sensori-neural hearing loss caused by a particular drug:

> Tim, age seven, was being treated for tuberculosis and had been on streptomycin for the year previous to his hearing evaluation. Streptomycin is often used for treatment of tuberculosis because of its great effectiveness against this disease. Audiological evaluation revealed a bilateral, sensori-neural hearing loss as shown in Figure 45. There was mild to moderate loss in the lower test frequencies, with a severe loss in the higher frequencies. Understanding of speech was markedly reduced even when it was presented at intensity levels well above that at which conversation normally occurs.

> In addition to his problem with tuberculosis, Tim was now in need of rehabilitation for his hearing loss because of the injudicious use of an ototoxic drug. His hearing loss might have been avoided or held to a much milder degree had monitoring audiometry been performed while he was on the drug.

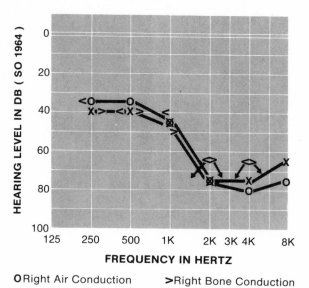

O Right Air Conduction   > Right Bone Conduction
X Left Air Conduction   < Left Bone Conduction
✓ No Response

Figure 45   Drug-induced bilateral sensori-neural hearing loss.

Tim was fitted with a hearing aid and enrolled in special classes for the hard-of-hearing where he could receive training in the use of a hearing aid, auditory training, and lipreading as well. In such cases it becomes a challenge to prevent a child from adding an educational handicap to the already existing hearing handicap.

The so-called "childhood diseases," that many people think have no serious consequences often cause hearing loss. Mumps, measles, chicken pox, scarlet fever, diptheria, and whooping cough can attack the end organ of hearing and cause sensori-neural hearing loss. Fortunately, it is now no longer inevitable that a child undergo these diseases. Only recently vaccines have been developed to immunize children against measles, rubella, and mumps.

Hearing loss resulting from these diseases is usually bilateral, except for mumps. Mumps is the most common cause of unilateral hearing loss, and the loss is usually total. The following case illustrates hearing loss from mumps:

John, age seven, is presently enrolled in therapy for an articulation problem that consists mainly of substitutions of one sound for another. At the age of five, he came down with a case of mumps that resulted in a profound loss of hearing in his right ear. His left ear was normal. His audiogram is typical of unilateral deafness due to this disease.

In this youngster's case it would have been a mistake to think that his articulation problem was in any way related to his hearing loss. People with unilateral hearing are able to function fairly normally, although the sense of direction of sound may be somewhat impaired. With a child, however, even this tends to be something they are able to compensate for. In John's case, the important thing was to prevent any damage to his good ear either by illness or accident. All his teachers in school were told of his loss, and he was given preferential seating. Speech therapy was continued, the clinician making sure she was working from his unimpaired side.

Effects of Noise   A kind of hearing loss which is receiving a great deal of attention at this time is noise-induced hearing loss. Noise-induced hearing loss produces a gradual loss of hearing, and is due to exposure to loud noise over a long period of time. It should not be confused with "acoustic trauma," which is a sudden loss of hearing due to one exposure to a loud noise such as an explosion.

Since man is becoming concerned over pollution of his environment, the topic of "noise pollution" is a timely one. There is a growing concern over environmental noise as indicated by the Conference on Noise as a Public Health Hazard held in Washington, D. C., on June 13–14, 1968.[5] We should also be concerned about the noise generated by the new "jumbo" jets, increased traffic, and new industry.

A more subtle danger to the ears of youth also exists. A number of studies have indicated that "hard rock" music can cause noise-induced hearing loss.[6] Another study has indicated that the potential for damage is there, but that there is not the great danger that our youth is going deaf as many popular articles in the mass media would lead one to think.[7] This last study indicated that "rock" musicians who are exposed the most do not incur hearing losses of any great magnitude. Since this type of music does exceed the 85 to 90 decibels of sound that is considered safe, the exposure time is probably a critical factor. Young people just do not listen to loud music eight hours a day, five days a week, for years. However, the man working in the noisy environment of a foundry may be exposed to noise that exceeds safe intensity levels for a full working day for many years. The following case study illustrates this point:

> J. V., age forty-seven, stated that he was no longer able to hear birds sing or the tick of his watch. He complained of a "high-pitched ringing" in both ears. He also complained of difficulty hearing in group situations or in the presence of background noise. J. V. had worked in a drop forge for twenty-three years and was exposed to extremely loud noise for most of the working day. He had spent the last twelve years as a "hammerman" operating a huge hammer used to flatten steel bars. A subsequent hearing evalutaion revealed the high-frequency, sensori-neural hearing loss shown in Figure 46.

> J. V. was fitted with a hearing aid that gave a high-frequency

[5] W. D. Ward and J. E. Fricke, (eds.), "Noise as a Public Health Hazard: Proceedings of the Conference," *American Speech and Hearing Association Reports,* IV (1969).

[6] C. P. Lebo, K. S. Oliphant, and J. Garrett, "Acoustic Trauma from Rock-and-roll Music," *California Medicine,* CVII (1967), 378–80; D. M. Lipscomb, "High Intensity Sounds in the Recreational Environment," *Clinical Pediatrics,* VIII (1969), 63–68; R. R. Rupp and L. J. Koch, "But, Mother, Rock 'n' Roll Has to be Loud: The Effect of Noise on Human Ears," *Michigan Hearing* (Spring, 1968), 4–7.

[7] W. F. Rintelmann and J. F. Borus, "Noise-induced Hearing Loss and Rock-and-roll Music," *Archives of Otolaryngology,* LXXXVIII (1968), 377–85.

emphasis and a special vented earmold that further emphasized the higher frequencies. Since he had worked in an environment which made normal communication almost impossible, he had become rather adept at speechreading. He was advised to wear ear-protective devices while working in order to prevent any further damage to his ears.

Noise-induced hearing loss causes damage to the higher frequencies first. The point of greatest loss is usually at 4000 Hertz, and this is referred to as an "acoustic trauma dip." Men such as J. V. usually get along quite well while they are working, since communication with fellow employees is difficult at best. However, upon retirement, they often find it impossible to enjoy a movie or the theater, and social groups also present difficulty. Thus, this person tends to withdraw from social contacts of any kind, and the well-known loneliness of the hearing impaired begins to take hold.

Presbycusis   The hearing loss that people incur with advancing age is called *presbycusis*. It is the most common kind of sensori-neural hearing loss. The incidence of presbycusis seems to be increasing, but this is understandable when one considers that people live much

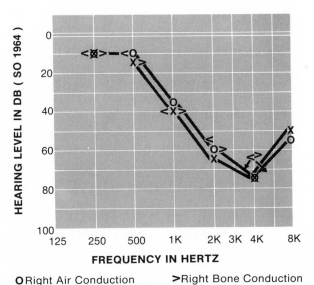

O Right Air Conduction   > Right Bone Conduction
X Left Air Conduction   < Left Bone Conduction
↙ No Response

Figure 46   Noise-induced hearing loss.

longer than they used to and that we now have a substantial percentage of senior citizens in this country. The loss of hearing by presbycusis is a rather slow, insidious process and probably starts early in life, although the symptoms of hearing loss are usually not manifested until the person is over sixty years of age. The higher sound frequencies are affected first, and as the disorder gradually progresses, the person has trouble in hearing lower frequency sounds as well. Comprehension of speech may be affected to a much greater degree than would be expected from thresholds on a pure-tone audiogram. Even in the presence of a mild loss in pure-tone thresholds, the person may have extreme difficulty understanding speech. It is for this reason that an older person may be labeled as being inattentive or senile, when actually he just has presbycusis.

The causes of presbycusis are complex and little is known about them. There is apparently a degeneration of structures not only in the inner ear, but along the central pathways and in the cerebral cortex of the brain. It has also been stated that the hearing loss is due to the wear and tear on the ear from everyday living in our noisy society; studies on primitive tribes in Africa do not reveal nearly the amount of loss with age. Aging, of course, does not affect every person in the same way, and some people have relatively good hearing even into very old age. The following case is typical of the problems involved in presbycusis:

> Mr. J. D., age sixty-seven was referred for an audiological evaluation and hearing-aid evaluation and selection following otologic consultation for his hearing problem. He was originally examined by the otologist upon the insistence of his daughter with whom he had been living since the death of his wife two years previously. The otologist diagnosed his disorder as presbycusis.

> Mr. J. D. stated that he had noticed a decrease in hearing sensitivity for a number of years, but that it had become much worse during the past two years. He complained of difficulty hearing the radio and television, and he had to have the volume turned up beyond the comfort level of other family members. Consequently, he had gradually lost interest in watching television. Conversation was also difficult for him to follow, and he found himself more and more frequently having to ask what was said. He felt that if other family members would not mumble or speak so fast he would be able to hear them without difficulty.

An interview with Mr. J. D.'s daughter revealed that she had become concerned for her father since he was showing an increasing tendency to isolate himself from other people. She also felt guilty. She worked outside the home and was usually tired in the evening. Talking with her father was a strain. She had to speak louder and often repeat what she said. This was annoying to her, so she found herself avoiding conversation with her father. It was at this point that she decided to seek professional advice and thought that perhaps a hearing aid might help them.

Audiological evaluation revealed the moderate, bilateral, sensori-neural hearing loss shown in Figure 47. Fortunately, Mr. J. D.'s understanding of speech, when it was presented at a fairly loud level, was good. A subsequent hearing-aid evaluation indicated that he received substantial benefit from wearing amplification.

The foregoing case, although it has its unique aspects, is typical not only of the hearing loss, but also of the family dynamics that are often involved. A hearing aid was not the total answer to this man's problem. He needed to have a greater understanding of his problem and so did the other family members. Rehabilitation in this type of

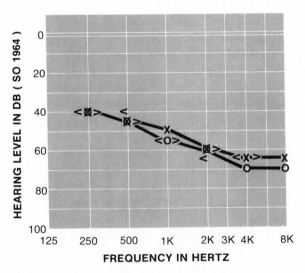

O Right Air Conduction   > Right Bone Conduction

X Left Air Conduction   < Left Bone Conduction

Figure 47   Bilateral sensori-neural hearing loss diagnosed as Presbycusis.

case should involve family counseling so that its members can do their share in improving communications. For example, we often find improvement in communication by pointing out to the family that shouting at the hard-of-hearing person does no good, and that instead they should talk more slowly and distinctly. It is also important that the family realize the advantages and disadvantages of hearing aids and how they operate.

Central Auditory Impairments

The terms *central hearing loss* or *central deafness* are used to describe a hearing loss due to some problem in the auditory pathways in the brain stem or the auditory cortex itself. Audiologically this type of disorder shows itself as a sensori-neural problem on the pure-tone audiogram. However, even though the pure-tone audiogram may be normal, the person may be unable to use the incoming stimuli meaningfully. He may hear speech, but be unable to understand it.

One example of this type of auditory disorder is called *auditory agnosia*. As we have seen in our chapter on aphasia, in auditory agnosia the person hears but is unable to recognize meaningful sounds. Auditory agnosia often accompanies receptive aphasia and is a complicating factor in the rehabilitation of an aphasic patient. This type of auditory disorder is thus quite different from the hearing losses previously described that affect the peripheral hearing mechanism. When a central problem occurs in a child before the development of speech, it is extremely difficult to distinguish it from a peripheral hearing loss. Not enough is understood about these central problems, and their treatment is extremely difficult.

Hearing Impairment

Many persons use the term "deafness" to refer to any degree of hearing impairment. They say, for instance, that they are "just a little deaf in one ear." What they mean, of course, is that they have some amount of unilateral hearing loss. Again, if they say "The man is a deaf mute" they probably make two mistakes, first believing that he is completely without any hearing at all (which is very rare) and, secondly, that he cannot produce any sound at all (which is completely false). As Newby (1972) writes, "Actually there are very few individuals whose auditory mechanism is completely dead. Most persons classified as deaf have some shreds of hearing remaining, that is, some level of hearing that is demonstrable on an audiometric test. It is the *usefulness* of this residual hearing which determines whether the person is deaf or hard of hearing." (p. 308)

The Deaf   A crude cutoff point that distinguishes the profoundly deaf from the hard of hearing is a loss of 90 dB or more. Even though these persons occasionally may be able to hear a few extremely loud sounds, they cannot rely on their hearing for communicative purposes. They live in a very silent world. Based upon the time of their hearing loss, they are divided into two groups, the *congenitally deaf* and the deafened *(adventitiously deaf)*. The latter were born with normal hearing but later lost their sense of hearing through illness or accident. The reason for the distinction is that if the hearing loss occurred after the child had learned to talk his communication problems and training will differ markedly from that of the congenitally deaf child.

The Hard of Hearing   The degree of hearing loss shown by the other group, the hard of hearing, is usually classified as *Mild* (a loss of 30–50 dB), *Moderate* (50–70 dB), and *Severe* (70–85 dB). Persons with mild hearing losses usually have fairly normal speech and can understand normal conversation if the other speaker is not too far away, but they may have trouble hearing the teacher in school or others who speak faintly or indistinctly. Persons with moderate hearing losses can understand you only if you talk to them loudly. They have difficulty participating in group discussions or hearing you in the presence of noise. According to Silverman (1971) their language and vocabulary is usually limited and they show their hearing loss by their articulation errors and voice deviations. The severely impaired often resemble the deaf. They may be barely able to hear the sound of a very loud voice from about a foot away, but they probably cannot understand what is said. Even with a very powerful hearing aid they tend to have trouble distinguishing the consonant sounds. Their comprehension and language, voice and articulation problems are so obvious that they are often called the "border-line deaf."

Prevalence   We are not sure how many persons of all ages have hearing impairments, but we do have fairly good estimates for school children because of the auditory screening tests which have been administered in that setting all over the country. About five to ten percent of all school children appear to have some degree of hearing loss and a large number of the aged show some impairment of hearing. It has been estimated that there are about 188,000 deaf persons in this country and about 8,500,000 individuals with a lesser degree of hearing loss.[8]

Hearing Rehabilitation

As in the organic speech disorders, the effective rehabilitation of a person with a hearing disorder is dependent on the skill, knowledge, and cooperation of a number of different specialists. Let us describe some of these professionals.

The Otologist   The otologist is concerned with the medical aspects of hearing impairment. He is first of all a physician who is concerned with the total well-being of a patient, and secondly, a specialist in the area of pathological hearing. The otologist is interested in determining if a hearing loss is present and in differentiating between conductive and sensori-neural impairments. He may use various tuning fork tests or perform an audiometric evaluation. He may also check vestibular functioning by means of caloric tests since ear problems often manifest themselves through spells of dizziness or vertigo. He also has at his disposal the information that can be gained by laboratory procedures such as X-rays, blood tests, bacteriological tests, neurological examinations, and so on. In addition to the specialized techniques used to determine the medical status of a patient's ears, the otologist treats any aural pathologies he may find. This treatment may take the form of prescribing medication such as antibiotics for a middle-ear infection, or it may entail some type of ear surgery.

The Audiologist   Once the otologist has completed his medical treatment, or has determined that medical treatment is not feasible for a particular hearing loss, his basic responsibility is finished except for making the proper referral. It is precisely at this point that the audiologist becomes the primary person responsible for the patient's well-

[8] From *Human Communication and Its Disorders: An Overview*, Report of the National Advisory Neurological Diseases and Stroke Council, 1969, p. 11–13.

being. The audiologist's chief role is one of rehabilitation. This does not rule out the important job he may play in detecting hearing losses or referring patients for otologic consultation. He also supplies information based on certain special audiological tests which may help to determine the site of the lesion and thus aid the otologist in his differential diagnosis. The audiologist is also often able to obtain information about the hearing function of very young children or other difficult-to-test patients. He can detect malingering and pseudohypocusis, or hypocusis. He may also work closely with the otologist in determining the amount of sensori-neural reserve in an ear when middle-ear surgery is being contemplated. In some settings the foregoing may, in fact, be his primary responsibilities.

The habilitation and rehabilitation aspects of hearing impairment are the essential domain of the audiologist. Through extensive clinical testing he is able to describe how a person's peripheral hearing functions and to plan the therapy needed to help the patient cope with his everyday communicative demands. This plan may incorporate hearing-aid evaluation and selection procedures as well as activities involving auditory training and speechreading. These will be discussed more thoroughly in the next section.

A complete program of aural rehabilitation would include auditory training, speechreading, hearing-aid orientation, speech correction, speech conversation, vocational guidance, and counseling. Any one hard-of-hearing person may not need all of these services, and we usually find that auditory training and speechreading form the core of the therapy with the hard-of-hearing.

Auditory Training   Auditory training teaches the hearing-impaired person to make the best possible use of his residual hearing. Even among those individuals classified as profoundly deaf there is usually some residual hearing for low-frequency sounds. Most hard-of-hearing persons often have a great deal of residual hearing that encompasses a relatively broad frequency range, and they may not be making full use of the hearing they possess. Auditory training is training in listening. Recently, we have begun to recognize that listening skills can be improved by training not only in the hard-of-hearing but even among normally hearing children and adults. To cite a simple example—a person learning to play the guitar usually has a difficult time tuning it since this requires the ability to tell when two strings sound exactly alike when they are held in a certain manner by one hand and plucked with the other. With a bit of persistent practice, the person is usually able to tune the guitar quite readily, since he becomes able to hear even a slight discrepancy between the tones and to make the proper adjustment. We don't usually refer to this discriminatory process as auditory training, but that is exactly what it is; and it illustrates the point that the discriminating ability of the ear can be improved.

Auditory training with the hard-of-hearing must vary according to the age of the person, the age of the onset of hearing loss, and with severity of the loss. It need not be as intensive with adults who have previously had normal communication skills as it would be with a child who must learn to send and receive verbal messages despite a hearing loss. With children, auditory training may start at the level of gross sound discrimination. At this level the child is first taught to differentiate bells from whistles or whistles from horns by the noises they make. Identification training is begun by using only two objects at one time, and then gradually other noisemakers are added. This type of training is continued until the child is quite aware of the importance of sound in making the identification, and until he can make correct differentiations consistently without the aid of visual clues.

From this stage we progress to what is often referred to as "gross speech discriminations." Depending on the skill of the child, the discrimination of speech sounds can begin by first distinguishing between such words as *ball* and *car* and then proceeding to the more difficult contrasts of *bell* and *ball*. In the latter instance, although the discrimination is finer, we would still consider this gross speech discrimination since the distinctive differences are produced by dissimilar vowels. Finer speech discriminations are called for when two words such as *same* and *came* are contrasted because consonants do not have as much acoustic power or duration as do the vowels. The acoustic differences between them are even less detectable when such words as *same* and *shame* are contrasted. This pair of words would be particularly difficult for persons having a high-frequency hearing loss because much of the energy necessary for the intelligibility of [s] and [sh] is found in the frequency range of greatest loss. Nevertheless, through skillful auditory training most persons can make real gains.

After he is proficient in making discriminations of single words, the hard-of-hearing person should go on to sentences and paragraphs. Many clinicians feel that therapy should begin with the larger wholes and then work toward the finer discriminations in single words, the argument being that there are more helpful clues in a sentence. Single unrelated words are harder to identify than sentence strings. Therefore, key words are often used, and the patient is asked to repeat the sentence or write down what he hears. To be correct, he must hear the key words in the sentences.[9] Paragraphs can also be prepared that concern subjects or activities suitable for children or adults. After reading the paragraph, the clinician can ask prepared questions in order to determine how well the person was able to follow running speech. Since many hard-of-hearing persons have difficulty understanding speech in group situations or in the presence of a background noise, all of the above levels can be repeated by introducing varying levels of background noise. The clinician can make tape recordings of various types of noise or the babble of conversation and present this noise at gradually increasing intensity levels until the patient has increased his discrimination proficiency.

Speechreading   The term *speechreading* has now generally displaced the older term *lipreading*, doubtless because there is much more involved in comprehension through visual cues than in just watching lips. Facial expressions, head movements, gestures—all of these can furnish important clues as to what is being said. Even normally hearing people use visual clues to a greater extent than they realize.

Numerous approaches in teaching speechreading have been advocated, but basically they can be divided into two broad categories: those advocating the analytic and the synthetic approaches. The analytic approaches stress careful analysis of phonetic elements, whereas the synthetic approaches advocate grasping the "whole" rather than one part at a time. Anyone who specializes in work with the hard-of-hearing will need to familiarize himself with the methods advocated long ago by Nitchie, Bruhn, the Kinzies, and Bunger.[10] Few audiologists adopt only one of these approaches since our research does not seem to show that any one method is any better than the others. The better contributions of each method can be adapted to specific individuals in therapy by the hearing clinician.

Whatever approach is used, there are certain principles that must be followed. The stimulus material must be presented in a *natural* manner much as it would be encountered in a normal communication situation. Whenever material is presented pantomimically

[9] Examples of these types of sentences are given in H. Davis and S. R. Silverman, (eds.) *Hearing and Deafness*, 3d ed. (New York: Holt, Rinehart & Winston, Inc., 1970), p. 491.

[10] E. B. Nitchie, *Lip-reading, Principles and Practice* (New York: Frederick A. Stokes Company, 1921); M. E. Bruhn, *The Mueller-Walle Method of Lipreading for the Hard of Hearing* (Washington, D. C., 1949); C. E. Kinzie, and R. Kinzie, *Lip-reading for the Deafened Adult* (Chicago: Winston, 1931); A. M. Bunger, *Speech Reading—Jena Method* (Danville, Ill.: Interstate, 1952).

without voice, there is a tendency to exaggerate mouth movements. This is why we use a voice when stimulating the hard-of-hearing person in speechreading. However it is important, especially at the beginning of speechreading training, that the visual channel be emphasized as much as possible; for if the client can hear the clinician, he may be depending on his hearing too much and not obtaining enough practice in observing visual clues. For this reason we often speak very softly or whisper in the periods of speechreading. Through sufficient practice in front of a mirror, the clinician can learn to speak without exaggerated movements of his articulators even when pantomiming. Remember also, that in group work the patients must be seated so that all are able to see the clinician's face equally well.

Beginning lessons in speechreading for children should present the more visible speech sounds so that the child can experience some success right from the start. The child can be told how each sound is made, but care should be taken not to become too analytical. Each lesson should consist of (1) a list of vocabulary words with which children of certain age levels are familiar, (2) a series of practice sentences incorporating the words, and (3) a practice story or exercise that incorporates the words.

It must be remembered that speechreading alone is not a perfect substitute for hearing since many sounds of English are just not visible. For this reason a combination approach of auditory training and speechreading is usually recommended. Also, a truly effective program of speech reading must be geared to the interest of the patients involved. With children, lessons can be made enjoyable and interesting if they revolve around things which children tend to love, such as animals or fairy tales. School subjects such as arithmetic, history, and language can be incorporated into speechreading lessons. These kinds of lessons also have the advantage of preparing the child for the vocabulary encountered in the regular classroom.

Initially, speechreading lessons may revolve around matching the movements of the articulators to the names of common objects. However, progress must be made toward the goal of having the child grasp thoughts and concepts which are conveyed in more abstract language. Thus, speechreading progress is from the concrete to the more abstract. Where we begin depends a lot upon the age and severity of the hearing loss. With the hard-of-hearing child who has a good deal of residual hearing and can learn some language through the auditory channel, it may not be necessary to begin at the simple matching level. Determining the needs of the individual child is all-important in good therapy.

Hearing Aids

The modern hearing aid is an electronic device that changes acoustical energy into electrical current. The electric current is then amplified and changed back to acoustical energy with greater intensity.

A hearing aid consists of three major components: a microphone, a transistor amplifier, and a receiver. The microphone changes the sound waves into variations in electric current that are then fed into the amplifier where they are made more intense. The amplified current is then fed into the receiver, a miniature loudspeaker, where it is converted back to sound waves. The resulting acoustic energy is now, however, at a greater intensity level than originally. In the hearing aid, all three components mentioned above have been miniaturized; and with miniaturization, power and fidelity have usually been sacrificed for wearing comfort.

In addition to the main components, a hearing-aid must have a source of power, which is usually a small carbon-zinc, silver oxide, or mercury battery. The hearing aid must also feed into the ear, and this is accomplished by a custom earmold which is individually fitted. Hearing aids can be classified into two distinct types according to where they are worn. Those aids worn on the head can be built into glasses, or suspended from the ears (auricle aids), or actually inserted into the ear. All of those which are worn on the head are collectively called ear-level aids.

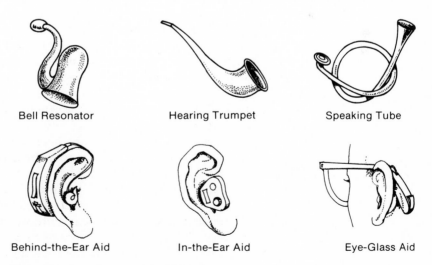

Bell Resonator   Hearing Trumpet   Speaking Tube

Behind-the-Ear Aid   In-the-Ear Aid   Eye-Glass Aid

Figure 48 Some hearing aids: Old and new.

437

Body hearing aids are usually larger and more powerful, and they are used with more severe hearing losses. The fairly large grill in the center of the case serves as the microphone, and the large button receiver is connected to the earmold. The cord connecting the receiver to the case is also readily visible. Since the cord plugs into each component, it can be disconnected, and different receivers can be used with the same instrument to achieve various frequency responses. Body-type aids also tend to have certain additional components not always found in ear-level aids. They usually have an on-off switch, whereas the ear-level aid may not, and a hinged battery compartment is swung out to break the battery contacts. The body-type aid also has a tone control whereby two or three settings enable one to change the frequency response characteristics of the instrument; the changes are usually made to obtain a low- or high-frequency emphasis or a flat response across the frequency range amplified by the instrument. A telephone pickup coil is also found on the body-type instruments. This enables the user to hear over a telephone without using the microphone of the aid.

Hearing aids are effectively used by people having various kinds of hearing losses. Some years ago it was a common belief that a sensori-neural hearing loss could not be helped by a hearing aid. This was probably quite true with the old carbon-type amplifiers because they introduced so much distortion into the instrument. Today, however, with the much more efficient transistor amplifier, some people with sensori-neural hearing losses derive substantial benefit from wearing hearing aids. In fact, the number of hearing aids used by people with conductive losses has declined because modern surgical techniques are often able to restore conductive hearing losses to a level where amplification is not needed.

After obtaining a hearing aid a person with a hearing loss is in need of some hearing-aid orientation sessions. In these he learns how to care for and use his hearing aid. This would include such things as changing batteries, cleaning the earmold, adjusting the volume control, and so on. He must also come to realize right from the beginning that he is not getting his ears back. For one thing, the quality of sound reproduction is not very good because a hearing aid is essentially a low-fidelity instrument, and hearing aid users often expect too much from their instruments. We must help such a person understand that a hearing aid is not usually the total answer to his problem. Difficult listening situations such as those involving groups or background noise will also be difficult when wearing a hearing aid. In fact, he will learn that in some situations the hearing aid may even add to the confusion. Then too, the hearing aid may seem so unnatural to the person that he may tend to reject it too hastily. One reason for this is that with the instrument, he is now hearing sounds he hasn't heard for a long time, and so he feels bombarded by noise. This is especially true of the adult who has gradually lost part of his hearing over a period of time. Just as a person with normal hearing has to adapt to noise and to direct his attention to what he desires to hear, the hard-of-hearing person must also learn to ignore extraneous noises and to devote his attention to what is being said. At times a child or adult may complain that his hearing aid squeals whenever he turns the volume control up to where he is getting effective amplification. This particular squeal is due to amplified sound reaching the pickup microphone. It is the result of sound leaking out around a poorly fitting earmold. Either the earmold was not properly fitted in the first place, or the ear has changed so that the mold no longer fits. In the case of young children, the earmold may have to be changed every few months or even sooner, depending on growth patterns. A properly fitted earmold should allow the person to turn his aid up to full volume without obtaining the squeal that results from feedback.

The first few weeks of using a hearing aid will probably be the most difficult for the hard-of-hearing person. However, if he is helped to understand more about his particular problem, can manipulate the controls of the aid, and understands that the hearing aid is only as good as the effort he puts forth in learning to use it, he is well on his way to becoming an effective hearing-aid user.

Although you may feel that we have overloaded you with too much information in this chapter, we have really only skimmed the surface features of audiology as a field in itself, the sister field of speech pathology.[11] You yourself will probably suffer some hearing loss if you live long enough. In any case, you will meet many individuals with hearing problems, and be able to serve them better because of the knowledge you have acquired.

References

BENNETT, C. "Speech Pathology and the Hearing Impaired Child." *Volta Review*, 76 (1974), 550–56.

BLATCHFORD, C. H. "A Hearing in Deafness." *Volta Review*, LXXVI (1974), 208–12.

DAVIS, H. and S. R. SILVERMAN. (eds.) *Hearing and Deafness* (3rd Ed.) New York: Holt, Rinehart & Winston, Inc., 1970.

[11] The author's mild feelings of guilt for so belaboring you are fortunately assuaged by his sublime confidence in your ability to forget.

DI CARLO, L. M. *The Deaf.* Englewood Cliffs, N.J.: Prentice-Hall, Inc., 1964.

EMERICK, L. L. *A Workbook in Clinical Audiometry.* Springfield, Ill.: Charles C. Thomas, 1971.

GIOLAS, T. G., E. J. WEBSTER, and L. M. WARD. "A Diagnostic Therapy Setting for Hearing Handicapped Children." *Journal Speech Hearing Disorders,* XXXIII (1968), 345–50.

GOODHILL, V. and P. GUGGENHEIM. "Pathology, Diagnosis, and Therapy of Deafness." in L. E. Travis (ed.) *Handbook of Speech Pathology and Audiology.* Englewood Cliffs, N.J.: Prentice-Hall, Inc., 1971.

HARDY, R. E. and J. C. CULL. (ed.) *Educational and Psychosocial Aspects of Deafness.* Springfield, Ill.: Charles C. Thomas, 1974.

HARTBAUER, R. E. *Aural Rehabilitation: A Total Approach.* Springfield, Ill.: Charles C. Thomas, 1975.

LING, D. *Speech and the Hearing Impaired Child: Theory and Practice.* Washington, D.C.: Alexander Graham Bell Association for the Deaf, 1976.

MARTIN, F. N. *Introduction to Audiology.* Englewood Cliffs, N.J.: Prentice-Hall, Inc., 1975.

NEWBY, H. A. *Audiology* (3rd ed.) Englewood Cliffs, N.J.: Prentice-Hall Inc., 1972.

——"Clinical Audiology." in L. E. Travis (ed.) *Handbook of Speech Pathology and Audiology.* Englewood Cliffs, N.J.: Prentice-Hall, Inc., 1971.

O'NEILL, J. J. *The Hard of Hearing.* Englewood Cliffs, N.J.: Prentice-Hall, Inc., 1964.

PLESTER, D., A. EL-MOFTY, and H. ROSEN. "High-frequency Audiometry in Presbycusis: A Comparative Study of the Mabaan Tribe in the Sudan with an Urban Population." *Archives Otolaryngology,* LXXX (1964), 18–32.

QUIZLEY, S. R. "The Deaf and Hard-of-Hearing." *Review of Educational Research,* XXXIX (1969), 103–24.

ROTTER, P. "Working with Parents of Young Deaf Children." in R. E. Hardy and J. C. Cull (eds.) *Educational and Psychosocial Aspects of Deafness* (Springfield, Ill.: Charles C. Thomas, 1974).

SANDER, D. A. *Aural Rehabilitation.* Englewood Cliffs, N.J.: Prentice-Hall, Inc., 1971.

SILVERMAN, RICHARD S. "The Education of Deaf Children." in L. E. Travis (ed.) *Handbook of Speech Pathology and Audiology.* Englewood Cliffs, N.J.: Prentice-Hall, Inc., 1971.

—— and D. J. WARK. "Communication Problems Associated with Unilateral Hearing Loss." *Journal Speech Hearing Disorders,* XXXII (1967), 336–42.

11

THE PROFESSION OF SPEECH PATHOLOGY

By now you should have acquired a fairly good picture of the field of speech pathology and the different problems with which speech pathologists must cope. Some of you may be intrigued enough to consider entering this profession, but even those who are not so vocationally inclined should know something about the qualifications and training of its workers if only because when they encounter a person with a speech handicap they will want to make sure that the person to whom you make the referral is qualified and competent. Moreover, since most of you will probably work closely with a speech pathologist in your own career, you should know something about his training and experiences. Often he can be of great help to you and to those you serve.

Professional Most (but not all) speech pathologists belong to the American
Organizations Speech and Hearing Association (ASHA). As its name suggests, this organization includes both speech pathologists and audiologists, though the former constitute the large majority of its membership. Also, because the backbone of the field is research, it includes speech and hearing scientists as well. ASHA's membership has shown an outstanding and continuing growth, from a mere 1600 members in 1950 to 13,000 in 1970 and 23,000 in 1975, and this despite a continuing upgrading of the membership requirements.

The American Speech and Hearing Association, through its board of examiners, is the accrediting agency both for the college centers which train speech pathologists and audiologists and for the service centers in which they work. It administers the comprehensive examinations which lead to the awarding of its valued Certification of Clinical Competence, and it monitors and evaluates the Clinical Fellowship Year (one of paid employment under supervision) that

442

must precede the taking of the national examination for the certificate.[1]

The association publishes four journals, the *Journal of Speech and Hearing Disorders*, the *Journal of Speech and Hearing Research*, *Language, Speech and Hearing Services in the Schools*, and *Asha* as well as other monographs and materials. A House of Delegates made up of representatives from the various state speech and hearing associations serves as the legislative body for the profession, while the executive business is carried out by the officers and committees of the association. National, regional, and state conventions are held each year in different parts of the country to provide opportunities for continued in-service education through short courses, seminars, and research reports. Any student who is interested in entering this young and vigorous profession should try to attend one of these meetings. There he will find not only a pervasive feeling of comradeship but also a real hunger to learn and grow professionally.

Training Centers   There are approximately 300 colleges and universities presently training speech pathologists, 200 of which have been accredited by the Education and Training Board as providing the requirements of A.S.H.A. One of these requirements is the Master's degree, and this seems to be the national trend. Even though you are attending an institution whose training program terminates at the B.A. level, we would not advise you to enter this field if you could not do graduate work successfully, even if you could get a job without the Master's degree. Besides the fact that you would be deprived of the status and advantages of membership in the professional organization to which the large majority of speech pathologists belong, there is a growing number of states which now require a license to practice speech pathology and usually the requirements for licensure are the same as for membership in A.S.H.A. Again, if you hope to work in any clinical setting other than some of the public schools you will need the A.S.H.A. Certificate of Clinical Competence since Medicaid and Medicare funds often support these programs as they do any successful private practice, and these agencies require certification of the speech pathologists whose services they reimburse. There are some excellent training centers that do not offer the Master's, but anyone from these institutions who plans to make speech pathology a life-long career should plan to go elsewhere later for graduate work.

[1] The academic background, casework experiences, and other requirements for membership and certification, together with the Code of Ethics to which all members subscribe, may be found in the current A.S.H.A. Directory.

Varieties of Professional Employment: Public Schools
A survey by Willis and Willis (1976) showed that the public schools employ 41 percent of the 23,000 speech pathologists who belong to A.S.H.A. For many clinicians, the school setting provides not only excellent salaries, vacation time, and security, but also a unique opportunity for service. Although she is employed as a teacher, she is a very special kind of teacher—a teacher-clinician. Her job is more like that of a school nurse than of a classroom teacher. Other teachers refer children to her for diagnostic and remedial services, or she discovers them through screening tests. She works with these children individually or, more often, in small groups. The case loads seem (and often are) very large. Many public-school speech clinicians see over fifty children each week, and they therefore work with most of them in groups ranging from three to about seven children in a group. Fortunately, the majority of these children do not present very difficult problems. Most of them have mild articulatory defects and improve swiftly. A few of them need individual therapy and parental counseling. Usually one day each week is set aside for these purposes and for general coordination of the clinician's program with other school activities. One of the basic advantages of this setup is that it permits the child to have therapy in a natural rather than a clinical setting, and it makes possible a transfer of new skills from the therapy room into the child's daily life in the school. For the speech clinician, too, there are advantages. She is not frozen in the same room of the same school with the same children under the same principal day after day and month after month. She moves from school to school, often shifting midmorning from one to another. She prepares her own schedule, selects her own cases, designs her own therapy, and does not have to put on overshoes or collect the milk money. Somehow, her regime keeps her from having to wear the teacher's mask. She remains a pretty free agent. A good clinician can usually dismiss over a third of her cases each year, and most of the rest show improvement. Thus she has a sense of real achievement, which is augmented by the appreciation of parents, teachers, and the children themselves.

Speech Therapy in the Hospital Setting
It is difficult to describe any typical program for this type of practice since programs vary widely. The hospital speech pathologist generally sees the more severely impaired cases, especially those of organic origin. She works with patients such as those with aphasia, cleft palates, cerebral palsy, laryngectomees, stuttering, voice problems, and dysarthrias. A portion of her work is solely diagnosis; the rest is therapy, both individual and in small

groups. The case load is small. Therapy is usually difficult, however, and often the prognosis may be poor. At times the amount of real improvement may be slight. Hospital therapy demands real competence on the part of the speech pathologist. He (or she) must show that professional competence in the white glare of the hospital walls under the scrutiny of other specialists in rehabilitation. But hospital speech therapy is also very rewarding. One constantly learns more and more about the human being. There are ward rounds and staffings of cases of all types. There is close collaboration with the physiotherapist, as well as with the medical profession.

Speech Therapy in Schools for Crippled Children   In the orthopedic schools, we find a blend of the two types of therapy settings described above. The case loads are small and the problems are usually difficult. Much of the work is individual therapy, although small groups are also employed when socialization is needed. The therapist often must coordinate her own therapy with that of the other special teachers. For example, if the classroom teacher is having a social science project on the farmer's life, the speech clinician will use this theme in the communication used to work on smooth breathing in a child with cerebral palsy, or on the final sounds of the words *cows* and *chickens* as spoken by a postpolio child with a partially paralyzed tongue and a lateral lisp. Each child is studied very intensively from every angle by the staff members of such a school, and the speech clinician is a member of a team.

Speech Therapy in Community Speech and Hearing Centers   Fairly recently we have seen the establishment of speech and hearing clinics supported not by the schools, hospitals, or colleges but by the community health and welfare organizations. Preschool children are thereby provided with services, as are the aged adults, and these centers often provide a professional setting in which the practice of speech pathology and audiology can be very rewarding. They also serve as diagnostic agencies to which workers in the public schools may refer their more difficult cases.

Private Practice   Once a speech pathologist has satisfied the clinical certification requirements of the American Speech and Hearing Association (not only certain strict academic requirements but also a professional examination and therapy experience under the supervision and sponsorship of a designated professional speech pathologist) he may do private practice in this field. In this setting, the speech pathologist often works with cases referred by physicians or other speech pathologists and is paid for his work by the patient, insurance company, or the government. He may have an office in a medical arts building or clinic, or may do the work in his own home. Many female speech pathologists do some private practice in their homes once they are married and have small children of their own. There also seems to be a growing trend for private summer speech clinics operated by public-school speech clinicians in which intensive therapy is offered to the more severely handicapped children who could not be adequately served during the school year. The majority of the cases seen in private practice are those with delayed speech, stuttering, or the organic speech disorders. There are many problems that arise in private practice that should be seriously considered by individuals who plan such a career. It is no bed of roses.

Audiology We have already indicated that there are many other settings in which speech therapy is flourishing. However, most professional speech pathologists begin their work either in the clinic or the public schools and then diverge later. So we will not describe these other types of work here. However, we must not forget to describe the way in which speech therapy serves as a beginning for other careers, especially those of audiology and special education. All speech pathologists take some courses in hearing during their undergraduate preparation, and they take more when they continue in graduate school. Some of them find in audiology a smell of scientific certainty (illusory or not) which contrasts markedly with that of speech therapy where one must constantly deal with probabilities and the intangible. They find in audiometry and the research on hearing loss a definiteness which they crave. Audiology is a very fast-growing field, and the demand for workers is even greater than in speech therapy. All beginning students should give it serious consideration.

Special Education In much the same way, beginning speech pathologists usually take courses in special education as part of their undergraduate preparation, and those who later work in the public schools often come into close contact with other special teachers. As a result, some of them (the males especially) find themselves active in such professional organizations as the Council for Exceptional Children,

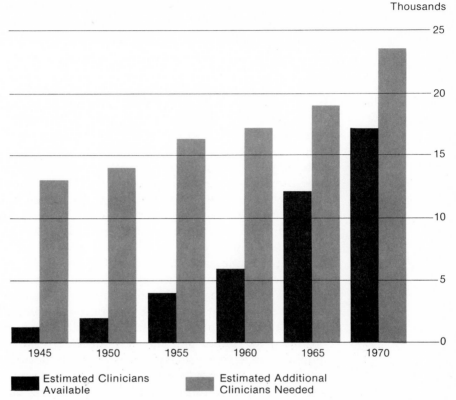

Thousands

Figure 49 Job opportunities. (From *Career Information: Speech Pathology and Audiology,* Published by The American Speech and Hearing Association, 9030 Old Georgetown Road, Washington, D.C. 20014.)

which serves all the fields of special education including the gifted child. Perhaps because of his experience in organizing and administering the speech therapy program and the public-relations work which it often entails, the speech pathologist becomes a marked man in the school system. He knows all the principals and the superintendent. He works with all the special teachers. Moreover, he already has an extensive background in not one but two fields of rehabilitation: speech and hearing. These experiences and qualifications often lead superintendents to encourage the speech pathologist to do graduate work in special education in the areas in which his preparation was scanty so that he can be promoted to the directorship of all special education services. Those of us in speech therapy often regret our own profession's loss when a competent clinician becomes an administrator, but when this occurs (and it has been happening more frequently each year), at least his newly hired replacement can find sympathetic understanding and support.

Career   Most students enter a career in speech pathology because
Satisfactions   they want to help others, because they are compassionate, and certainly their ability to help communicatively deprived persons solve their problems is one of their major satisfactions. We need meaningfulness in our lives. Having status and power and material possessions and belly pleasures are not enough to constitute a good life. Surely there should be something more. Most clinicians find that extra something in their fellow man, in seeing some twisted life become untangled as the result of their efforts.

But there are other satisfactions as well. For one thing, the work itself is usually pleasant work. Our clients come to us feeling that speaking is unpleasant, that communication is full of threat. They are often hesitant to enter a close relationship. Accordingly, one of our first tasks is to change these attitudes; we must make conversing pleasant rather than punishing. With little children much of our work is done through play and even with adults our interaction is usually flavored with humor and comradeship. The best clinicians we have known have shared several traits in common: they cared deeply about others and they were very sensitive to human needs and feelings. They were genuine, open, and reasonably well-adjusted. And they were gay spirits!

References

AMERICAN SPEECH AND HEARING ASSOCIATION. *Guide to Clinical Services in Speech Pathology and Audiology.* 9030 Old Georgetown Road, Washington, D.C., 20014.

ASHA COMMITTEE ON REHABILITATIVE AUDIOLOGY. "The Audiologist: Responsibilities in the Habilitation of the Auditorily Handicapped." *ASHA,* XVI (1974), 68–70.

BLACK, M. E. "The Origins and Status of Speech Therapy in the Schools." *ASHA,* VIII (1966), 419–25.

BLAKELY, R. *The Practice of Speech Pathology: A Clinical Diary.* Springfield, Ill.: Charles C. Thomas, 1972.

BRAUNSTEIN, S. and S. BIEDERMAN. "From Speech Pathologist to Language Classroom Teacher: What Does It Take?" *Language, Speech Hearing Services in the Schools,* V (1974), 245–52.

Brown, J. C. "The Expanding Responsiblities of the Speech and Hearing Clinician in the Public Schools." *Journal Speech Hearing Disorders,* XXXVI (1971), 538–42.

Curlee, R. F. "Personal Incomes in the Speech and Hearing Profession." *ASHA,* XVII (1975), 21–30.

Dickson, S. (ed.) *Communication Disorders: Remedial Principles and Practices.* New York: Scott, Foresman, 1974.

Emerick, L. L. and J. T. Hatton. *Diagnosis and Evaluation in Speech Pathology.* Englewood Cliffs, N.J.: Prentice-Hall, Inc., 1974, 223–49.

Freeman, G. C. "Innovative School Programs: The Oakland Schools Plan." *Journal Speech Hearing Disorders,* XXXIV (1969), 220–25.

Frick, J. E. "Personal Incomes in the Speech and Hearing Profession." *ASHA,* XIV (1972), 10–16.

Haller, R. M. and N. Sheldon. *Speech Pathology and Audiology in Medical Settings.* New York: Stratton Intercontinental Medical Book Corporation, 1976.

Handy, J. C. and D. T. Counihan. "The Certificate in Clinical Competence." *ASHA,* XIII (1971), 601–6.

Johnson, W. "Communicology." *ASHA,* X (1968), 44–58.

Knight, H. S. "Function of the School Clinician." *ASHA,* XII (1970), 12–17; 20–23.

Knight, P. D. "Private Practice in Speech Pathology." *ASHA,* X (1968), 436–44.

Moll, K. L. "Issues Facing Us. Licensure and Certification." *ASHA,* XVI (1974), 488.

Newman, P. W. *Opportunities in Speech Pathology.* New York: Vocational Guidance Manuals (235 East 45th St., N.Y.C.), 1968.

Nicolais, J. P. "Summary of 18 State Laws Licensing Speech Pathologists and Audiologists." *ASHA,* XVII (1975), 99–102.

O'Toole, T. J. and E. L. Zaslow. "Public School Speech and Hearing Programs: Things Are Changing." *ASHA,* XI (1969), 499–501.

Paden, E. P. *A History of the American Speech and Hearing Association.* Washington, D.C.: American Speech and Hearing Association, 1974.

Panagos, J. M. and S. J. Hanna. "A Speech and Hearing Program in Appalachia." *Rehabilitation Literature,* XXIX (1968), 2–7.

Perkins, W. H. "Our Profession: What It Is." *ASHA,* IV (1962), 339–44.

Perkins, W. *Speech Pathology: An Applied Behavioral Science.* St. Louis: C. V. Mosby, 1971.

——, R. Shelton, G. Studebaker, and R. Goldstein. "National Examinations in Speech Pathology and Audiology: Philosophy and Operations." *Asha,* XII (1970), 175–81.

Sheehan, J. G., R. G. Hadley, and L. Lechleidner. "Career Satisfaction and Recruitment in Speech Pathology and Audiology." *Asha,* VI (1964), 277–83.

Travis, L. E. (ed.) *Handbook of Speech Pathology and Audiology.* Englewood Cliffs, N.J.: Prentice-Hall, Inc., 1971.

Van Hattum, R. (ed.) *Clinical Speech in the Schools: Organization and Management,* Springfield, Ill.: Charles C. Thomas, 1969.

WALLE, E. L. and P. W. NEWMAN. "Rehabilitation Services for Speech, Hearing, and Language Disorders in an Extended Care Facility." *Asha*, IX (1967), 216–19.

WESTON, A. J. (ed.) *Communicative Disorders: An Appraisal.* Springfield, Ill.: Charles C. Thomas, 1972.

WILLIS, C. R. and J. B. WILLIS. "Survey of Training Programs in Speech Pathology and Audiology." *Asha*, XVI (1974), 200–2.

WINGO, J. W. and G. F. HOLLOWAY. [EDS.] *An Appraisal of Speech Pathology: A Symposium.* Springfield, Ill.: Charles C. Thomas, 1973.

GLOSSARY

Abracadabra: A magical set of words or sounds used as an incantation.

Acalculia: Loss of ability in using mathematical symbols due to brain injury.

Acoustic: Pertaining to the perception of sound.

Adenoids: Growths of lymphoid tissue on the back wall of the throat (nasopharynx).

Affricate: A consonantal sound beginning as a stop (plosive) but expelled as a fricative. The *ch* /tʃ/ and the *j* /dʒ/ sounds in the words *chain* and *jump* are affricates.

Agnosia: Loss of ability to interpret the meanings of sensory stimulation; due to brain injury; may be visual, auditory, or tactual.

Air wastage: The use of silent exhalation before or after phonation on a single breath.

Alaryngeal: Without a larynx.

Alexia: Difficulty in reading due to brain damage.

Allergy: Extreme sensitivity to certain proteins.

Allophone: One of the variant forms of a phoneme.

Alveolar: The ridges on the jaw bones beneath the gums. An alveolar sound is one in which the tongue makes contact with the upper-gum ridge.

Anomia: Inability to remember familiar words due to brain injury.

Anoxia: Oxygen deficiency.

Antiexpectancy: A group of devices used by the stutterer to distract himself from the expectation of stuttering.

Aphasia: Impairment in the use of meaningful symbols due to brain injury.

Aphonia: Loss of voice.

Approach-avoidance: Refers to conflicts produced when the person is beset by two opposing drives to do or not to do something.

451

Approximation: Behavior which comes closer to a standard or goal.

Apraxia: Loss of ability to make voluntary movements or to use tools meaningfully; due to brain injury.

Articulation: The utterance of the individual speech sounds.

Aspirate: Breathy; the use of excessive initial airflow preceding phonation as in the *aspirate* attack.

Assimilation: A change in the characteristic of a speech sound due to the influence of adjacent sounds. In *assimilation nasality*, voiced sounds followed or preceded by a nasal consonant tend to be excessively nasalized.

Asymmetry: Unequal proportionate size of the right and left halves of a structure.

Ataxia: Loss of ability to perform gross motor coordinations.

Athetosis: One of the forms of cerebral palsy characterized by writhing, shaking, involuntary movements of the head, limbs, or the body.

Atresia: The blockage of an opening or canal.

Atrophy: A withering; a shrinking in size and decline in function of some bodily structure or organ.

Attack: The initiation of voicing.

Auditory memory span: The ability to recall a series of test sounds, syllables, or words.

Aural: Pertaining to hearing.

Auricle: The visible outer ear.

Autism: An emotional disturbance in children resulting in a detachment from their environmental surroundings; almost complete withdrawal from social interaction.

Avoidance: A device such as the use of a synonym or circumlocution to escape from having to speak a word upon which stuttering is anticipated; also a trick to escape from having to speak in a feared situation.

Babbling: A continuous, free experimenting with speech sounds.

Basal fluency level: A period of communication in which no stuttering appears. See *Desensitization therapy*.

Baseline: An initial level of response prior to conditioning.

Base-rate: The presumably stable rate of responding to a stimulus or stimuli.

Bicuspid: The fourth and fifth teeth, each of which has two cusps or points.

Bifid: Divided into two parts, as in a cleft or bifid uvula.

Bilabial: A sound produced with both lips as the main articulators.

Binaural: Pertaining to both ears.

Bliss symbols: A set of pictographs for the non-verbal person.

Bone conduction: The transmission of sound waves (speech) directly to the cochlea by means of the bones of the skull.

Bradylalia: Abnormally slow utterance.

C.A.T.: Children's Apperception Test, a projective test of personality.

Catastrophic response: A sudden change in behavior by the aphasic characterized by extreme irritability, flushing or fainting, withdrawal or random movements.

Catharsis: The discharge of pent-up feelings.

Cerebral palsy: A group of disorders due to brain injury in which the motor coordinations are especially affected. Most common forms are athetosis, spasticity, and ataxia.

Clavicular breathing: A form of shallow, gasping speech-breathing in which the shoulder blades move with the short inhalations.

Cleft lip or palate: See Chapter 9.

Cluttering: A disorder of time or rhythm characterized by unorganized, hasty spurts of speech often accompanied by slurred articulation and breaks in fluency.

Cochlea: The spiral-shaped structure of the inner ear containing the end organs of the auditory nerve.

Cognate: Referring to pairs of sounds which are produced motorically in much the same way, one being voiced (sonant) and the other unvoiced (surd). Some cognates are /t/ and /d/; /s/ and /z/.

Commentary: The verbalization of what is being perceived as in self-talk or parallel talk.

Conductive hearing loss: Hearing loss due to failure of the bone levers in the middle ear to transmit sound vibrations to the cochlea.

Configurations: (in articulation therapy) Patterning of sounds in proper sequence.

Contact ulcers: A breakdown in the tissues of the vocal folds, usually near their posterior attachments to the arytenoid cartilages.

Content words (Contentives): Words such as nouns and verbs that carry the major burden of meaningfulness.

Contingent: Following as a consequence of some preceding behavior.

Continuant: A speech sound which can be prolonged without distortion; e.g., /s/ or /f/ or /u/.

Corpus: A collection of terms.

Covert: Hidden behavior; inner feelings, thoughts, reactions.

Creative dramatics: An improvised, unrehearsed playlet acted spontaneously by a group of children with the unobtrusive aid of an adult leader.

CV: A syllable containing the consonant-vowel sequence as in *see* or *toe* or *ka*.

CVC: A syllable containing the consonant-vowel-consonant sequence, as in the first syllable of the word *containing*.

Decibel: A unit of sound intensity.

Deep testing: The exploration of an articulation case's ability to articulate a large number of words, all of which include one specific sound, to discover those in which that sound is spoken correctly.

Delayed auditory feedback: The return of one's own voice as an echo.

Denasality: A lack of, or reduced nasality.

Dental: Pertaining to the teeth. A dentalized *l* sound is made with the tongue tip on the upper teeth.

Desensitization: The toughening of a person to stress; increasing the person's ability to confront his problem with less anxiety, guilt, or hostility; a type of adaptation to stress therapy used for beginning stutterers. See Chapter 8.

Diadochokinesis: The maximum speed of a rhythmically repeated movement.

Differential diagnosis: The process of distinguishing one disorder from another.

Differentiation: The functional separation of a finer movement from a larger one with which it formerly coexisted.

Dipthong: Two adjacent vowels within the same syllable which blend together.

Distortion: The misarticulation of a standard sound in which the latter is replaced by a sound not normally used in the language. A lateral lisp is a distortion.

Dysarthria: Articulation disorders produced by peripheral or central nerve damage.

Dyslalia: Functional (nonorganic) disorders of articulation.

Dysphasia: The general term for aphasic problems.

Dysphemia: A poorly timed control mechanism for coordinating sequential utterance. It is variously conceived as being due to a constitutional and hereditary difference or to psychopathology. It reflects itself in stuttering and cluttering.

Dysphonias: Disorders of voice.

Ear training: Therapy devoted to self-hearing of speech deviations and standard utterance.

Echolalia: The automatic involuntary repetition of heard phrases and sentences.

Echo speech: A technique in which the patient is trained to repeat instantly what he is hearing, following almost simultaneously the utterance of another person. Also called "shadowing."

Egocentric: Self-centered; pertaining to the self and its display.

Ego strength: Morale or self-confidence.

Electroencephalogram (E.E.G.): The record of brain waves of electrical potential. Used in diagnosing epilepsy, tumors, or other pathologies.

Embedding: The placement of words, phrases, or clauses within the basic subject-predicate sentence structure.

Embolism: A clogging of a blood vessel as by a clot.

Empathy: The conscious or unconscious imitation or identification of one person with the behavior or feelings of another.

Encephalitis: A disease characterized by inflammation or lesions of the brain.

Epiglottis: The shield-like cartilage that hovers over the front part of the larynx.

Epilepsy: A neurological disease characterized by convulsions and seizures.

Esophageal speech: Speech of laryngectomized persons produced by air pulses ejected from the esophagus.

Esophagus: The tube leading from the throat to the stomach.

Etiology: Causation.

Eunuchoid voice: A very high-pitched voice similar to that of a castrated male adult.

Eustachian tube: The air canal connecting the throat cavity with the middle ear.

Expressive aphasia: The difficulty in sending meaningful messages, as in the speaking, writing, or gesturing difficulties of the aphasic.

Falsetto: Usually the upper and unnatural range of a male voice produced by a different type of laryngeal functioning.

Fauces: The rear side margins of the mouth cavity which separate the mouth from the pharynx.

Feedback: The backflow of information concerning the output of a motor system. Auditory feedback refers to self-hearing; kinesthetic feedback to the self-perception of one's movements.

Fixation: In stuttering, the prolongation of a speech posture.

Flaccid: Passively uncontracted, limp.

Fluency: Unhesitant speech.

Frenum: The white membrane below the tongue tip.

Fricative: A speech sound produced by forcing the airstream through a constricted opening. The /f/ and /v/ sounds are fricatives. Sibilants are also fricatives.

Function words (functors): Words which indicate action, arrangement, and relationship. Example: prepositions, articles, adverbs, and conjunctions.

Generative (Transformational) Grammar: A system of rules for producing all the well-formed sentences of a language.

Gibbegedong: A voiced velar-tongue click.

Glide: A class of speech sounds in which the characteristic feature is produced by shifting from one articulatory posture to another. Examples are the *y* /j/ in *you,* and the /w/ in *we.*

Glottal catch (or stop): A tiny cough-like sound produced by the sudden release of a pulse of voiced or unvoiced air from the vocal folds.

Glottal fry: A ticker-like continuous clicking sound produced by the vocal cords.

Glottis: The space between the vocal cords when they are not brought together.

Gutteral voice: A low-pitched falsetto.

Hard contacts: Hypertensed fixed articulatory postures assumed by stutterers in attempting feared words.

Harelip: A cleft of the upper lip.

Hemiplegia: Paralysis or neurological involvement of one side of the body.

Hemorrhage: Bleeding.

Hierarchy: A series of items graded according to difficulty.

Hyperactivity: Excessive and often random movements as often shown by a brain-injured child.

Hypernasality (Rhinolalia aperta): Excessively nasal voice quality.

Hyponasality: Lack of sufficient nasality, as in the denasal or adenoidal voice.

Identification: In articulation therapy, the techniques used to recognize the essential features of the correct sound or its error.

Idioglossia: Self-language with a vocabulary invented by the child.

Incidence: Frequency of occurrence.

Incisor: Any one of the four front teeth in the upper or lower jaws.

Infantile swallow: A form of swallowing in which the tongue is usually protruded between the teeth.

Inflection: A shift in pitch during the utterance of a syllable.

Interdental: Between the teeth. An interdental lisp would show itself in the substitution of the *th* for the *s* as in *thoup* for *soup.*

Interiorized stuttering: A form of stuttering behavior in which no visible contortions or audible abnormalities are shown, but a hidden struggle usually in the larynx or breathing musculatures is present. Also characterized by clever disguise reactions.

Isolation techniques: Activities used to locate the defective sound in utterance.

Jargon: Continuous but unintelligible speech.

Kernel sentences: The early primitive sentence forms from which other transformations later develop.

Kinesthesia; The perception of muscular contraction or movement.

Kinetic analysis: The analysis of error sounds in terms of their movement patterns.

Labial: Pertaining to the lips.

Lalling: An articulatory disorder characterized by distortions of the /l/, /r/, /t/, /d/, or /s/ largely due to inactivity or sluggishness of the tip or blade of the tongue.

Lambdacism: Defective /l/ sound.

Laryngeal: Pertaining to the larynx.

Laryngectomy: The surgical removal of the larynx.

Laryngologist: A physician specializing in diseases and pathology of the larynx.

Larynx: The cartilaginous structure housing the vocal folds.

Lateral: A sound such as the /l/ in which the airflow courses around the side of the uplifted tongue. One variety of lateral lisp is so produced.

Lesion: A wound; broken tissue.

Lexicon: The stock of terms in a vocabulary.

Lingual: Pertaining to the tongue. A lingual lisp is identical with an interdental lisp.

Lisp: An articulatory disorder characterized by defective sibilant sounds such as the /s/ and /z/.

Malleus: The bone of the middle ear which rests against the eardrum.

Malocclusion: An abnormal bite.

Mandible: Lower jaw.

Maxilla: Upper jaw.

Medial: The occurrence of a sound within a word but not initiating or ending it.

Median: Midline, in the middle.

MMPI: Minnesota Multiphase Personality Inventory, a test of personality problems.

Monaural: Hearing with one ear.

Monitoring: Checking and controlling the output of speech.

Monopitch: Speaking in a very narrow pitch range, usually of one to four semitones.

Motokinesthetic method: A method for teaching sounds and words in which the therapist directs the movements of the tongue, jaw, and lips by touch and manipulation.

Mucosa: The mouth and throat linings which secrete mucous.

Multiple sclerosis: A progressive and deteriorating muscular disability produced by overgrowth of the connective tissue surrounding the nerve tracts.

Muscular dystrophy: A disease of unknown origin characterized by progressive deterioration in muscle functioning and also by withering of the muscles.

Mutism: Without speech. Voluntary mutism: refusal to speak.

Myasthenia: Muscular weakness.

Nares: Nostrils.

Nasal emission: Airflow through the nose.

Nasal lisp: The substituting of a snorted unvoiced /n/ for the sibilant sounds.

Nasendoscopy: A technique for viewing the velo-pharyngeal closure structures from above.

Nasopharynx: That part of the throat, pharynx, above the level of the base of the uvula.

Negative practice: Deliberate practice of the error or abnormal behavior.

Negative reinforcement: The cessation of unpleasantness when applied contingently.

Nerve deafness: Loss of hearing due to inadequate functioning of the cochlea, auditory nerve, or hearing centers in the brain.

Nonfluency: Pause, hesitation, repetition, or other behavior which interrupts the normal flow of utterance.

Nucleus: A central core. Nucleus situations are those in which the client tries especially hard to monitor his speech so as to improve it.

Obturator: An appliance used to close a cleft or gap.

Occluded lisp: The substitution of a /t/ or a /ts/ for the /s/, or the /d/ and /dz/ for the /z/.

Omission: One of the four types of articulatory errors. The standard sound is replaced usually by a slight pause equal in duration to the sound omitted.

Operant conditioning: The differential reinforcement of desired responses through the systematic control of their contingencies.

Opposition breathing: Breathing in which the thorax (chest) and diaphragm work oppositely against each other in providing breath support for voice.

Optimal pitch level: The pitch range at which a given individual may phonate most efficiently.

Orthodontist: A dentist who specializes in repositioning of the teeth.

Oscillations: Rhythmic repetitive movements, repetitions of a sound, syllable, or posture.

Otologist: A physician who specializes in hearing disorders and diseases.

Overt: Clearly visible or audible behavior.

Palpation: Examining by tapping or touching.

Panendoscope: A device which permits direct observation of the velo-pharyngeal closure through the mouth.

Parallel talk: A technique in which the therapist provides a running commentary on what the client is doing, perceiving, or probably feeling.

Paraphasia: Aphasic behavior characterized by jumbled, inaccurate words.

Perseveration: The automatic and often involuntary continuation of behavior.

PFAGH: An acronym representing penalty, frustration, anxiety, guilt, and hostility.

Pharyngeal flap: A tissue bridge between the soft palate and the back wall of the throat.

Pharynx: The throat cavity.

Phonation: Voice.

Phonemic: Refers to a group of very similar sounds represented by the same phonetic symbol.

Phonetic placement: A method for teaching a new sound by the use of diagrams, mirrors, or manipulation whereby the essential motor features of the sound are made clear.

Phonology: The linguistic area dealing with speech sounds and their characteristics.

Pitch breaks: Sudden abnormal shifts of pitch during speech.

Plosive: A speech sound characterized by the sudden release of a puff of air. Examples are /p/, /t/, and /g/.

Polygraph: An instrument for recording breathing, heart beat, and other functions.

Preparatory set: An anticipatory readiness to perform an act.

Presbycusis: The hearing loss characteristic of old age.

Primary reinforcer: A stimulus which satisfies a basic need and is not dependent upon learning. Examples: water, food, sex.

Proboscis: Nose.

Prognosis: Prediction of progress.

Propositionality: The meaningfulness of a message or utterance; its information content.

Proprioception: Sense information from muscles, joints, or tendons.

Prosthesis: An appliance used to compensate for a missing or paralyzed structure.

Prosthodontist: A dental specialist who makes prostheses.

Pubertal: Pertaining to the period during which the secondary sexual characteristics begin to appear.

Pyknolepsy: A mild form of epilepsy characterized by stoppages in speech, among other things.

Receptive aphasia: Aphasia in which the major deficits are in comprehending.

Reciprocal inhibition: The mutual cancellation or inhibition produced by pairing incompatible response tendencies such as anxiety and anger.

Rhinolalia: Excessive nasality.

Rhotacism: Articulatory errors involving the production of the *r* sounds.

Rorschach: A test of personality involving the use of ink blots.

Schedules of reinforcement: The program for administering reinforcements. May be total (100 percent) in which reinforcement is given after each desired response, or partial (e.g., given for every five responses, etc.).

Secondary reinforcer: A stimulus which has been previously associated with a primary reinforcer.

Secondary stuttering: Refers to the advanced forms of stuttering in which awareness, fear, avoidance, and struggle are shown.

Self-talk: An audible commentary by the person describing what he is doing, perceiving, or feeling.

Semitone: A half-tone, a half-step on the musical scale.

Septum: The partition between the right and left nasal cavities formed of bone and cartilage.

Shadowing: See *Echo talk*.

Sibilant: A class of fricative consonant sounds characterized by high-pitched noise. Examples are /s/ and /z/.

Sibling: Brother or sister.

Sigmatism: Lisping.

Sonant: A voiced sound.

Spastic: *(noun)* An individual who shows one of the varieties of cerebral palsy. *(adjective)* Characterized by highly tensed contractions of muscle groups.

Spastic dysphonia: A voice disorder in which phonation is produced only with great effort and strain.

Stabilization: The process of making a response permanent and unfluctuating.

Stapedectomy: Surgical removal of the stapes.

Stapes: The innermost bone of the middle ear.

Stigma: A mark or sign of defect or disgrace.

Stoma: The hole in the neck through which the person must breathe after laryngectomy.

Stop consonant: A sound characterized by a momentary blocking of airflow. Examples are the /k/, /d/, and /p/.

Strident lisp: Sibilants characterized by piercing, whistling sounds.

Strident voice: Harsh voice quality.

Surd: Unvoiced sound such as the *s* as opposed to its cognate *z* which is voiced or sonant.

Syntax: The grammatical structure of a language.

Tachylalia: Extremely rapid speech.

Tempo: Rate of utterance.

Thorax: Chest.

Time-outs: Intervals of silence administered contingently by the experimenter when an undesired speech response such as stuttering occurs.

Tinnitus: Ringing noises in the ears.

Tooth prop: A small wooden or plastic peg to be held between the teeth.

Toxemia: A condition in which toxins produced by infection are present in the blood.

Trachea: The windpipe.

Trauma: Shock or injury.

Tremor: The swift, tremulous vibration of a muscle group.

Tympanic membrane: The eardrum.

Unilaterality: One-handedness; preference for one hand as contrasted with ambidexterity.

Uvula: The hanging portion of the soft palate. The velar tail.

Velum: Soft palate.

Velopharyngeal closure: The more or less complete shutting off of the nasopharynx.

Ventricular phonation: Voice produced by the vibration of the false vocal folds.

Vocal fry: See *Glottal fry.*

Vocal play: In the development of speech, the stage during which the child experiments with sounds and syllables.

Xanthippe: Why Socrates became a philosopher.

INDEX

A

Affricates, 80
Aglossia, 348
Agnellography, 361
Agnossia, visual and auditory, 374–375, 430
Agraphia, 125, 374
Alaryngeal aphonia, 340–348
Alexia, 125, 374
Allophones, 84, 166
American Speech and Hearing Association, 15, 442–443, 444, 445
  Certificate of Clinical Competence, 443, 444
Anomia, 374
Anxiety, 26–29
Aphasia, 12–13, 31–32, 40, 68–69, 82, 87, 124–127, 373–377
  causes of, 378–379
  prognosis, 380
  tests for, 377–380
  treatment of, 381–389
    psychotherapy, 389
  types of, 379
Aphonia, 62, 218n, 242. *See also* Spastic dysphonia
  alaryngeal, 340–348
  functional vs. organic, 64
  hysterical, 220–223
Apraxia, 82, 375
Aronson, A. E., 225
Articulation disorders, 93, 122. *See also* *specific disorders, e.g.* Lisping
  causes of, 48–52, 164–173

Articulation disorders *(cont.)*
  conditions predisposing to, 163–164
  diagnosis of, 48–52, 157–164
  kinetic analysis of, 161–163
  organic factors in, 167–169
  tests for, 158–164. *See also specific tests*
  treatment of, 173–214
    cleft-palate speech, 370
    at isolated word level, 182–195
    at the sentence level, 205–214
    at the syllable level, 196–198
    at the word level, 199–205
Asai technique, 341n
Asha (periodical), 443
Asoka, King (India), 35
Assimilation nasality, 65
Ataxia, 391–392
Attila the Hun, 34
Audiology, 15–16, 432–433
  employment in, 446
Audiometry, 408
  pure tone, 408–410
  speech, 410–412
Auditory memory span, 165
Auditory stimulation, 189–190
Auditory training, 433–435
Autism, 130–131
Autism theory of speech acquisition, 101–102

B

Babbling, 93–96
Baby-talk, 51, 137

S

Saint Francis of Assisi, 35
Sander, E. K., 321n
Sandow, 275
Schizophrenia, childhood, 129–130
Schuell, H., 377
Schultz, A. R., 398n
Self-hearing. *See* Self-listening
Self-listening, 95, 185–187
Self-talk, 141–142, 330
Semantics, 85
  development in, 108–111
Sensori-neural hearing loss, 412, 421–423
Sentence formation, 102–105
Senturia, 218n
Shakespeare, Wm., 34
Shames, G., 285n
Shanks, J. C., 236
Sheehan, J. G., 265–266
Silverman, R. S., 431, 435n
Simonson, J., 380n
Skinner, B. F., 144n
Sloane, H. N., 148
Slobin, D., 102
Slow-motion speech method, 207
Smith, M. E., 109
Smith, S., 95
Snidecor, J. C., 345
Social babbling. *See* Babbling
Sokolowsky, R. R., 222–223
Sound-modification method, 192
Sound production. *See* Phonation
Sound sequences. *See* Morphemes
Sound shaping, 187–189
Spastic dysphonia, 64, 67, 223–225. *See also* Aphonia
Speech and language, 75–89
  development of, 91
  babbling, 93–96
  deterrents to, 121–135
  inflected vocal play, 96–98
  learning theories of, 99–105
  phonological, 105–111
  reflexive utterance, 92–93
  sentence formation, 102–105
Speech audiometry, 410–412
Speech disorders, 4–8. *See also specific types*
  anxiety and, 26–29

Speech disorders *(cont.)*
  classification of, 45–48
  culture and. *See* Speech disorders, society and
  definition of, 43–44
  diagnosis of, 40–42, 46–48. *See also under specific disorders*
  fear and, 262–268, 297–298, 302, 304–305
  frustration and, 17–18, 23–26, 269–271, 295–296, 301, 306, 317–320
  guilt and, 29–31, 271, 296, 301, 305–306, 320
  hearing defects and, 15–16, 81, 94, 120, 122–124, 165, 405–440
  hostility and, 22–23, 31–32
  parents and, 11–12, 16–17, 19, 26, 30, 41–42, 140–144, 211, 316–336
  penalties of, 18–22
  society and, 7, 21–22, 43. *See also* Handicapped, history of
Speech Foundation of America, 289n, 308n, 312n
Speech mechanism, 77–82
Speech pathology, 42, 53
  employment opportunities in, 444–448
  professional organizations, 442–443
  role of, 8–17, 40–72
  training centers for, 443
Speech Reading—Jena Method (Bunger), 435n
Speech reception threshold (SRT), 410
Speech therapy, 40. *See also under specific disorders and methods*
  cognitive approach to, 149–150
  designing, 174–182
  distinctive approach, 177–179
  linguistic approach to, 136–141, 177–179
  operant conditioning in, 145–149, 176–177
  parental role in, 30, 140–144, 211, 316–336
  professional diagnosis for, 48–52, 134–135, 157–164
  proprioceptive feedback in, 213
  traditional, 179. *See also* Phonetic placement
Speech Therapy and the Bobath Approach to Cerebral Palsy (Crickmay), 393n
Speechreading, 435–436
Spondee words, 410

U

Unison speech method, 207–208

V

Van Riper, C., 171, 250–251, 261n, 276n, 277n
Vander-Reiden, G. C., 398n
Ventricular dysphonia, 64
Verbal Behavior (Skinner), 144n
Vigotsky, 150
Voelker, C. H., 245–246
Voice disorders, 218–220. *See also*
  Phonation *and specific disorders, e.g.,*
  Hypernasality
  intensity. *See* Aphonia; Spastic
    dysphonia
  pitch, 60–62, 228–240
  quality, 65–68, 240–253
  treatment of, 221–223, 226–228, 238–240, 246–253
Voice quality, disorders of:
  assimilation nasality, 65, 241–242
  breathy voice, 66, 242–244
  denasality, 66–67, 78, 242
  diagnosis and treatment of, 246–253
  hoarseness, 66, 245–246

Voice quality *(cont.)*
  hypernasality, 65, 78, 241
  stridency, 65–66, 67, 244–245
Voluntary mutism, 28, 40–42

W

Walsh, H., 178n
Ward, W. D., 426n
Weber, J. L, 178n
Webster, L. M., 281n
Wechsler Intelligence Test, 130
Weir, R., 94
Wepman, J. M., 166n, 377
Westlake, H., 358, 360
Wilkinson, E. M., 353n
Williams, D., 269
Willis, 444
Wilson, 218n
Winitz, H., 98, 159, 167, 170
Wood, B. S., 102
Wood, N., 118–119, 126–127
Wright, G., 342n

Z

Zwitman, D. H., 341n